Exploring the Dirty Side of Women's Health

D1458913

Women leak, inevitably and often bountifully. In this book, a selection of international contributors examine bodies, leakage and boundaries, illuminating the contradictions and dilemmas in women's healthcare.

Using the concept of pollution, *Exploring the Dirty Side of Women's Health* highlights how women and health issues are categorised and health workers and women are confined to roles and places defined as socially appropriate. The book explores current and historical practices, such as:

- childbirth and midwifery practice;
- policies and social practices around breastfeeding;
- gynaecological nursing, female incontinence and sexually transmitted infections;
- miscarriages and termination of pregnancy.

Exploring the Dirty Side of Women's Health addresses things out of place, from the idea of 'dirty work' to feeling 'dirty', from diagnoses that disrupt our self-image to beliefs and practices which undermine health service provision. This book uses the contradictions in our thinking around pollution and power to stimulate thinking around women's health. It will appeal to students and academics researching midwifery, anthropology, gender studies and nursing as well as midwives and breastfeeding counsellors.

Mavis Kirkham is Professor of Midwifery at Sheffield-Hallam University. She has been a midwife and a researcher for over 30 years and maintains a clinical practice mostly doing home births.

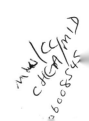

Exploring the Dirty Side of Women's Health

Edited by Mavis Kirkham

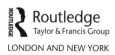

Routledge
Taylor & Francis Group

LONDON AND NEW YORK

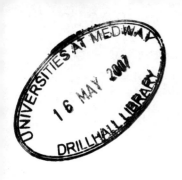

First published 2007
by Routledge
2 Park Square, Milton Park, Abingdon, Oxon OX14 4RN

Simultaneously published in the USA and Canada
by Routledge
270 Madison Ave, New York, NY 10016

*Routledge is an imprint of the Taylor & Francis Group,
an informa business*

© 2007 selection and editorial matter, Mavis Kirkham;
individual chapters the contributors

Typeset in Baskerville by BC Typesetting Ltd, Bristol
Printed and bound in Great Britain by
TJ International, Padstow, Cornwall

British Library Cataloguing in Publication Data
A catalogue record for this book is available from the British Library

Library of Congress Cataloging in Publication Data
A catalog record has been requested for this book

ISBN10: 0–415–38324–2 (hbk)
ISBN10: 0–415–38325–0 (pbk)
ISBN10: 0–203–96734–8 (ebk)

ISBN13: 978–0–415–38324–0 (hbk)
ISBN13: 978–0–415–38325–7 (pbk)
ISBN13: 978–0–203–96734–8 (ebk)

Contents

Contributors

Helen Callaghan is Clinical Nurse/Midwife, Family and Ambulatory Services, Nambour General Hospital, Queensland, Australia.

Pamela J. Wood is Associate Professor, Graduate School of Nursing, Midwifery & Health, Victoria University of Wellington, New Zealand.

Maralyn Foureur is Clinical Professor of Midwifery, Graduate School of Nursing, Midwifery & Health, Victoria University of Wellington, New Zealand.

Rachel C. Newell was formerly Midwifery Lecturer, School of Nursing & Midwifery, University of Dundee.

Kuldip Bharj is Senior Lecturer in Midwifery, University of Leeds.

Ruth Deery is Reader in Midwifery, Division of Midwifery, University of Huddersfield.

Fiona Dykes is Reader in Maternal and Infant Health and leader, Maternal & Infant Nutrition and Nurture Unit (MAINN), Faculty of Health, University of Central Lancashire, Preston.

Susan Battersby is an independent midwifery researcher/lecturer.

Cheryl Benn is Associate Professor, School of Health Sciences, Massey University, New Zealand.

Suzanne Phibbs is Lecturer, School of Health Science, Massey University, New Zealand.

Alison Spiro is Health Visitor, Harrow PCT.

Mary Smale is Breastfeeding Counsellor and Tutor, National Childbirth Trust.

Janet Chawla is Director, MATRIKA Charitable Trust, India.

Subhadhra Rai is Associate Professor, School of Nursing, Laurentian University, Ontario, Canada.

Margaret Chesney is Director of Midwifery Education, University of Salford.

Sharon C. Bolton is Reader in Organisational Analysis and Director, MA Human Resource and Knowledge Management Programme, Lancaster University Management School.

Joanne Jordan is Lecturer, School of Nursing and Midwifery, Queen's University Belfast.

Julia Frost is Research Fellow, School of Nursing and Community Studies, Faculty of Health and Social Work, University of Plymouth.

Hilary Piercy is Lecturer in Nursing, School of Nursing & Midwifery, University of Sheffield.

Simon Dyson is Reader in Applied Social Sciences, Unit for the Social Study of Thalassaemia and Sickle Cell, De Montfort University, Leicester.

Acknowledgements

Many people have made this book possible. I am grateful to the authors for fitting this writing into their busy and committed lives. I would also like to thank those who gave papers at the conference which, for differing reasons, do not appear here: Trudy Stevens, Lesley Barclay and Mary Stewart. Their work has influenced our thinking.

Anna Fielder, Nadine Edwards, Lis Garratt, Lesley Taylor, Helen Stapleton and Liz Perkins have stimulated my thinking in the editing of this book. I appreciate their ideas and their support.

I would like to thank Jane Flint for organising the conference and Joanne Mirfield for her support in the editing of this book. Their competence and endless support makes my work possible.

Introduction

Women leak, inevitably and often bountifully. Menstrual blood, birth fluids, breast milk and sometimes tears lead us to be seen as leakier than men at a physical level. Women are often seen to work through a network of relationships, a web, rather than the hierarchy of male decision-making (Gilligan 1982). Within such a web of relationships, emotions, knowledge and other personal attributes flow, often freely, sometimes unconsciously. Dirt is defined by Mary Douglas as 'matter out of place' (Douglas 1966). In any context, appropriate place is clearly a matter of categorisation, which is usually done by the socially powerful. What leakage is dirty or threatening, and what is bountiful and fruitful, is clearly a matter of categorisation.

I wanted to call this book 'Leaky Ladies' because a book about social pollution is about leakage, of many sorts. 'Ladies' is a term applied to women when they are being categorised, especially in health care. Midwives often speak of 'my ladies' when referring to their caseload. A term of apparent respect, which also puts us firmly in our place, inevitably leads to leakage, in many dimensions. Such a title, however, would not fit modern search techniques.

This book is the fruit of many labours. Margaret Chesney, Kuldip Bharj and I have spent a long time seeking to understand the complexities of dirt and pollution in the context of birth in India and Pakistan. Midwifery is dominated by the dilemmas, in traditional and modern settings, of the seeming contradiction that life originates from that which is seen as most dirty and low in status.

The subject of midwives' work in modern maternity units as 'dirty work', and the persistence of 'birth dirt' in an Australian medicalised setting, was opened up for me when I first read Helen Callaghan's PhD thesis (Callaghan 2002). Subsequent conversations with Helen, Lesley Barclay and colleagues during our research exchange with the University of Technology, Sydney, made us all eager to think further about these matters. These discussions led to a conference held in Sheffield in 2004 called 'Pollution and safety: exploring the "dirty" side of women's health'. This gathering stimulated our thinking further and linked up researchers who had not previously known of each other. This book follows from that conference and includes a number of chapters that were not given as conference papers. The book could not be called by the title of the conference, since that could lead to it being wrongly classified as a book about pollution of the physical environment.

This book falls into four sections. 'Mothers, midwives and dirt – past and present' explores birth dirt in different times and places. Helen Callaghan provides a theoretical context before discussing her own study. She used videotapes of labour together with analysis of textbooks to examine modern Australian hospital practices around birth and the containment of dirt. Her resulting theory of birth dirt is about the power relationships in childbirth. Labouring women are dirty, leaking and 'kept in their place'. Midwives manage and contain the dirt of birth and have a subordinate, though mediating, role relative to doctors. Pamela Wood and Maralyn Foureur present a historical study of a New Zealand hospital and the efforts, douches and disinfectants used to ensure 'a clean front passage' to protect both the hospital wards and their patients' uteri from approaching infection. The nuances of birth dirt, its management and associated discourses and their changes over time are carefully considered. Rachel Newell's historical study examines the end of the post-partum period as marked by the Anglican rite of the churching of women. Newell examines the physiological and epistemic dimensions of this ritual and links it with the modern postnatal examination. Kuldip Bharj interviewed Muslim childbearing women and their interpreters concerning their experiences in maternity hospitals in the north of England. A view expressed in this study shows how hospital staff can be seen as defiling women, though this is the opposite of how these staff would see themselves. Ruth Deery and I examine 'emotional toxic waste' amongst community midwives in the north of England. The midwives felt emotionally drained and that other peoples' troubles were 'dumped' upon them, with little opportunity to offload such burdens. With no concept of recycling such waste to increase their knowledge or professional resources and no experience of safe space for reflection, the midwives resisted the provision and use of clinical supervision. All these chapters are about stopping things crossing boundaries and different concepts of where and what the boundaries are.

'Breastfeeding as pollution' addresses the dilemmas and contradictions of breastfeeding in societies where official rhetoric extols breastfeeding as a superior form of infant nutrition, but where bottle feeding is the norm and many breastfeeding women feel very isolated. Exposure and leakage are major concerns, as women struggle to keep their milk, their breasts and their relationships with their babies in their socially ordained right place, well out of sight. Fiona Dykes examines women's experiences of breastfeeding in hospital in the north of England, which she finds to be beset by dualisms and associated dissonances. Susan Battersby examines how English mothers and midwives can experience breastfeeding as embarrassing and dirty work when carried out in public. The location of facilities for breastfeeding within or adjacent to toilets compounds the view of breastfeeding as dirty and highlights the isolation experienced by many breastfeeding mothers. Cheryl Benn and Suzanne Phibbs interviewed New Zealand women who saw themselves as having an excessive milk supply. These mothers had to make many adjustments in feeding their babies and experienced considerable personal challenges, loads of washing and social isolation 'for their own good'. Alison Spiro studied Hindu and Jain Gujarati families in London and in India. Breast milk is seen by them as pure and able to convey elements of the mother's identity and heritage to her child. The liminality of the process of breastfeeding and the milk itself, as it passes between two bodies, increases the danger associated with it. For these women, the danger of the evil eye, not the exposure of the breast, prevents them breastfeeding in the presence of any but close family. Mary Smale looks at breastfeeding knowledge and the danger of leakage of personal embodied understanding into professional 'scientific' work. Resulting dilemmas and contradictions are examined which limit the experience of professionals and mothers and ensure professional dominance. Breastfeeding thus provides a clear example of the potential for leakage, not just of milk, but of social, emotional and professional matter out of place. Breastfeeding is recommended by health services, but the realities of this activity involve negotiating the values, beliefs and embodiments of its social context, which are usually beset by contradictions.

The work of the dai, the traditional birth attendant in the Indian subcontinent, is the subject of three chapters. Here concepts of caste, gender and family duties highlight what is seen as dirty work. Janet Chawla draws on the Motherhood and Traditional Resources, Information, Knowledge and Action Project (MATRIKA) in north India. Matrika are also a diverse group of female, collective and semi-divine figures associated with mothering. The workshops in this action research were underpinned by explicitly stated values very different from those that underpin professional health care: empathy and active listening. The resulting understanding of '*narak*' has connotations of filth but also signifies the fertility and fruitful potential held in common by the earth and women. What is labelled polluting is here approached with reverence and, with this understanding, contradictions between modern teaching and traditional beliefs are examined. From this basis communication between systems could be possible.

Subadhra Rai's chapter is also concerned with listening to dais, in Gujarat, India. These dais are of low caste and therefore considered appropriate to undertake the dirty and polluting work around birth. Within this context, however, they describe themselves as doing work of selfless duty for those in need. The image of their work as dirty and polluted gives them a degree of economic and social monopoly and enables them to create a boundary around their authoritative knowledge. Margaret Chesney examines concepts of shame, honour and pollution for Pakistani women who gave birth in Pakistan, some of whom later moved to northern England. The social vulnerabilities of women and of dais are explored. The relationships between families, the dai and the medical system suggest that, whilst family decision makers rather than the dai take key economic decisions such as transfer of a labouring woman to hospital, in the view of health professionals, the dai now contains blame as well as pollution.

The last section of this book looks at 'Leakage and labelling' in health care more widely than just concerning birth. Sharon Bolton explores the world of gynaecological nurses in a hospital in northern England. Their status as women carrying out 'dirty work' is seen as special, requiring distinctive womanly knowledge and skills. 'In their celebration of women's work and "dirty work" they actively define a distinctive kind of "other" with which they can challenge the status quo.' This chapter makes salutary reading for me as a midwife. The gynaecological nurses' descriptions of their caring and respectful work around reproduction without the joy and gratitude surrounding live births highlighted for me the many levels and aspects of 'dirty work'. Joanne Jordan addresses female urinary incontinence and the views of specialist continence nurses. These nurses seek to change the view that incontinence is inevitable as women age, and help women to achieve continence. This could be seen as empowering women, though some avoid this self-help approach, or it could be seen as medicalisation of the deteriorating female body. The interactions between women and health professionals are seen, again, to be complex. Julia Frost interviewed women over 35 years of age who had experienced miscarriage, and explores theoretical debates and empirical examples to examine the utility of concepts of leakiness. Where women experienced 'individualised' and 'flowing care' and specific space was provided, such as an Early Pregnancy Assessment Unit, this was perceived as acknowledgement of the continuities and ruptures of their experience of themselves as women and as mothers. More commonly, their experience was of inappropriate placing.

Hilary Piercy examines the association between sexually transmitted infections (STI), particularly genital chlamydia, and the concept of dirt. She traces the process by which STIs became synonymous with women of lower classes, especially prostitutes who were seen as 'contaminated, separate and distinct from other women'. Despite changes in sexual mores, the women she interviewed felt 'dirty' when diagnosed to have chlamydia. They experienced painful dissonance when diagnosis placed them in a 'dirty category' which they located in 'otherness'. This work has considerable implications in the context of proposed changes in screening for chlamydia. Simon Dyson examines genes as matter out of place for 'White English' carriers of sickle cell and thalassaemia traits. Many feel themselves 'tainted' by genes, which they see as 'black'. The adjustment of clients to a status largely problematised by their racism is skilfully contained and 'cooled' by counsellors who are themselves black. Coping with the self, categorised as other, is a recurring theme in these and other chapters.

In the final chapter I attempt to draw threads together.

References

Callaghan, H.M. (2002) Birth dirt: relations of power in childbirth. Unpublished PhD, Faculty of Nursing, Midwifery and Health, University of Technology, Sydney, Australia.

Douglas, M. (1966) *Purity and Danger*. London: Routledge.

Gilligan, C. (1982) *In a Different Voice*. Cambridge, MA: Harvard University Press.

Section 1

Mothers, midwives and dirt – past and present

1 Birth dirt

Helen Callaghan

Introduction

This chapter is a brief overview of the theory on birth dirt and is based on the work 'Birth dirt: relations of power in childbirth' (Callaghan 2002). The term 'birth dirt' was coined to describe the theory which explains the power and/or dirt relationships in childbirth. Birth dirt exists, but its nature will vary depending on the time, the place and the culture. Who and what is clean or dirty similarly varies and will depend on and similarly create the discourses surrounding birth in the particular time, place and culture.

The study from which this theory was developed was about women, both birthing women and midwives, and their experiences of birth in Australia. The aim of the research was to examine the discourses and related practices surrounding birth and how these discourses shaped the power relationships between the women, their families and their care-givers. The focus of the study was the interactions, particularly communication patterns, the use of language and the practices, that occurred between the woman, her support people and health professionals. Data collection consisted of videotaping women in labour in a tertiary level public hospital in a major regional Australian city. Twenty-two couples were videotaped; all except one couple were having their first baby. Discourse analysis was the method used to analyse the tapes.

Due to various disciplinary approaches, there are many ways of 'doing' discourse analysis and no agreed method or methodology. The common thread in all the approaches, however, is the privileged position of language and its structuring effect together with an interpretative and reflexive analysis (Burman and Parker 1993). As analysis of the data progressed, the importance of Foucault's understanding of power (1972/1982, 1967/1997, 1980, 1994) and the clinical gaze (1975) became central to the thesis. Preliminary analysis of the videotapes led to an examination of my midwifery education through professional and consumer texts, casebooks and memory, with the concepts of 'clean and dirty' also being explored. As the study evolved, the focus sharpened and the study narrowed to the discourses surrounding who and what was considered clean or dirty and how this is constructed and played out in childbirth. Critical incidents were transcribed in detailed with a focus on the 'clean and dirty' aspects, then analysed using both texts and visual data. The incidents focused on various aspects of labour: one woman's desire to protect her modesty and conceal her genitalia ('the naughty bits'); a vaginal examination; the manner in which the midwives and the doctor dressed for birth; the hard physical work of the labouring woman; what is 'yuck' about birth and how both the midwives and the women and their families used very similar terms to describe this; breastfeeding and authorita-tive knowledge; and treatment of the dirty baby. The interpretations from each labour were synthesised into a unified socio-political analysis.

Pollution and dirt

Discussion on pollution inevitably leads to an examination of Mary Douglas's seminal work, *Purity and danger* (1966/1992), in which she focused on the sym-bolic interpretation of the rituals associated with pollution. Both Douglas (1966/1992: 35, 73) and Clark and Davis (1989: 651) defined 'ritual pol-lution' (within a religious system) and 'secular defilement' (within a civil system) as a state of uncleanliness derived via contact with a 'dirty' or 'pollut-ing' person, object or activity. However, the terms are used interchangeably, with 'pollution' the most commonly used term. For example, in discussions about the non-religious human, or the natural environment, the term used is usually 'pollution', or sometimes 'contamination', rather than 'defilement'. In health systems the term used, in the sense of the item or person being dirty, is 'contamination'.

'Dirt' is defined 'as matter out of place' (Douglas 1968/1999: 109), or 'dis-order', or 'it exists in the eye of the beholder' (Douglas 1966/1992: 35, 2), or a 'fantasy' (Kubie 1937), or what 'comes out of the skin or touches it and clings' (Enzensberger 1972: 9), or 'the object jettisoned out of that boundary' (Kristeva 1982: 69). Douglas (1966/1992: 120) considered the bodily orifices as vulnerable and whatever came from them symbolised both 'danger and power'. She considered that contact with the refuse from the body orifices was also dangerous and carried a 'symbolic load' (Douglas 1966/1992: 3).

Weaver (1994: 77) has pointed out the difficulty of defining dirt: ' "dirt" does not mean clean, good, clear, fresh, brightness of colour, hygienic, inno-cent, morally pure'. These various states are neither 'natural' nor 'inherently stable', while the person must fight to maintain these states through various methods: 'cleaning, washing, confessing', all of which indicate that there must be 'ritualistic practices' to maintain cleanliness (Weaver 1994: 77–78). A clean/dirty hierarchical structure was noted by various authors (Clark and Davis 1989; Derrida 1981; Enzensberger 1972; Kubie 1937; Ross *et al.* 1968). Weaver (1994: 78) noted 'clean and dirty are not equal, dichotomous, mutually exclusive categories with independent and inherent meanings'. The role of dirt in society is explained:

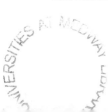

all dirt relationships . . . [should be] reinterpreted as power relationships. Anyone carrying dirt is powerful, and anyone in power utilizes dirt
for purposes of control. The one who can defile others, whether clean
himself or not is the boss.

(Enzensberger 1972: 47)

Pollution, for Enzensberger (1972: 22–23), originates or is derived from four
sources of dirt:

1 'Contact and excretion'
2 Intermingling
3 Decay and a reversal of order
4 'Mass'

Enzensberger (1972: 32) included human social behaviour when discussing
pollution and he wrote about dirt as being essential when there is 'structure
and order'. Dirt, for him, was the negation of the structure and order. He
described the characteristics of dirt:

1 Dry objects
2 Spots and splashes
3 'The wet and fatty'
4 Anything sticky and that makes threads
5 Any form of coagulation or wobbling
6 Anything that 'ferments, putrefies, sours . . .'
7 An increase 'of mud clay slime slush ooze . . .'
8 'Everything that crawls creeps writhes wriggles . . . slithers or spurts . . .'

(Enzensberger 1972: 16–17)

Although the list describes the physical characteristics of dirt, these characteristics are freely applied to people and their behaviours. For example, we
speak of individuals as being 'a worm', or 'a creep', or they are 'a fuck wit'.
Many of these colourful, but derogatory, terms are 'sex-elimination amal-
gam[s]' (Clark and Davis 1989: 657).
   Kubie (1937: 391) is explicit in that he considers the body a 'mobile dirt
factory, exuding filth at every aperture'. He suggested a hierarchy of dirt,
that is, humans react to dirt as if it possesses different degrees of 'dirtiness'
(Kubie 1937: 394). He contended that there would also be a universal rank-
ing of body products from the 'cleanest' to the 'dirtiest' (Kubie 1937). This
assumption was confirmed (Dimond and Hirt 1974; Hirt *et al.* 1969; Kurtz
et al. 1968; Ross *et al.* 1968). Milk was either the cleanest or the second
cleanest item, while semen was one of the cleaner items. An important
suggestion by Kurtz *et al.* (1968: 13) is that the hierarchy of body products
may be interpreted as products which are 'natural' and in harmony with
the body – 'body-syntonic' (tears, milk, and semen) – or those considered

foreign, diseased, unnatural, or 'waste' products of the body – 'body-alien' (faeces, phlegm, and pus). The latter group would include menstrual blood and the placenta.

Kubie (1937: 395) admitted that the *'most important single consequence of this hierarchy of fantasies is an unconscious but universal conviction that woman is dirtier than man'* (original emphasis). Although Kubie does not mention it, it is clear from his assumptions that the female genitalia are also considered dirtier than the male genitalia. Based on Kubie's hierarchy, the female genitalia are dirty, not just because of their surroundings, but because of their physiology and their anatomical shape. He does discuss his belief in women's obsessive conviction of having 'one aperture too many and that a dirty one' (Kubie 1937: 398).

The functions of pollution

Douglas (1966/1992: 3) believed pollution functions at two levels in society: an expressive level and an instrumental level. At the first or expressive level, the commonly held beliefs and social pressures are used to influence other people's behaviour. For example, the dominant societal belief in the contagiousness of blood and body substances is continually being promoted by various health institutions and the media. There is an expectation from the community, institutions, and professional bodies that protective apparel will be used if there is any risk of contamination. The second or instrumental level at which pollution functions occurs when there is a violation of the law which threatens what is considered the ideal in society, with the violation itself being a danger both for the society and the transgressors (Douglas 1966/1992). Douglas considered this produced two effects: (1) the threat of danger forces the person to maintain the desired social order; and (2) the enforcer is also reminded of the necessity to maintain the social order.

Douglas (1966/1992) considered that because we want to avoid dirt, we become creative and organise our environment so that avoidance of dirt is easier, by creating environments that suit the desired function and minimise the need for purification rituals. Douglas (1978) commented that pollution and purification are linked by ritual, while the nature of the rituals will define the seriousness of the pollution. This concept can be applied to the health care system where dirt 'specialists' undertake the ritual purification or cleansing.

Dirt and work

Hughes (1971: 312), a sociologist, believed that all occupations contained tasks which could be labelled as 'dirty', and provided a partial definition of 'dirty work' – it was 'drudgery . . . requires no skill. It has to be done, but is a low-prestige item.' Work is 'dirty' in several ways: by being 'physically disgusting', or it may symbolise degradation, or it may be contrary to 'our moral conceptions' (Hughes 1971: 343). According to White (1973: 288), a 'poor-man's work' means low pay levels, the worker is close to dirt and grime, is unable to determine when, where, and what he works at, often doing 'hard, dirty, night-time jobs'. Various authors have labelled work as 'dirty', covering a variety of jobs in different occupations or groups, and varying levels of skill or knowledge. Some examples are: housework (Davidoff 1979); physically heavy, tough work (Reed and Kramis 1996); repetitive, unskilled manufacturing work, shift work (Probert 1989); sanitary work (Perry 1978; Prashad 1995); care of people considered on the margins of society – deviants, drunks, people who have overdosed, homeless persons, welfare and disability recipients (Brown 1989; Jeffery 1984); and body work. Body work includes nursing, midwifery, and hospice care (Hunt and Symonds 1995; Lawler 1991; Lawton 1998; Murcott 1993; Wood 2001). Littlewood (1991: 178) has used the term 'sick dirt' to describe the demarcation of 'dirt' work in hospitals between nurses and domestic staff where the nurses remove one type of pollutant, excretions from the body, such as vomit, urine and faeces, while the domestics remove dust, tidy the spillage from flowers, and do other similar work.

Dirt and the health system

Clinical waste is defined as:

> that which has the potential to cause injury, infection or offence, and includes sharps, human tissue waste, laboratory waste, animal waste resulting from medical, dental or veterinary research or treatment that has the potential to cause disease; or any other waste, arising from any source, as specified by the establishment.
>
> (National Health and Medical Research Council 1999: 7)

This definition is mirrored in other documents (NSW Health Department 1998, 1999a, 1999b) and they all use the phrase 'potential to cause . . . offense'. These definitions support Douglas's (1966/1992) claim that western concepts of dirt are actually what we have rejected from various symbolic systems and are related to matters of hygiene, or etiquette, or aesthetics. This is made explicit in the *National guidelines for waste management in the health-care industry* (National Health and Medical Research Council 1999: 9) when it is stated that the disposal of clinical waste is guided by 'public expectations and *aesthetic considerations*' (my emphasis). A similar comment is made in an infection control policy document (NSW Health Department 1992).

Birth dirt

'Sick dirt' (Littlewood 1991: 178) is insufficient to explain the dirt of child-birth as in most instances the woman is not ill, and even if the process is abnormal it is rare for the dirt of abnormal childbirth to be the same as the dirt of a sick person. The childbirth process is limited by the physiological process and definite time constraints. The period of gestation, the labour and delivery period, and the postpartum period in which the woman adapts to her new body and role are also predetermined and known. The last is a minimum of six weeks, but is extended depending on the time the woman breastfeeds. The exact time frame may vary in different cultures and different times, but it is constructed around the physical reality of childbirth. The rare instances when 'birth dirt' would overlap with 'sick dirt' would occur when the woman experienced an illness related to the pregnancy – for example, hyperemesis,[1] endometritis,[2] breast abscess,[3] abdominal abscess, wound infection.

Birth dirt exists, but its nature will vary depending on the time, the place and the culture. Who and what is clean or dirty similarly varies and will depend on, and similarly create, the discourses surrounding birth in the particular time, place and culture. Most importantly, the power relationships are reflected in who is 'clean' (powerful) and who is 'dirty' (powerless). In the 1970s, the dirt of birth was about 'germs', or bacteria. In addition to the care of the parturient woman, the midwifery focus of care, which was directed by the obstetricians, was on searching for infections, or potential infections, or preventing infection, with many ritualistic practices based around controlling the pregnant woman. Currently, body substances and fluids are considered 'dirty' or contaminating. The midwives' work now incorporates controlling, containing and cleansing the new dirt of birth. Although the focus of the health professionals in each era examined in the study is different, 'the relations of power' remain the same – the control and surveillance of the childbirth process, and of the women, including the midwives.

The dirt of birth

Although during the labour and delivery process all body products are assumed to be contaminating, or dirty, there are particular body parts, or organs, or individuals which are treated as if they are particularly dirty. These are derived from or are unique to the woman's body. In the video-tapes the woman, her baby, and her family are seen as contaminating to varying degrees. Because of the continual potential severity of the contaminating ability of the woman, she is the person who needs to be most constrained. The baby, while dirty at birth, and a source of continual contamination, simply because of size and developmental age, is not a huge contamination problem. The baby can also be seen as a product of the hospital, as it was the management of the woman in labour and birth by the medical and/or midwifery staff which resulted in the birth of the baby. The baby formally becomes a patient at birth and begins a lifetime relationship with medicine.

Female genitalia and modesty

During labour the woman's reproductive passages, but particularly the genitalia, are a primary focus of the health professionals' attention or gaze. This
is a cause of embarrassment for some women – one participant described
and demonstrated how her breasts and genitalia were 'naughty bits' or
'dirty', and should be hidden. The need of the labouring woman for modesty
and privacy during labour is sometimes forgotten by health professionals in
modern Australia. Yet, for those women who are shy, or young, or private,
or come from a different ethnic background, or a particular religious community, modesty is an essential part of their normal life. Examinations in
childbirth, particularly those related to the woman's breasts and vagina,
can be a source of distress, discomfort and embarrassment for some women
(Henslin and Biggs 1995; Menage 1993; Schott and Henley 1996). This was
validated in the study.

The famous sexologist and psychologist Havelock Ellis (1936: 80) considered modesty was related to the woman's 'fear of arousing disgust . . . due
to the close proximity of the sexual centre to the points of exit of those
excretions which are useless and unpleasant'. For Carter (1995: 113) women
are responsible for maintaining their modesty and privacy through 'careful
"reading" of individual situations'. In the study, using Carter's terms, both
labouring women and midwives read the situation and maintained the
woman's modesty and privacy by carefully positioning individuals in the
birthing rooms so that their genitalia were not unnecessarily exposed.

Baby dirt

Although all the women videotaped during the birth were happy and eager
to touch and hold their baby, this was not true for most of the fathers. On
the videotapes, enfolding of the baby by the father and the support people
only occurred when the baby had been wiped clean and wrapped. The baby
is considered dirty but not from their dirt and so they wait until he or she is
cleaned, either partially or totally.

A newborn baby is covered in material which corresponds to many of
the characteristics of dirt provided by Enzensberger (1972: 16–17). For
example, the baby is always born wet and may be slippery or greasy from
the vernix; he may be covered in splashes of urine or in threads of bloody
mucus; from the intestinal tract, the baby may excrete meconium, which is
a thick, sticky, dark greenish, black, tar-like substance; the newborn baby
may be described as 'spitty', that is, drooling mucus from his mouth and
sometimes his nostrils; the baby's hair is often saturated with liquor, mucus,
blood, and sometimes meconium; the newborn baby has a distinctive smell
and, while not offensive, it is often a strange new smell to some of those
present at the birth; and finally, the baby could be considered to have

wormed his way out of a hole, the vagina, while babies are known to wriggle and twist.

The newborn baby can be considered dirty for several less obvious reasons. He is a prime example of Enzensberger's (1972) pollution whose origin is intermingling: first by the intercourse of his parents, then secondly by living inside his mother for approximately nine months. A similar argument is presented by Martin (1999: 126): the pregnant woman is a 'paradigm case of boundary transgression as well as the forbidden mixing of kinds'. The baby may be exposed to maternal faeces during the birth. 'Expulsion', the technical term, has connotations of driving out, or being rid of. Thus, the newborn baby must be driven out or got rid of, supporting Enzensberger's (1972) views of the newborn baby as polluted because of contact with his mother and because he is excreted from her body.

The newborn baby may have experienced trauma from the birth resulting in abrasions, bruising, swellings or other marks. Although these blemishes are usually either temporary, or a variation of normal, often even the most loving of parents will bemoan their presence and the resulting negative appearance of their baby. Even so, if permanent defects occur, the infants and their parents are often stigmatised (Darling and Darling 1982). These blemishes and permanent defects fit both Enzensberger's (1972) eighth characteristic of dirt and Goffman's (1963/1973) spoiled identity.

The placenta

Currently, all body products are treated as dirty; however, the placenta is also treated as a waste product which has a 'use by date'. At the study site, following the delivery of the placenta and its examination, it was disposed of in a machine, a placenta 'mucher', which vitamises the organ and sends the pieces into the sewerage system. The other method of disposal in Australia is incineration. Both processes clearly indicate how dirty the placenta is perceived to be. The dirtiness of the placenta was also reflected in how the placenta was treated for one couple who took their placenta home. It was placed in a plastic bag. However, the midwife was not content that the placenta was secure in the plastic bag and stated: 'And then I'll put it in another bag [pause] just in case.' Presumably, in case there was a hole in the first bag. The second bag was not a normal plastic bag, but a contaminated waste bag which is of extra strength, not so flexible, a bright yellow in colour, labelled 'contaminated waste' together with the internationally recognised black biohazard symbol on it. This behaviour is powerfully symbolic as another ordinary plastic bag would have served the same purpose. However, by providing the couple with a yellow contaminated waste bag, they are implying several things. The placenta is officially labelled as 'contaminated waste' and unless the couple remove it from this bag they will be constantly reminded of how the placenta is perceived by the majority of Australians and by the various governmental institutions. By using the contaminated waste bag with its official label, the Health Department and the medical profession, through the actions of the midwives, are demonstrating their power by shaping the community's world view of the placenta. By labelling the placenta as 'waste' the midwives are implying that the placenta is waste material, or rubbish, and does not need to be treated with respect. Similarly, the 'contaminated' in the label implies that the placenta is contaminated, while the reality is that for the majority of women there is only a slight risk of it actually being contaminated or infectious. The impression gained from the videotape is that the midwives appear to be acting in a magnanimous fashion in returning the placenta to the woman, as it is normally part of their role to contain its contaminating powers by destroying it. It is as if the placenta has been transformed by the institution from something that is the woman's to something that belongs to the institution, and, therefore, the state. The use of the yellow contamination bag supported the partner's reaction to the placenta: it was something he did not want to look at or touch. It is worth noting that one of the contradictions of the midwife's action was that although the placenta was officially labelled as 'contaminated waste', the parents were given neither gloves for when they were handling the placenta, nor any instructions on how to deal with the 'contaminated' item when they returned to their home.

The dirtiness of the placenta and menstrual fluid in comparison to 'normal' blood was noted in Laws's (1990) study. It is possible that the image of where they have come from is enough to classify them as 'dirty'. The shedding of the lining of the uterine wall is the reason given by Angier (1999) for our perception of menstrual blood as dirty. So a possible reason for describing the afterbirth as dirty is that the placenta and membranes are also attached to the uterine wall and are shed following the birth of the baby. Nathanielsz (1992: 65) considered the placenta to be 'thrown away' as it is no longer useful, and described it as 'the body's only throw-away organ'.

An alternative view of the afterbirth, particularly in non-western cultures, is that it and the baby have a special relationship. Angier (1999: 91) considers that the uterus and the placenta 'mother' the baby in a way that will never be repeated; while the afterbirth is referred to as the baby's 'life force' in Bangladesh (Jackson 1999: 58). In many cultures the afterbirth is considered a person (Trevathan 1987) and is described as companion (Waikato Polytechnic 1999), or grandmother (Parvati 1983), or 'friend' (Body Shop Team 1991; Trevathan 1987), or sibling (Priya 1992; Trevathan 1987; Watterson 1998). Perhaps more importantly, the correct disposal of the placenta is linked to the future of the baby, or the woman's childbearing abilities (Kitzinger 1993; Priya 1992; Trevathan 1987).

Colostrum, breast milk and lactating breasts

Midwives who assist women who are breastfeeding are expected to wear protective apparel. This may be gloves only, but if there is a risk of milk spraying the midwife, she is required to wear protective eye-wear. Breastfeeding is dirty work and the colostrum is a contaminating fluid, as was demonstrated by the midwife facilitating the breastfeeding by using the same gloves for cleaning equipment and the feeding. Since the improved understanding of the modes of transmission of hepatitis and HIV colostrum and breast milk are no longer seen as 'clean' body fluids, but are considered to be as potentially contaminating as all other body substances (National Occupational Health and Safety Commission and Worksafe Australia 1995).

Kitzinger (1979: 207) has expanded upon the links between breast milk and 'unclean secretions': the flow of breast milk is often uncontrolled during the early phases of lactation (like pus or mucus); it may jet out at 'socially inconvenient' times; it is a 'waste product' and requires removal; and it is a body fluid excreted like sweat. There is a taboo against seeing things coming out of our bodies, but there is no problem with eating in public (Giles 1997). Clearly, breastfeeding is a bodily function which is excretory for the woman, but it is a consuming function for the infant. Normally these functions are mutually exclusive.

Breastfeeding may be considered to belong to the private sphere of life and as such it is inappropriate and 'indecent' (Montagu 1986: 72) to do it in public. Publicly breastfeeding is evidence that the baby has 'stolen' the woman's body from his father (Kitzinger 1985: 227). Breastfeeding has been considered as an act of humiliation by some Christians and was considered a reminder of 'the Fall from Grace' (Potts and Short 1999: 158). As it may be considered dirty, or animalistic, or undignified, breastfeeding women are often expected to express their breast milk or feed their baby in the toilets or nappy-change rooms, if there is no mothers' room available. Even women who breastfeed in private, but leak milk from their breasts in public, are often embarrassed (Britton 1998). This may be due to the stain on their clothes, as all stains are considered 'dirty'. The women may perceive it as evidence of their lack of control of their body which is on display to everyone who sees the stain. There are few workplaces which provide facilities for women to either breastfeed their babies or express their breast milk. Women can be asked to cease feeding their baby, or to remove themselves from public places (O'Rourke 1994). Lomer's (1999: 49) Adelaide study noted that some members of the public want to impose on-the-spot fines for women who breastfeed in public!

In western society the breasts are considered as sexual objects, the property of the woman's partner, and therefore they should be hidden from sight except when on display in the 'right' place, such as in the media, on the beach, in the pool, or in the privacy of the home. Lomer (1999) has suggested that because the breasts of a lactating woman do not fit the ideal image of desirable breasts, they are seen as distasteful. Others in the community may consider artificial feeding as the 'norm' and breastfeeding as abnormal.

From this discussion, it is obvious that the lactating breasts, the colostrum, and/or the breast milk issuing from them are perceived as 'dirty', or harmful or offensive, by many in the community. Several decades ago, when the 'germ' theory was paramount, health professionals considered the breasts had to be cleaned before the baby was fed (Bailey 1975; Towler and Butler-Manuel 1973) and the equipment used during this process had to be sterile (Royal Women's Hospital Melbourne 1970). The 'symbolic load' attached to colostrum, breast milk and breastfeeding is complex and at times difficult to determine and this complexity was confirmed in this study.

Power relationships exhibited in labour

The study demonstrated the hierarchical nature of power in the Australian birthing room. The doctor is in charge, with the midwife working as assistant and in charge only in the absence of the medical staff. The woman is controlled by the midwife, while the partner and family are usually on a lower level again. This was seen in all the videotapes. The midwives considered the birthing room their space to organise as they wished.

The concept of touch as never being neutral (Kitzinger 1997) and expressing hierarchical status was important in this study. Kitzinger's (1997: 215) seven different forms of authoritative touch were used in the analysis: blessing touch, comfort touch, physically supportive touch, diagnostic touch, manipulative touch, restraining touch, and punitive touch. In the videotapes, it is evident that there is another form of authoritative touch, which I have referred to as 'directive touch'. Directive touch occurs when the care-giver uses touch to give the woman directions or commands, for example, applying pressure or traction to a part of the woman's body in order to get her to change her position. For the women in the research, of the eight forms of touch, they experienced all forms except punitive touch. The partner and support people used the blessing, comfort, and physically supportive touch frequently. The midwives and doctors used physically supportive touch occasionally, and diagnostic, manipulative, restraining and directive touch regularly, thus indicating a high level of power and control over the women. The health professionals usually provided physically supportive touch only for brief periods prior to the woman being supported by her partner or family. The women, like the newborn baby who is unwashed, are rarely touched without the barrier of gloves.

During the study, the most commonly worn uniform by medical and midwifery staff was the theatre scrub suit. This is recognised and standardised globally wherever western-style medicine is practised. It is a specialised form of uniform, worn by a small percentage of hospital staff. It bestows a certain amount of status and prestige on the wearer because of its association with operating theatres, the centre of modern medicine. The midwife's uniform can also be considered 'a vehicle of collective hygiene' (Roche 1994: 232), as the midwife is the health worker most closely linked to maintaining the cleanliness of the delivery room. Intriguingly, Roche (1994: 239) considered that the underlying principles relating to wearing a uniform provided a mechanism which has great similarity to Douglas's (1966/1992: vii) 'gestures of separation, classifying and cleansing' and is a means of creating social order.

From the discussion on dirty work and the hierarchical structure of Australian childbirth, it is clear that, as Enzensberger (1972) noted, dirt relationships are power relationships. Those who control childbirth in Australia are the medical profession and institutions, who together have determined who and what is contaminated or contaminating, and how this contamination should be contained. At a local level, that is, the hospital, the hospital medical staff and other health professionals, including midwives, carry out the dictates of these two groups. The labouring woman is vulnerable and dangerous, as was suggested by Frazer (1978) and Douglas (1966/ 1992). She has become powerful because contemporary conceptions of dirt make all the current rituals (wearing of protective clothing, management of the 'dirty' body fluids and substances) surrounding birth necessary to protect the health professionals. This powerfulness is recent, new, and reverses previous constructions. The subordinate position of the women and their families was evident in the critical incidents, while a major focus of the work of the midwife is the controlling, containing and cleansing of the 'dirt' surrounding birth.

Pollution and purification in childbirth

Historically, doctors had to create a space for themselves in maternity care, an area not previously recognised as theirs and considered by their medical colleagues as a 'dirty' area (Donnison 1988; Oakley 1976). To become acceptable to the women and their medical colleagues, this group had to prove that they were as good as the doctors who worked in medicine and surgery, and better than the midwives. They developed their own ways of seeing (the clinical gaze), and standards, then marketed them as superior. Although they might not agree on the causes of puerperal sepsis, they were fairly united in their opposition to the midwives who were labelled as 'dirty' (Castiglioni 1927/1941; O'Hara 1989). They promoted themselves as 'scientific', with the ability to perform life-saving procedures due to their ownership of the obstetric forceps. There was a proliferation of hospitals, including lying-in hospitals, in which they could develop their science, especially if they had access to a morgue. While the conditions in the hospitals were often poor and unhygienic, the doctors could study puerperal sepsis and other diseases. With the acceptance of the 'germ theory' the doctors continued being scientific and became 'clean', while the denigration of midwives continued. Because concepts of asepsis were believed to have produced improved outcomes for childbirth, policies and procedures relating to them became entrenched.

During my midwifery training in the 1970s, the maternity units and hospitals were built and organised in such a way as to enhance unity of form and function. The focus was on searching for sepsis, preventing its entry into the hospital, the women, the babies and the midwifery staff. The doctors were keen to extend their clinical gaze through the use of interventions in childbirth, especially labour. Rituals were developed which coped with the demands of keeping the women, the babies and the environment 'clean'. The labour wards were built with admission and/or preparation rooms, first stage rooms, operating theatres and delivery rooms; the wards had separate nurseries which included infant milk storage areas and milk formula rooms; the antenatal clinic had cubicles in which the women were seen. The labour ward was treated, and kept clean, as if it was an operating theatre. The women and their families were segregated and directed to particular areas depending on their perceived 'dirtiness' or 'cleanliness', or their vulnerability to 'dirt'. The babies were isolated from their families, with restricted access only for the parents, but they were freely accessible to the hospital staff. The baby could be seen at set times during the visiting hours, but only through the glass of the nursery windows. The rituals associated with the required functions of each area were quickly learnt and internalised – for example, the continual scrutiny of the women and their babies, the shaves and enemas of the labour ward, the breast trays and cord trays on the postnatal wards. To facilitate unity, it was necessary for everybody to know their relative position of importance and status within the hospital. As student midwives we soon learnt where we fitted in that hierarchical structure.

More recent hospital designs have included maternity wards without ordinary nurseries, only special care or intensive care nurseries, and birth centres, either attached to the main hospital or as free-standing units. The study site is designed in this way. The focus in this era of universal/standard precautions is the prevention of contamination by blood and body substances, and a continuation and extension of the clinical gaze on the women and their babies. The focus is no longer on preventing sepsis, it is on preventing cross-infection, especially to the health care workers. The hospital equipment is designed to make it easy to keep the birthing area free from material which would increase the risk of cross-infection. For example, the trolleys used in the delivery suite for the birth are made of stainless steel and are easily wiped clean. Much of the equipment is disposable and therefore does not require cleaning. There are mobile linen trolleys, and easily moved contaminated and normal rubbish bins. These are all lined with the appropriate plastic bag, so that the contents can be disposed of without touching the contaminated or dirty items. There are plastic covers for the mattresses and pillows so that these do not become contaminated or dirty with blood or body substances and are easily cleaned. Although these existed during my midwifery training, they were used sporadically. There are disposable draw-sheets and under-pads to minimise the need to wash the blood and body substances from the linen and to aid in the collection of these products. The floors and walls are made of materials which are easily cleaned. The staff wear theatre clothes so that if by chance they do become contaminated with blood or body substances, they can easily change into a clean outfit.

The midwife: mediator and paradox

The midwife is the dirty worker, so can consider herself as dirty. This was demonstrated throughout the study in different cultures and different times. She incorporates the dirty work into her midwifery work. She controls, con-tains and cleans the dirt that occurs during the birth. Because of the focus on dirt, there is a corresponding focus on protecting the health care worker from the dirt. Because of the midwives' role in relation to dirt, they act as a protective layer for those health professionals who have more status and power than they do. Yet, the midwife simultaneously has a role as being the mediator between the childbearing woman and the institutional rituals surrounding pollution and cleansing. According to McDonald (1992: 160), the midwives 'are the front line, representing the institution's efficiency, sterility and high seriousness'. The midwives protect the institution and its staff from the dirt of birth. Within the institution the midwife has an impor-tant role, but her position in the hierarchical structure is subordinate. In the context of providing care to women, she is sometimes more powerful than at other times, but this depends on the absence or presence of medical staff. This is the paradox: the midwife is both dirty and clean, powerless and powerful. She is the manager of the dirt and is responsible for controlling, containing and cleansing the dirt of birth.

Sanitising the birth

The woman's labour and birth can be sanitised in several ways. This sanitis-ing may be described as any method that 'cleans up' the birth process, that is, removes or reduces the dirt of birth, and/or the dirty work aspects of labour. In the videotapes the midwives continually, almost automatically, clean the birthing area. This is the most obvious way in which the birth is sanitised. The ultimate method of sanitisation, however, is an elective caesarean section. The woman does not experience the pain and distress of labour, and has a general, spinal or epidural anaesthetic. The surgery is performed through an adhesive dressing containing pockets which collect the body substances. At the completion of the surgery, the captured body substances are discarded; thus, the uncontrollable flow of blood and body substances usually seen during a vaginal birth is prevented.

Like an operative delivery, an instrumental delivery (forceps or vacuum extraction) will reduce the amount of work done by the woman. The use of analgesia can 'clean up' the labour by reducing or removing the work, distress and pain elements for the woman. If the woman does not use pharmacological methods of pain relief, the midwife will need to support her in the non-pharmacological methods she has decided to use. This can be taxing work. As one student midwife noted: 'pain relief, you'd love them to take something . . . they make your job more difficult' (Begley 2001: 31). For this midwife, the use of analgesia can reduce the woman's need for and dependence upon the midwives, thus reducing the midwives' workload.

There is a literal sanitisation of labour which occurs in many mainstream textbooks by either ignoring or minimising the woman's work as an aspect of labour; instead they focus on the clinical aspects of labour and birth, such as the stages of labour, the anatomy and physiology as it relates to the progress of labour, the mechanisms of labour, pain relief, and the strength, frequency and duration of the contractions (Beischer and Mackay 1986; Brucker and Zwelling 1997; Hickman 1985; Humphrey 1995; O'Brien and Cefalo 1996; Oxorn 1986; Rosevear and Stirrat 1996; Ross and Hobel 1992). It is as if by focusing on the work done by health professionals in managing labour, the work women do to deliver their baby can be ignored. One text does not even acknowledge the woman's role in pushing in the second stage and considers uterine contractions as the 'source of power' during the birth process (Burroughs 1992: 171). Another textbook continually uses the terminology of production and never mentions the woman, but instead relates the discussion to the uterus and the uterine contractions: 'uterine work', 'not working at maximum capacity', 'contractions become more efficient and uterine work increases' (Liu and Fairweather 1985: 22). This literal sanitisation of the women's labour is another way of emphasising the knowledge and power of the medical profession and the women's need of their skill and expertise. It emphasises the powerlessness of the women during the childbirth process.

Women, both giving birth and as midwives, continue to be constructed as the dirtier sex. Because of women's different anatomy and physiology – including the ability to give birth, and, therefore, the ability to produce body products such as menstrual blood, baby, lochia, liquor, colostrum that are also unique to women – they are considered dirtier than men. Anatomically, there is no denying that women have an extra orifice. Some may even consider that the lactating breasts provide multiple 'exit holes' for body products. The result is that labour and birth are dirty work for women, both as the mothers and as midwives. This research would seem to indicate that regardless of what women do or achieve they will always be the dirty workers, and seen as the most appropriate group to do the dirty work related to the home and the body. For the midwives, being focused on managing the dirt of birth means that they are less likely to focus completely on the women they provide care for. Instead of being with women, they are more aligned 'with dirt'.

Because of the way Australian society, and most western societies, perceive disease, dirt, contamination, pollution and impurities, we have constructed a health system that is aimed at coping with disease and dirt originating from the body. The failure of antibiotics to cope with serious infective illnesses, such as hepatitis and HIV/AIDS, together with the evolution of antibiotic-resistant bacteria, has led to the development of containment strategies directed at the prevention of the transmission of diseases, and the protection of healthcare workers.

Conclusion

The theory of birth dirt was developed following an analysis of videotapes of the interactions between health professionals, labouring women and their families, and the practices and discourses surrounding childbirth in Australia. This was followed by an analysis of textbooks from the beginning of obstetrics, and my midwifery training in 1970, and consumer material. The concepts of pollution, defilement, contamination and dirt and the work of theorists from a variety of disciplines have been crucial to this study and the development of the theory, although the work of Mary Douglas (1966/1992) was the starting point for the discussion. An underlying assumption in western philosophy of the categorisation of 'clean' and 'dirty' is that women are dirtier than men. Understanding these concepts, it became evident how each culture 'sees' their 'dirt', how it protects itself from pollution, and how it manages purification rituals.

The theory of birth dirt is about the power relationships in childbirth. Childbirth in Australia is hierarchical with the doctor as the person in charge. The midwife is his assistant when he is present, but she is in charge in his absence. The midwife is in charge of controlling, containing and cleansing the dirt of birth. She is the dirt manager and as such she is a dirty worker. The subordinate position of the midwife has not altered from when I undertook my midwifery education.

The discourses and discursive practices surrounding the women and the midwives as the labour progresses show that the woman is dirty for several reasons: she is continually leaking throughout her labour; she is on the margins; she is about to deliver/excrete a dirty being who will also be on the margins; and she is doing hard physical work. Because of their perceived dirtiness, the women and their families are kept in their place. Birth dirt exists but its exact nature will vary depending on the time, the place, the culture and the discourses which surround birth. However, whoever does the dirty work will be in a subordinate position. The midwife is a mediator and in a paradoxical position of being powerful and powerless in relation to birth dirt. The methods of sanitising birth have been made evident in this research and require subordination of women, as mothers and midwives, through dress, behaviour, discourses and practices to keep the most powerful safe.

Acknowledgements

Without the co-operation of the women and their families and the midwifery, medical and nursing personnel who agreed to be videotaped during labour this study would not have occurred. The Family Health Research Unit, which was jointly funded by the University of Technology, Sydney and South East Sydney Area Health Service, supported this study through the loan of equipment. Grants which supported this study were from: 1. Australian College of Midwives Inc.; 2. Upjohn Pty Ltd; 3. Beckton Dickinson; and, 4. NSW Nurses' Registration Board. I thank them all and I am indebted to them.

Notes

1 Hyperemesis gravidarum is excessive vomiting in pregnancy requiring treatment.
2 Endometritis is an infection of the endometrium, the lining of the uterus.
3 An abscess is a collection of pus and may be found in any body space or cavity (Sweet 1992).

References

Angier, N. (1999) *Woman: an intimate geography*. London: Virago.
Anon (1994) Magistrate slated on breastfeeding order. *Newcastle Herald*. Newcastle: Newcastle Herald, p. 4.
Bailey, R.E. (1975) *Obstetric and gynaecological nursing*. London: Baillière Tindall.
Begley, C.M. (2001) 'Giving midwifery care': student midwives' views of their working role. *Midwifery* 17: 24–34.
Beischer, N.A. and Mackay, E.V. (1986) *Obstetrics and the newborn: an illustrated textbook*. Sydney: W.B. Saunders.
Body Shop Team (1991) *Mamatoto: a celebration of birth*. London: Virago.
Britton, C. (1998) 'Feeling letdown': an exploration of an embodied sensation associated with breastfeeding. In S. Nettleton and J. Watson (eds) *The body in everyday life*. London: Routledge.
Brown, P. (1989) Psychiatric dirty work revisited: conflicts in servicing nonpsychiatric agencies. *Journal of Contemporary Ethnography* 18: 182–201.
Brucker, M.C. and Zwelling, E. (1997) The physiology of childbirth. In F.H. Nichols and E. Zwelling (eds) *Maternal-newborn nursing: theory and practice*. Philadelphia: W.B. Saunders.
Burman, E. and Parker, I. (1993) Introduction – discourse analysis: the turn to the text. In E. Burman and I. Parker (eds) *Discourse analytic research: repertoires and readings of texts in action*. London: Routledge.
Burroughs, A. (1992) *Maternity nursing: an introductory text*. Philadelphia: W.B. Saunders.

Callaghan, H.M. (2002) Birth dirt: relations of power in childbirth. Unpublished PhD thesis, Faculty of Nursing, Midwifery and Health University of Technology, Sydney.

Carter, P. (1995) *Feminism, breasts and breast-feeding*. Basingstoke: Macmillan.

Castigilioni, A. (1927/1941) *A history of medicine*. New York: Alfred A. Knopf.

Clark, P. and Davis, A. (1989) The power of dirt: an exploration of secular defilement in Anglo-Canadian culture. *Canadian Review of Sociology and Anthropology* 26: 650–673.

Darling, R.B. and Darling, J. (1982) *Children who are different: meeting the challenges of birth defects in society*. St Louis: C.V. Mosby.

Davidoff, L. (1979) Class and gender in Victorian England: the diaries of Arthur J. Munby and Hannah Cullwick. *Feminist Studies* 5: 87–141.

Derrida, J. (1981) *Positions*. London: Athlone.

Dimond, R.E. and Hirt, M. (1974) Investigation of generalizability of attitudes towards body products as a function of psychopathology and long-term hospitalization. *Journal of Clinical Psychology* 30: 251–252.

Donnison, J. (1988) *Midwives and medical men: a history of the struggle for the control of childbirth*. New Barnet, Herts: Historical Publications Ltd.

Douglas, M. (1966/1992) *Purity and danger: an analysis of the concepts of pollution and taboo*. London: Routledge.

Douglas, M. (1968/1999) *Implicit meanings: selected essays in anthropology*. London: Routledge.

Douglas, M. (1978) Introduction. In J.G. Frazer (author) and S. MacCormack (ed.) *The illustrated golden bough* (abridged edn). London: Macmillan.

Ellis, H. (1936) *Studies in the psychology of sex*, Vol. 1. New York: Random House.

Enzensberger, C. (1972) *Smut: an anatomy of dirt*. London: Calder and Boyars Ltd.

Foucault, M. (1967/1997) *Madness and civilization: a history of insanity in the Age of Reason*. R. Howard (trans.). London: Routledge.

Foucault, M. (1972/1982) *The archaeology of knowledge, and The discourse on language*. A.M.S. Smith (trans.). New York: Pantheon Books.

Foucault, M. (1975) *The birth of the clinic: an archeology of medical perception*. New York: Vintage Books.

Foucault, M. (1980) *Power/knowledge: selected interviews and other writings 1972–1977*. C. Gordon (ed.). New York: Pantheon Books.

Foucault, M. (1994) Sex, power and the politics of identity. In P.E. Rabinow (ed.) *Essential works of Foucault 1954–1984. Ethics: Subjectivity and truth*, Vol. 1. London: Penguin Books.

Frazer, J.G. (1978) *The illustrated golden bough*. S. MacCormack (ed.) (abridged edn). London: Macmillan.

Giles, F. (1997) Two breasts, twelve weeks. In D. Adelaide (ed.) *Mother love 2: more stories about births, babies and beyond*. Milsons Point, NSW: Random House.

Goffman, E. (1963/1973) *Stigma: notes on the management of spoiled identity*. Harmondsworth: Pelican Books.

Henslin, J.M. and Biggs, M.A. (1995) Behaviour in pubic places: the sociology of the vaginal examination. In J.M. Henslin (ed.) *Down to earth sociology: introductory readings*. New York: Free Press.

Hickman, M.A. (1985) *Midwifery*. Oxford: Blackwell Scientific Publications.

Hirt, M., Ross, W.D., Kurtz, R. and Gleser, G.C. (1969) Attitudes to body products among normal subjects. *Journal of Abnormal Psychology* 74: 486–489.

Hughes, E.C. (1971) Work and self. In *The sociological eye: selected papers on work, self, and the study of society*. Chicago: Aldine Atherton Inc., pp. 338–347.

Humphrey, M.D. (1995) *The obstetrics manual*. Sydney: McGraw-Hill.

Hunt, S. and Symonds, A. (1995) *The social meaning of midwifery*. Basingstoke: Macmillan.

Jackson, D. (1999) *Eve's wisdom: traditional secrets of pregnancy, birth and motherhood*. London: Duncan Baird.

Jeffery, R. (1984) Normal rubbish: deviant patients in casualty departments. In N. Black, D. Boswell, A. Gray, S. Murphy and J. Popay (eds) *Health and disease: a reader*. Milton Keynes: Open University Press.

Kitzinger, S. (1979) *The experience of breastfeeding*. Harmondsworth: Penguin Books.

Kitzinger, S. (1985) *Woman's experience of sex*. Harmondsworth: Penguin Books.

Kitzinger, S. (1993) *Ourselves as mothers*. Toronto: Bantam.

Kitzinger, S. (1997) Authoritative touch in childbirth: a cross cultural approach. In R.E. Davis-Floyd and C.F. Sargent (eds) *Childbirth and authoritative knowledge: cross-cultural perspectives*. Berkeley: University of California Press.

Kristeva, J. (1982) *Powers of horror: an essay on abjection*. New York: Columbia University Press.

Kubie, L.S. (1937) The fantasy of dirt. *The Psychoanalytic Quarterly* 6: 388–425.

Kurtz, R., Hirt, M., Ross, W.D., Gleser, G. and Hertz, M.A. (1968) Investigation of the affective meaning of body products. *Journal of Experimental Research in Personality* 3: 9–14.

Lawler, J. (1991) *Behind the screens: nursing, somology, and the problem of the body*. Melbourne: Churchill Livingstone.

Laws, S. (1990) *Issues of blood: the politics of menstruation*. Basingstoke: Macmillan.

Lawton, J. (1998) Contemporary hospice care: the sequestration of the unbounded body and 'dirty dying'. *Sociology of Health and Illness* 20: 121–142.

Littlewood, J. (1991) Care and ambiguity: towards a concept of nursing. In P. Holden and J. Littlewood (eds) *Anthropology and nursing*. London: Routledge.

Liu, D.T.Y. and Fairweather, D.V.I. (1985) *Labour ward manual*. London: Butterworths.

Lomer, K. (1999) Bosom buddies. *Sun-Herald. Good Weekend (supplement)*, 26 June. Sydney, p. 49.

McDonald, V. (1992) *Speaking of birth: an Australian midwife talks with parents about childbirth*. Newham, Victoria: Scribe Publications.

Martin, E. (1999) The fetus as an intruder: mothers' bodies and medical metaphors. In R. Davis-Floyd and J. Dumit (eds) *Cyborg babies: From techno-sex to techno-tots*. New York: Routledge.

Menage, J. (1993) Letters to the Editor. Women's perceptions of obstetric and gynaecological examinations. *British Medical Journal* 306: 1127–1128.

Montagu, A. (1986) *Touching: the human significance of the skin*. New York: Harper & Row.

Murcott, A. (1993) Purity and pollution: body management and the social place of infancy. In S. Scott and D. Morgan (eds) *Body matters: essays on the sociology of the body*. London: Falmer Press

Nathanielsz, P.W. (1992) *Life before birth: the challenges of fetal development*. New York: W. H. Freeman and Co.

National Health and Medical Research Council (1999) *National guidelines for waste management in the health care industry*. Canberra: AGPS.

National Occupational Health and Safety Commission and Worksafe Australia (1995), Vol. 2000. Sydney: Worksafe Australia, p. 4.

NSW Health Department (1992) *NSW infection control policy for HIV, AIDS and associated conditions* (State Health Publication No. (AIDS) 92-57). Sydney: AIDS Bureau, NSW Health Department.

NSW Health Department (1998) *Waste management guidelines for health care facilities* (State Health Publication No. EH 980098). Sydney: NSW Health Department.

NSW Health Department (1999a) Health care workers infected with HIV, hepatitis B or hepatitis. *Circular* 99/88, 1–12.

NSW Health Department (1999b) Re: Clinical waste definition, Section 3.1 – Waste management guidelines for health care facilities. *Circular*, 99/13, 1–2.

Oakley, A. (1976) Wisewoman and medicine man: changes in the management of childbirth. In J. Mitchell and A. Oakley (eds) *The rights and wrongs of women.* Harmondsworth: Penguin Books.

O'Brien, W.F. and Cefalo, R.C. (1996) Labor and delivery. In S.G. Gabbe, J.R. Niebyl and J.L. Simpson (eds) *Obstetrics: normal and problem pregnancies.* New York: Churchill Livingstone.

O'Hara, G. (1989) *The world of the baby: a celebration of infancy through the ages.* New York: Doubleday.

O'Rourke, J. (1994) Breast-feed mum thrown out of court. *Daily Telegraph Mirror*, 18 May. Sydney, p. 5.

Oxorn, H. (1986) *Oxorn-Foote: human labor and birth.* Norwalk, Conn.: Appleton-Century-Crofts.

Parvati, J. (1983) Lotus birth fully bloomed. In J.I. Ashford, P. Morganstern, S. Ritchie and M. Scott (eds) *The whole birth catalog: a sourcebook for choices in childbirth.* Trumansburg, NY: Crossing Press.

Perry, S.E. (1978) *San Francisco scavengers: dirty work and the pride of ownership.* Berkeley: University of California Press.

Potts, M. and Short, R. (1999) *Ever since Adam and Eve: the evolution of human sexuality.* Cambridge: Cambridge University Press.

Prashad, V. (1995) Between economism and emancipation: untouchables and Indian nationalism, 1920–1950. *Left History* 3: 5–30.

Priya, J.V. (1992) *Birth traditions and modern pregnancy care.* Shaftesbury, Dorset: Element.

Probert, B. (1989) *Working life: arguments about work in Australian society.* Ringwood, Victoria: Penguin Books.

Reed, T. and Kramis, A. (1996) Trinity at Dubna (reunion of the Soviet nuclear empire, May 1996). *Physics Today* 49: 30–35.

Roche, D. (1994) *The culture of clothing: dress and fashion in the 'ancien régime'.* Cambridge/Paris: Cambridge University Press/Fondation de la Maison des Sciences de l'Homme.

Rosevear, S.K. and Stirrat, G.M. (1996) *Handbook of obstetric management.* Oxford: Blackwell Science.

Ross, M.G. and Hobel, C.J. (1992) Normal labor, delivery, and the puerperium. In N.F. Hacker, J.G. Moore, J.S. Berek, R.J. Chang and C.J. Hobel (eds) *Essentials of obstetrics and gynecology.* Philadephia: W.B. Saunders.

Ross, W.D., Hirt, M. and Kurtz, R. (1968) The fantasy of dirt and attitudes toward body products. *Journal of Nervous and Mental Disease* 146: 303–309.

Royal Women's Hospital Melbourne (1970) *Neonatal paediatric notes for student midwives*. Melbourne: The Royal Women's Hospital Melbourne.

Schott, J. and Henley, A. (1996) *Culture, religion and childbearing in a multiracial society: a handbook for health professionals*. Oxford: Butterworth Heinemann.

Sweet, B.R. (1992) *Baillière midwives' dictionary*. London: Baillière Tindall.

Towler, J. and Butler-Manuel, R. (1973) *Modern obstetrics for student midwives*. London: Lloyd-Luke (Medical Books) Ltd.

Trevathan, W.R. (1987) *Human birth: an evolutionary perspective*. New York: Aldine de Gruyter.

Waikato Polytechnic (writer), Citizen, J. and Nicholson, D. (directors) (1999) Placenta: the child's companion [Video VT090 PAL]. J. Orange (producer). Hamilton, New Zealand: The Waikato Polytechnic.

Watterson, B. (1998) *Women in ancient Egypt*. Stroud, Glos: Wrens Park.

Weaver, A. (1994) Deconstructing dirt and desease: the case of TB. In M. Bloor and P. Taraborrelli (eds) *Qualitative studies in health and medicine*. Aldershot, Hants: Avebury.

White, D. (1973) Those who do the butt-end jobs. *New Society* 23: 288–291.

Wood, P.J. (2001) In R. Hawley and B. Leelarthaepin (eds) *Stories from the Field 2 Conference. Program and abstracts*. Sydney: University of Sydney, p. 44.

2 A clean front passage: dirt, douches and disinfectants at St Helens Hospital, Wellington, New Zealand, 1907–1922

Pamela J. Wood and Maralyn Foureur

In response to a growing concern about New Zealand's maternal and infant mortality rates at the beginning of the twentieth century, the 1904 Midwives Act established formal midwifery training and registration, and enabled the setting up of St Helens hospitals throughout New Zealand. These hospitals trained midwives and provided a state maternity service, delivered primarily by midwives, for working-class married women whose husbands earned less than £3 a week.

In June 1905, the Wellington St Helens Hospital was the first to be established. Our analysis of the first fifteen years of its existing case-notes, 1907–1922, numbering 3,670 patient records, reveals midwives' ideas about 'dirt' in relation to mothers who gave birth there.[1] This chapter offers an historical perspective to the current reflection on ideas about dirt in midwifery, childbearing and women's health today. It explores how the notion of dirt was constructed in these Wellington St Helens Hospital records and considers how ideas about dirt shaped understandings of the nature of midwifery practice. In particular, it examines how the locus of a concern for dirt extended almost seamlessly between the woman's internal body and the hospital environment – and even, at times, to the home beyond. Attention slid between the primary bodily locus of dirt, the woman's vagina or 'front passage' as women modestly called it, to the front passage of the hospital and its adjoining rooms. Midwives responded to identified dirt with douches and disinfectants, tackling the front passages of the internal and external environment with equal energy.

Women as a bodily locus of dirt

Midwives wrote notes about the woman on her admission to hospital, following the birth and during the puerperium, in the large volumes of the patient record books. These case-notes provide a sound basis for examining midwives' various and changing constructions of dirt in relation to childbearing women.

Midwives carefully observed and recorded the woman's general appearance on admission. Frequently embedded in these observations were descriptions of women as a general bodily locus of dirt. When Mrs B entered the Wellington St Helens in March 1909 to give birth to her first baby, for example, the midwives noted that her body and limbs were covered with a rash and she had a 'pus-like mould in the right groin'. By the time she was discharged her condition had 'much improved'.[2] Mrs D, admitted in October 1909, was described as 'swarming with pediculi [head lice]', her very low condition being due to 'dirt and poor unsuitable diet'.[3] Mrs GM, in November 1913, was considered 'anaemic', in a 'generally weakened condition' and 'neglected', with 'running sores on [her] head and pediculi'. She was treated with a 'special diet, malt and cleanliness'.[4]

As the woman's stay progressed, the notes focused on her body's recovery from the birth process and recorded any bodily change or untoward event, such as infection. Mrs JM, for example, a 33-year-old woman admitted in May 1908 to give birth to her fifth child, was 'poorly nourished', had 'cardiac and pulmonary trouble', venereal disease and signs of toxaemia.[5] On the fourth day after the birth her 'badly inverted' left nipple began to 'suppurate'. This was treated with boracic compresses and her milk supply was suppressed by applying belladonna and glycerine and a tight binder, and by giving saline aperients. The 'small and sickly' baby girl, who had weighed just 4 lbs 10 ozs at birth, was fed by bottle. Mrs JM's underlying health problems were also treated and after three and a half weeks she was 'discharged almost well'.[6]

Without other details it is difficult to be sure whether this was actual suppuration or what would now be considered a misdiagnosis based on unusually thick, yellow colostrum secreted from the nipple, which could be visually mistaken for pus. The smell of it was not recorded. Nevertheless, this 'suppuration' marks Mrs JM's body, already undermined by ill health, as a site productive of bodily dirt in the form of pus, rather than as a healthy one productive of wholesome milk.

The notion of 'dirt' is a cultural construct. As Mary Douglas has pointed out, each culture creates a classification system to bring order to the world. If something does not fit into a category, ambiguously straddles the boundary between categories or crosses from one category to another, it is defined as 'dirt'. It is therefore 'matter out of place'. Because it violates cherished classification categories, it is considered dangerous and powerfully polluting. And it is at the margins of the body that the danger of pollution is greatest. Any matter crossing bodily boundaries is therefore 'matter out of place', a powerful form of dirt and particularly contaminating (Douglas 1975: 50–51).

While Douglas offers a useful approach to begin exploring the way dirt is constructed and experienced, more detailed research is needed to understand this in any particular context. Each culture determines what substances will be considered 'dirt' and these definitions can change through time, as Douglas herself acknowledges (1975: 60–61). Interpretations based on specific examples from cultures in specific times and places are therefore needed, rather than relying on a more general explanation. This chapter is therefore concerned with constructions of 'dirt' in the midwifery culture at the Wellington St Helens Hospital, 1907–1922.

According to Douglas's explanation, bodily secretions such as those from the breast or vagina would be regarded as potentially polluting as they have crossed a bodily boundary. The examples of breast milk and vaginal secretions, however, lead to a more complex construction of ideas around bodily substances than Douglas's explanation might suggest. Regarding breast milk as polluting is somewhat problematic, particularly when it was considered essential for the infant's welfare. St Helens midwives vigorously encouraged breastfeeding and recorded their success rates in annual reports. It was when this breast secretion changed from a readily recognised, wholesome form capable of nourishing the baby, to one associated with bodily decay, that the notions of 'dirt' and 'pollution' were engendered. The identification of Mrs JM's nipple discharge as 'pus' is an example. Pus represents decomposition of bodily tissue and is a substance to be treated with caution and control because of its capacity to contaminate. The midwives' energetic intervention perhaps had as much to do with their recoil from the apparent travesty of colostrum being replaced with pus as it did with their impulsion to treat an infection. And in regard to vaginal secretions, Douglas's argument holds only to the extent that it explains any commonly accepted standards of personal hygiene in which cleansing the body of these secretions is deemed desirable. Yet different forms of vaginal exudations were recognised as having varying degrees of power to pollute. These nuances require a more finely-grained analysis than Douglas's explanation allows, to distinguish in this time period between bodily secretions which were considered normal and those which were worrisome discharges identified as 'dirt'.

As others have noted, a substance identified as dirt is often unpleasant, slimy, sticky, difficult to remove and associated with decomposition and decay (Kristeva 1982). The key identifier, however, which is not included in these definitions, is that the substance must be considered problematic (Wood 2005: 8–9). Sputum, for example, meets all the above characteristics of form but its expectoration is seen as unproblematic by the person spitting on the footpath yet highly problematic by the nurse who collects it in patients' sputum mugs and carefully discards it. This fuller definition of dirt, which acknowledges the requirement for the substance to be considered problematic, is consistent with midwives' constructions of dirt in the Wellington St Helens case-notes. It was only when vaginal exudates were contaminated by external pollutants or resulted from infection that they were regarded as problematic and therefore dirty and requiring remedy.

The vagina was the passage between the external and internal environments. It was a dangerous passage through which the woman's bodily dejecta could pollute the outside environment, and external microbes lurking in the atmosphere, and on walls and floors, instruments and hands, could contaminate the woman's interior. This front passage was therefore of prime concern in the midwives' daily round in caring for women in the puerperium. The primary form of bodily exudate from the vagina after birth was the lochia. It shifted in its composition of blood and serum through the postnatal days and was described as containing dejecta, such as fragments of decidua and membranes, and cervical mucus. As lochia was considered normally free from bacteria and 'almost the same as the discharge from an aseptic wound' (Jellett 1929: 233), it was not seen as potentially contaminating, despite crossing bodily boundaries. Danger came in the other direction – from the environment's ability to contaminate the lochia.

Midwives were warned of this danger by Dr Henry Jellettt. He was the Consulting Obstetrician to the New Zealand Department of Health, formerly of the Rotunda Hospital in Dublin, and writer of midwifery textbooks used internationally. He explained to midwives that if care was not taken to maintain the aseptic condition of the vagina, 'putrefaction and pus-forming bacteria' would be found (Jellett 1929: 235). Despite normal lochia containing fragments of decidua and membranes, it was only at this point when bacteria caused tissue to putrefy that lochia became problematic. Midwives were trained to differentiate between normal and problematic lochia. They needed to prevent bacteria from entering the vagina and promote drainage from it following birth. The key to effective control was to keep the drainage flowing. Lochial discharge could not be allowed to collect in the vaginal passage where it would decompose. It could not be left on the outside of the vagina, keeping the perineum wet, or be allowed to soak dressings, draw sheets and mackintoshes. Contaminated pads had to be burnt immediately when removed. 'Fresh' lochia was therefore regarded as a normal bodily discharge following birth. It was when it was allowed to collect and decay that it became identified as problematic and therefore as troublesome dirt.

To assist lochial drainage, doctors advised 'early rising', although there was debate about the timing of this following the birth. By the end of the 1920s Jellett was advising midwives that the woman should get out of bed on the second or third day (Jellett 1929: 238), but in 1918 Matron H.C. Inglis of the Wellington St Helens had been shocked by a British doctor's suggestions for 'early rising'. If it meant sitting up in bed on the third day, she was 'very much in favour of it', but if it meant getting out of bed on that day, she had 'nothing but condemnation for such a scheme'. Her concern had more to do with life circumstances than lochia. It was also coloured by her evident belief that the British doctor's assumptions were based on a narrower view of life than her own. Earlier rising might be suitable for British women with 'plenty of leisure, plenty of maids and few children', but for the majority of women in New Zealand and for all those at St Helens, the fortnight or ten days in bed after confinement [was] the only rest these women [had] from one confinement to the next. Once a woman is allowed out of bed, she will be at work again, cooking her husband's dinner, running after the children, doing the washing, and, possibly, going to the pictures. . . . Let her sit up in bed as soon as possible after the first 24 hours, but tether her to the bed if she wants to leave it before ten days.[7]

State examinations for midwifery registration tested candidates' knowledge of vaginal anatomy and its changes in pregnancy and childbirth, and of sepsis, asepsis and the need for lochial vigilance. One examiner in 1921 was disappointed in candidates' answers to a 'straightforward' question about lochial changes. He warned that infection was not always 'accompanied by foul lochia'. Any midwife unacquainted with this fact might have a feeling of false security which was an absolute danger to her patient. 'A midwife who waits for putrid lochia as a cardinal symptom', he said, delayed the essential 'early recognition and vigorous treatment' ('State examination of midwives' 1921: 116). These comments indicate that midwives did indeed have a notion that lochia needed to show overt signs of decomposition, namely having a foul smell and putrid appearance, to be considered problematic and indicative of infection. Simply crossing a bodily boundary did not render it dirt.

It was vaginal discharge described as 'offensive', 'foetid' or 'purulent' that received the closest scrutiny. Midwives were vigilant in recording any offensive whiff of vaginal discharge or any worrisome sighting of yellow, green or bright red seepage. Any suspicion of 'dirt' in the form of mucky or smelly discharge was promptly recorded, reported and vigorously treated. Perhaps an extreme case was Mrs T, a 23-year-old woman requiring a forceps delivery for her first child in 1908 as her pelvis was considered to be 'undersized'. On the second day after delivery, midwives observed 'sloughing of the soft parts'[8] and a 'very offensive', 'pus-like discharge', both of which they attributed to the 'unusually prolonged' labour (fifty-seven hours). The perineum was noted as 'unhealthy and blue looking', with 'two or three sloughs' separating after Creolin douching.[9] Although we might now consider that the sloughing had more to do with the forceps delivery than the prolonged labour, midwives were basing their description on the belief, commonly held at that time, that sustained pressure from the baby's head during long hours of labour restricted blood supply to the vagina and perineum, consequently causing sloughing.[10] However, it is the association of bodily decomposition (slough and pus), olfactory offence and danger to the woman's well-being that concerns us here.

Descriptions of offensive discharges, pus and slough show midwives' constructions of the notion of bodily 'dirt'. They were also concerned with dirt in the birth environment, whether the hospital or home.

The hospital and home as a polluting locus of dirt

Cleanliness was an essential feature of the hospital environment. Midwives and others concerned with the condition of the hospital building regarded it as an almost seamless extension of the woman's internal bodily environment. Concern for the woman's 'front passage' as a site where dirt could contaminate in either direction extended as well to the front passage of the hospital. From its establishment in 1905 in a poorer inner area of the capital city, the Wellington St Helens Hospital occupied a series of rented wooden houses which soon became inadequate in size and convenience. In 1912 it shifted to a purpose-built hospital near the top of a hill in the same area, with pleasant views of hills and a glimpse of the sea. Reporters describing the interior gave as much attention to the dirt-rejecting or dirt-creating qualities of materials in the hospital's front passage, wards and delivery rooms, as midwives gave to the similar qualities of the woman's front passage. Smooth surfaces in both, whether polished floor or slippery mucous membrane, were considered conducive to a healthy environment. Wards arranged on one side of the 'wide corridor' of the hospital's front passage had smooth walls of Keane's cement and polished floors, while the bathrooms, labour ward, sterilising room and dispensary had smooth floors of Linotol ('St Helens Hospital, Wellington' 1912: 79–81).

While the building and finishing materials ensured unbroken surfaces where dirt could not collect and contaminate, keeping the hospital (and woman) free from dirt also depended on regular cleaning, fresh air and sunshine. Wards opened through French doors to wide balconies, and beds had rubber wheels so they could be wheeled smoothly outside ('St Helens Hospital, Wellington' 1912: 79–81). One newspaper reported in 1915 that the hospital was 'exquisitely kept, abounding in clean, fresh space, pleasant windows, and the whitest of linen', with one ward 'a veritable solarium'. The nursery was 'a place of shining floors, white screens, and absolute silence, notwithstanding there were in it twenty babies, in twenty little white bassionettes [*sic*]' ('St Helens Hospital, Wellington' 1915: 36).[11]

But dirt could also be brought into the hospital by the women coming to give birth. When women were admitted they first had a bath in a bathroom just inside the door of the hospital's front passage. This vigilance to protect the hospital and its temporary inhabitants from the polluting power of the woman's body mirrored the attention given to bathing, swabbing and disinfecting the outside of the woman's vagina so that introducing any instrument or probing fingers did not convey external contaminants. Both front passages could therefore contaminate, or be rendered dirty by external agents. Both required diligent attention.

Dirt as a mediator of midwifery practice

Dirt had the power to mediate midwives' understanding of midwifery practice and of its context, both physical and professional. Dirt represented
danger – to the woman, the newly established midwifery profession, the
St Helens hospitals and a country concerned about its maternal mortality
rate. Dirt therefore had the power to contaminate both physically and symbolically. Central to this power was the link between vaginal contamination
and puerperal sepsis, the chief cause of maternal deaths. For every 1,000
European babies born alive in New Zealand in 1900, more than three
mothers died but by 1903 the rate had risen to nearly six and reinforced the
perceived need for the Midwives Act.[12] This poor measure of the country's
health and threat to its standing as a robust young colony worried both
health officials and politicians, especially as families were becoming smaller
and the proportion of women giving birth was diminishing.[13] The country
wanted healthy mothers producing healthy infants to populate New Zealand
and the Empire. Maternal welfare was therefore an imperative.

At the time the St Helens hospitals were established, most maternal deaths
were due to puerperal sepsis. Its prevention formed a strong focus in the new
midwifery education. The danger of dirt issuing from, or introduced into,
the woman's vagina was therefore emphasised in lectures, textbooks, journal
articles and examinations. The state midwifery examination in 1920, for
example, questioned midwifery candidates on the causes and symptoms of
puerperal septicaemia and the precautions they would take to prevent its
occurrence. Although the examiner was disappointed that so many candidates avoided the question, he thought those who tackled it did so creditably
('State examination of midwives' 1920: 117–118).

The fear of puerperal sepsis lay in its threat to maternal well-being and, by
implication, to the well-being of St Helens hospitals, which had a reputation
to maintain as a safe environment for birthing. St Helens hospitals achieved
better birth outcomes for women and babies than any other hospital,
whether large or small, private or public[14] (Mein Smith 1986: 61–62, 72,
77–78, 118). Any encroachment on this record would cast a poor light on
the Department of Health, which had in the St Helens hospitals a testing
ground for new policies and practices designed to improve maternal and
infant health outcomes. It would similarly reflect on the doctors who had
nominal oversight of the hospitals, although little actual practice there.[15]
But perhaps it reflected particularly on midwives, who provided virtually
all the care in these hospitals and implemented any Department of Health
policies. As a group newly professionalised through legislation, regulation
and education, midwives perhaps felt the need to achieve and maintain a
high standard of care to dispel the widely recognised image of the un-
educated, unskilled and unclean lay midwife, an image which had in part
prompted, or justified, the 1904 legislation.[16] The description of dirtiness
was now applied by the mostly middle-class midwives to many of the

working-class women giving birth at St Helens.[17] With its power to pollute and cause puerperal sepsis, dirt also became a focus of policy and practical measures to safeguard maternal health and thereby, to a considerable extent, shaped and directed midwifery practice.

Midwives learnt the different forms of infection which could affect child-bearing women. Most were attributed to bodily decay, a key identifier of dirt, or to external microbes which were harboured in dirt and which caused bodily tissue to decompose into pus. Dirt was therefore the cause or effect of infection. As Jellett's textbook instructed them, sapraemia resulted from 'poisons' formed 'during the putrefaction or decomposition of dead animal matter', in this case blood clots or parts of the placenta left behind in the uterus. Bodily damage through 'the crushing and death of the soft tissues of the genital tract' in prolonged labour could also cause sapraemia, as believed to be the case with Mrs T (Jellett 1926: 325–326). Septic infection, on the other hand, referred to 'the invasion of the body by pus-forming organisms' (Jellett 1926: 328–329). Nevertheless, there was some argument over this distinction, particularly whether the body contained its own infective agents (as in the theory of autogenous or endogenous infection) or whether these were introduced (as in exogenous infection) by the careless midwife or doctor (Corkhill 1932: 381–382).[18] Whatever its origin, infection endangered the mother's life and could spread to others through contamination by hands or equipment. Midwives were urgently reminded by textbooks and examiners to be vigilant, as the bodily interior was a site where bacteria could readily multiply ('State examination of midwives' 1913: 93–96; 1921: 113–116).

In their case-notes, midwives used language which reflected the descriptions of puerperal sepsis they read in textbooks, in which the bodily interior was described as dangerously contaminated by dirt and decay. Besides the words used in explaining sapraemia and septic infection, Jellett's textbook described problematic vaginal exudates as 'foetid', 'abundant', 'frothy' and 'offensive fluid', or as 'putrid lochia' or a 'profuse and foul discharge'. A large, soft subinvoluted[19] uterus could contain 'pus-forming' 'dead tissue', 'decomposing matter', 'shreds of dead mucous membrane' and blood clots (Jellett 1926: 325–331). Many of these descriptors appear in the midwives' case-notes, especially in relation to problematic lochia.

The patient records of Wellington St Helens between 1907 and 1922 therefore show that a significant aspect of midwives' practice was controlling and minimising vaginal dirt. In this period before the development of anti-biotics, diligent and energetic treatment to prevent sepsis meant drainage and disinfectant douches. Treatment could be initiated by either midwife or doctor. Midwives had little confidence in the vagina's capacity to empty foetid lochia from the body, even when they positioned the woman in the bed to assist this. They therefore also sluiced the front passage with douches, often two or three times a day over several days, washing it out with a warm solution. Their confidence in this alternative measure is seen in the fact that so many women at the Wellington St Helens in this time period were douched. Moreover, the proportion douched increased from one-third (33 per cent) of all women in the first 1,000 records to almost a half (42.5 per cent) in the final 1,000 records. It is unlikely that such a proportion of women were actually infected but they showed the signs of at least a susceptibility to it. Prompt action was considered necessary if infections were to be prevented.

The reasons given often focused on the nature of the lochia. Problematic lochia was typically described as 'offensive', 'foul' or 'foetid' in smell, copious in amount and could sometimes be green or yellow in colour. Red or 'free' lochia several days after birth was also worrisome as it should by then have been brown or almost colourless and small in amount. Other discharges could be 'pus-like', 'putrescent' or 'putrid'. Other reasons for douching that were associated with signs of infection, though less evocative of stench and visible pollution, were subinvolution and recordings of a raised body temperature. Other miscellaneous reasons included after-pains, retained membranes, haemorrhage or scanty lochia.

Most reasons therefore related to dirt in various forms, or the fear of sepsis, but the proportion of douches given for each reason changed throughout the time period. Offensive lochia accounted for 58.8 per cent of douches in the first 1,000 records but just 6.8 per cent in the final 1,000 records. Subinvolution accounted for 21.6 per cent of douches in the first set of records but rose to 62.5 per cent in the final 1,000 records. Offensive lochia was readily associated through sight and smell with the ideas of decay, dirt and danger. Subinvolution, on the other hand, connected to dirt through its offering of (in Douglas's terms) an ambiguous surface, straddled the boundary between identifiable categories, in this case neither an expanded uterus nourishing or expelling the infant, nor one returned to its normal, contracted form. In Douglas's explanation, its danger lay in being an ambiguous bodily form and, to the midwives, in having a surface susceptible to infection. It was a bulky, warm, spongy, moist surface where bacteria contained in contaminating dirt could embed and grow.

It is unlikely that the change in reported reasons for douching represented a dramatic shift in the actual incidence of these conditions. It is more likely that it represented a change in the culture governing which aspects of women's bodies were given prominence in the case-note constructions – the boggy sponginess of the subinvoluted uterus or its foetid exudations.

Midwives' knowledge of the appropriate reasons and correct method of douching, and the choice and strength of antiseptic for it, was tested in the state examinations ('State examination of midwives' 1913: 93–96; 1920: 117–118). Midwives could sometimes exhibit too great a degree of vigour and diligence. The answers of some candidates indicated they would pour the solution from too great a height ('State examination of midwives' 1913: 96; 'Midwifery examination' 1917: 51) or use too strong a solution. The examiner noted that the strength of Lysol and perchloride of mercury suggested by some in 1913 would cause considerable pain to a woman with a lacerated vagina ('State examination of midwives' 1913: 96). Conversely, others in 1920 used a solution 'too weak to be of real service' ('State examination of midwives' 1920: 117).

Considerable thought went into choosing antiseptics or disinfectants for use in the St Helens hospitals for maintaining a clean environment, whether internal or external. Disinfectants of choice for douching were Creolin, Lysol and perchloride of mercury, usually administered at 118°F (47.7°C) and from a height no greater than the woman's knees when drawn up in bed ('State examination of midwives' 1913: 96). Matron Inglis reported to the Department of Health in 1914 that the Wellington St Helens was using 6 gallons each of Lysol and Creolin that year, as well as 20 lbs of boracic powder and 6 lbs of boracic lint, used in dressings.[20] Dr Thomas Paget, employed in the Department of Health from the mid-1920s, experimented with disinfectants in the St Helens hospitals by getting midwives to evaluate various kinds, particularly Cyllin and later Dettol, with Dettol being deemed the disinfectant of choice (Mein Smith 1986: 66).

The Wellington St Helens also used formalin to fumigate women's and infants' clothing before transferring the clothing to the wards. Although an attempt to control dirt, it was not always a safe method, as demonstrated in 1915 when a major fire was narrowly averted after clothing fell on to the formalin lamp. When the room was discovered in flames, the midwife ran to the fire hose and, although the fire brigade had recently declared the fire hose quite impossible for a woman to handle, she soon had the fire out. Patients were compensated for the destruction of their clothing ('A fire averted' 1915: 96).

While midwives had control over the cleanliness of the hospital environment, they had to find other ways to deal with the environment of the homes they were called to on 'outdoor cases'. The hospital's 'outdoor' or domiciliary service catered for a small number of working-class women throughout Wellington city and suburbs. Although Dr Agnes Bennett, the medical superintendent of the Wellington St Helens, exhorted women to have a domestic 'weekly turnout' in which, she said, sweeping with damp tea leaves, sunning, beating, rubbing and airing were better than vacuuming (Bennett 1921), a vacuum cleaner was hardly a reality of poorer working-class women's lives.

Midwives soon learnt how to create the clean environment they considered necessary for a safe birth in a woman's home. They covered the bed's under-sheet with a thick pad of newspapers, topped them with a piece of clean old linen secured with safety pins, replaced floor rugs under the bed with a sheet of newspaper to receive soiled swabs, washed the woman from waist to knees with Sinol soap and sterile water, removed her pubic hair, gave her a cup of warm milk and cleansed the rest of her body ('A district midwifery case' 1916: 167). Midwifery candidates could be examined on their knowledge of preparing the bedroom, as much as the woman. The 1911 examiner worried, however, that nearly all candidates imagining attending a woman whose labour had just commenced, 'erred through excess zeal' in stating they would 'wash [her] hair; scrub the floor and carbolise the walls and bed'. 'These things', he said, 'may be counsels of perfection, but are neither possible nor desirable when labour has commenced' ('Midwifery' 1911: 13).

Keeping the passages clean

The run of patient records used in this research ends in 1922, just at the time when New Zealand's maternal mortality rate had reached a level sufficient to spark official alarm in the Department of Health. For every 1,000 live births in 1920, more than six (6.48) women died. Although this rate appeared only slightly higher than that in 1903 (5.86/1,000) when the need for legislation was suggested, this time it was presented in the context of an international comparison. It ranked New Zealand as having the second highest rate in the western world.[21] Some commentators were less concerned with this statistic, asserting that there was no internationally uniform method for compiling statistics to permit reliable comparison,[22] but the level was still considered unacceptable. A Special Committee of the Board of Health in 1921 found puerperal sepsis was due to some mothers' lowered resistance to infection, unhygienic conditions in homes and private maternity hospitals, and excessive use of instruments and operative measures (such as forceps) at births.

It was at this point that the Department of Health appointed Thomas Paget and Henry Jellett, and the two doctors began a vigorous campaign to reduce the rate. A chief response was to initiate a standardised aseptic technique in childbirth, modelled through the St Helens hospitals, which played a significant part in achieving New Zealand's 1927 position as leading the world in the reduction of maternal mortality. At the same time, the aseptic technique reinforced the focus on the vagina as a passage of dirt, requiring aseptic measures as stringent as for a surgical operation.[23] Midwives wore gloves, masks and sterilised overalls, and the woman's body was shaved, bathed, emptied by enema, daubed with disinfectant and swathed in sterile drapes. Every attempt was made to render a sterile field that extended from the woman's front passage, if not to the front passage of the hospital, then at least to the edge of the delivery bed and the people surrounding it. Cleanliness of the remaining spaces in the hospital, however, including its front passage, and the environment in which midwives worked in people's homes, remained a constant concern. Dirt therefore had considerable power in shaping midwifery practice and in mediating midwives' understanding of their practice world.

Douglas's contention that dirt is matter which has crossed boundaries and is therefore dangerous and polluting does not offer an entirely precise or sufficient explanation of midwives' construction of dirt in the records of women giving birth at Wellington St Helens between 1907 and 1922. Certainly, the forms of dirt midwives identified were usually associated with matter crossing bodily boundaries, whether external contaminants introduced into the body or offensive vaginal discharges exuding from it, but not all bodily exudates were considered dirty and therefore problematic. Milk from the breast and lochia were regarded as normal bodily secretions following childbirth, even though they crossed the external margins of the body. It was the capacity of the exudate to contaminate which rendered it problematic and therefore 'dirty'. Offensive discharges, green vaginal ooze, lochia containing decomposing membranes, and sloughing perineal tissue were forms of bodily material that represented danger to the woman through their association with infection. These bodily dejecta also represented danger to others if not properly collected, channelled or controlled. Other women could be infected. The danger of puerperal sepsis lay not only in its threat to women's health but also in its threat to the reputation of midwife, hospital, medical policy-maker and colony. In this we see Douglas's contention that dirt has both the physical and symbolic power to pollute.

It was not only bodily dirt that was problematic. Dirt in the birth environment could contaminate a woman by entering her vagina on careless probing hands, unclean gloves or instruments. It was crucial that the environment be as smooth and sound as the vagina's mucous membrane. Anxiety over the woman's bodily interior extended in a continuum of concern to the external birth environment. Both needed to be scrupulously clean. Scrubbing and polishing floors, soaking the woman on admission to hospital and swabbing both with disinfectant helped ensure that the hospital corridor and the woman's vagina were rendered a clean front passage.

Notes

1 This research has been partially funded by grants from the Faculty of Humanities and Social Sciences at Victoria University of Wellington, and by a grant from the Capital Coast District Health Board, Wellington. We are grateful to Abbey McDonald for her work as research assistant in the initial phase of this research.
2 St Helens Wellington Patient Records, Case Number 471, March 1909.
3 St Helens Wellington Patient Records, Case Number 613, October 1909.
4 St Helens Wellington Patient Records, Case Number 1382, November 1913.
5 A serious condition believed to be caused by toxins or poisons circulating in the blood. It was marked by increased blood pressure, retention of bodily fluids and the presence of albumin in the urine. The condition could lead to convulsions and death. It was later known as pre-eclampsia.
6 St Helens Wellington Patient Records, Case Number 339, May 1908.
7 H.C. Inglis, letter to the editor, *Kai Tiaki*, October 1918, p. 182. She was responding to a suggestion by a Dr Haultain in an article printed in an earlier issue of a New Zealand nurses' professional journal. The journal had a number of titles in this period, but they were always accompanied by the additional title of *Kai Tiaki* which is used in this chapter.
8 Sloughing is a term to describe the death of bodily tissue which then separates from the damaged area.

9 St Helens Wellington Patient Records, Case Number 321, March 1908.

10 This argument was also put forward by later textbooks. See for example Jellett's 1926 edition of *Short Practice*, p. 326.

11 'St Helens Hospital, Wellington', *Kai Tiaki*, January 1915, p. 36. The article printed an excerpt from the *Evening Post* of the previous December.

12 The rates were 3.83 per 1,000 live births in 1900 and 5.86 per 1,000 in 1903. *New Zealand Official Yearbook 1906*, Wellington, 1906, p. 251. These statistics, expressed as maternal deaths per 1,000 live births, would today be referred to as a maternal mortality *ratio* and would more usually be expressed per 100,000. The maternal mortality *rate* is today calculated as the number of maternal deaths in a given period per 100,000 women of reproductive age, regardless of birth outcome.

13 The birth rate had fallen steadily from 34.35 per 1,000 population in 1885, to 29.44 in 1890 and 25.60 in 1900. In 1878 one-third of married women of child-bearing age gave birth whereas in 1901 the rate had fallen to one in four. *New Zealand Official Yearbook 1906*, pp. 208–209. Childbearing age was considered to be 15–45 years.

14 During the 1920s particularly, St Helens hospitals had the lowest rates for puerperal sepsis, forceps deliveries and, from 1927, maternal mortality.

15 Doctors were only called in if complications were anticipated or detected.

16 The report of the Inspector of Hospitals, Dr Duncan MacGregor, a year after the Midwives Act was implemented, declared that 'the day of the dirty, ignorant, careless woman, who has brought death or ill health to many mothers and infants will soon end'. 'Report of the Hospitals and Charitable Institutions of the Colony', *Appendices to the Journals of the House of Representatives*, 1906, H-22, p. 3.

17 As they paid a fee to train as midwives, they are likely to have been middle-class women. The fee was £10 for the six-month training for those who were already registered nurses, and £20 for other women who undertook the twelve-month training. In comparison, the upper limit weekly wage for working-class families, for women to be eligible for care at St Helens when giving birth, was £3 in 1905 and £4 from 1912.

18 Corkhill was a midwifery examiner for the Nurses and Midwives Registration Board.

19 These are drawn from Jellett, *Short Practice*, 1926, pp. 325–331. Subinvolution was a condition, detected by palpation, where the uterus did not return to its previous non-pregnant size and position in the pelvis in the expected time.

20 Memorandum from H.C. Inglis, Matron, St Helens Hospital Wellington, to Acting Chief Health Officer, Wellington, 19 September 1914, held at Archives New Zealand, H1, 111.

21 The US had a rate of 6.5/1000. New Zealand's rate would have been higher if statistics for the indigenous Maori population had been included, but these were not collected. 'Maternal mortality', *Kai Tiaki*, July 1921, p. 110. St Helens hospitals were reported as having a rate of 4/1,000 despite many serious cases being taken there at the last minute. Our research, however, shows a rate of 6/1,000 for the Wellington St Helens in the 1907–1922 period, but is based on incomplete records. See Pamela J. Wood and Maralyn Foureur, 'Exploring a New Zealand maternity archive, 1907–1922: a nurse historian and midwife collaborate', in B. Mortimer and S. McGann, eds, *New Directions in the History of Nursing*, London: Routledge, 2005, pp. 179–193.

22 See for example the comments by Dr Agnes Bennett, medical superintendent of the Wellington St Helens, in a lecture to 100 midwives on a refresher course in Wellington in 1922, printed in 'Practical asepsis in midwifery', *Kai Tiaki*, April 1922, pp. 57–58. See also the comments by Dr Elaine Gurr, the Department of Health's expert on antenatal care, in a lecture to midwives on a refresher course

in Wellington in 1928, printed in 'Ante-natal work', *Kai Tiaki*, July 1928, pp. 121–125.
23   Corkhill, *Lectures*, 1932, p. 76. See also 'Puerperal infection', *Kai Tiaki*, July 1921, p. 136. This view was also debated: see for example 'Maternal mortality', *Kai Tiaki*, October 1921, p. 186, which cited a *British Medical Journal* article asking, 'What is the exact mechanism by which a sterilised overall or a face mask prevents infection of a patient's uterus?'

References

'A district midwifery case' (1916) *Kai Tiaki*. July 1916: 167.

'A fire averted' (1915) *Kai Tiaki*. April 1915: 96.

Bennett, A. (1921) *Domestic Hygeine*. Pamphlet held at Alexander Turnbull Library, Wellington.

Corkhill, T.F. (1932) *Lectures on Midwifery and Infant Care: A New Zealand Course*. Christchurch: Coulls Somerville Wilkie.

Douglas, M. (1975) *Implicit Meanings: Essays in Anthropology*. London: Routledge & Kegan Paul.

Jellett, H. (1926) *A Short Practice of Midwifery for Nurses*, 7th edn. London: J. & A. Churchill.

Jellett, H. (1929) *A Short Practice of Midwifery for Nurses*, 8th edn. London: J. & A. Churchill.

Kristeva, J. (1982) *Powers of Horror: An Essay on Abjection*. New York: Columbia University Press.

Mein Smith, P. (1986) *Maternity in Dispute, 1920–1939*. Wellington: Historical Publications Branch, Department of Internal Affairs.

'Midwifery' (1911) *Kai Tiaki*. January 1911: 13.

'Midwifery Examination' (1917) *Kai Tiaki*. January 1917: 51.

'St Helens Hospital, Wellington' (1912) *Kai Tiaki*. July 1912: 79–81.

'St Helens Hospital, Wellington' (1915) *Kai Tiaki*. January 1915: 36.

'State examination of midwives' (1913) *Kai Tiaki*. July 1913: 93–96.

'State examination of midwives' (1920) *Kai Tiaki*. July 1920: 117–118.

'State examination of midwives' (1921) *Kai Tiaki*. July 1921: 113–116.

Wood, P. (2005) *Dirt: Filth and Decay in a New World Arcadia*. Auckland: Auckland University Press.

3 The thanksgiving of women after childbirth: a blessing in disguise?

Rachel C. Newell

The body is one of the places in which social concerns are symbolically enacted.

(Eilberg-Schwartz 1990: 117)

Forasmuch as it hath pleased Almighty God of his goodness to give you safe deliverance, and hath preserved you in the great danger of childbirth. You shall therefore give hearty thanks unto God and say . . .

(The Book of Common Prayer 1929: 173)

Introduction

This chapter is concerned with the Anglican rite of the 'Thanksgiving of Women after Childbirth commonly called the Churching of Women'. The ritual of churching was used by the Christian church as the rite of purifying women after childbirth. Although it was regarded as an act of thanksgiving, as an opportunity for the woman to receive a celebratory blessing, that characterization disguises the control that was exerted over parturient women and their midwives. This chapter discusses the place of notions of 'uncleanness' and 'pollution' within the postpartum experiences of women by exploring the relevance of churching for contemporary birth rituals. The churching of women had been in existence for hundreds of years before falling relatively rapidly into decline in the nineteenth century. There is a need to determine what insights such historical practices can provide for twenty-first-century perspectives on women's bodies, maternal roles and birth rituals. Focusing on elements of the practice of the thanksgiving of women after childbirth provides an excellent tool for this purpose. The aim of the chapter is, first, to outline a short history of churching; second, to provide a thick description of the biblical narrative as found in the Old Testament Book of Leviticus chapter 12: 1–8; and third, to discuss the possible relevance of the chapter content for contemporary birth rituals.

An outline of the 'churching rite'

The rite of the purification and thanksgiving of women after childbirth found its way into the Christian prayer books by the eleventh century (Bradshaw 1987; Coster 1990; McMurray Gibson 1996; Knodel 1997; Lee 1998). Produced by a male church of the past, the rite is the only ritual in the western Christian church to address women, and women of considerable significance: women who have recently given birth. Bradshaw (1987) demonstrates that the Levitical notions of postnatal defilement persisted in the early Christian church. His scholarly work on Hippolytus demonstrates that in the mid-fourth century AD, new mothers were considered unclean and were therefore required to sit with the catechumens (the unbaptized) during the forty days after childbirth prior to rejoining the worshipping community. Hippolytus included midwives in this prescription, but reduced their period of 'uncleanness' by half, that is, to a period of twenty days. In the medieval church, which licensed midwives in England (Forbes 1964; Donnison 1988; Gelis 1991), the medieval midwife emerges as the companion to the mother at her churching (Cressy 1993; McMurray Gibson 1996; Cressy 1997; Lee 1998). The post-Reformation sacramental Anglican church retained the churching rite but deleted the word 'purification' from the title. The rite emerged in the English church in the 1552 Prayer Book as the 'Thanksgiving of Women after Childbirth commonly called the Churching of Women' (Maltby 1998). Within the first 100 years following the English Reformation, the Puritan Henry Barrow, writing in 1590–1591 (see Carlson Leland 1966: 463), questioned the need for a special thanksgiving ceremony for something 'as natural as the birth of a child'. The rite was retained in the 1662 Anglican Book of Common Prayer. With the rise of modernity the practice of churching fell into decline. The Prayer Book remains in use today in the Church of England and in the Episcopal Church of Scotland. The short churching text or rubric has survived all Prayer Book reforms.

When the phrase a 'blessing in disguise' ends with a question mark, this may act as a sign, not of doubt but of multiplicity. It calls forth the notion of the multiple. So when the question 'what was going on?' is asked we are not seeking a singular answer as in 'what was the thing that was going on?' (as in a definitive interpretation or a truth claim), but rather multiple elements: what were the things that were going on? These things themselves are multiple. By multiple in this respect we do not mean simply the different parts of the same thing, but rather multiple things each of which may have parts or elements, which the word 'disguise' serves to augment, conceal or reveal.

It is important to note that the notion of disguise in this context is virtual rather than actual. This is to say that it is a concept by which the event called churching may be thought. Disguise in this respect is not a propositional referent applied to states of affairs. It is not accountable to external benchmarks of truth or falsity. It is a virtual tool for thinking the event of the body of a woman and bodies of women, and doing this in a manner that brings new insights and values to the event called churching.

It is out of the scope of this chapter to deal with the weight of evidence and insights presented by scholars over the past three decades concerning women's rituals. Notions of uncleanness and pollution lie at the very heart of the practice or event called churching. The main section of the chapter will discuss from a midwifery studies perspective what most scholars take to be the biblical background to the practice of churching, that is, the Jewish law of Leviticus 12: 1–8. The intention is to explore in detail and seek to identify elements in both the symbolism and the practice of the purification ritual for the postnatal woman.

Book of Leviticus

Mary Douglas (1966), writing from an anthropological perspective in her book *Purity and Danger*, puts it neatly: 'dirt' is the same as 'body matter out of place.' Douglas's work remains highly influential in her analysis of the meaning of purity in the study of religions. According to Jacob Neusner (1975), in his legal-religious construct of ideas of purity in ancient Judaism, conceptions of purity served the purpose of identification and differentiation of one cult from another. Both Neusner (1975) and Douglas (1966) agree that such ideas carry implications for the 'larger system', of which notions of purity are a part.

However, the reader is invited to consider the lived reality of being physically 'unclean' alongside the theocratic and intellectual notions of 'pollution' and 'impurity'. The lived reality of the recently delivered woman manifests itself in the form of the vaginal leakage of lochial blood. The vaginal discharge known as *lochia* is the outward sign that childbirth has taken place – blood which can be smelled, felt and observed on and from the body as it leaks out and may adhere to the skin of bruised and/or torn genitalia; what Julia Kristeva (1982: 65) calls 'secular filth'. It is only when the 'secular filth' becomes sacred impurity that exclusion on the basis of 'religious prohibition is made up'.

Most authors (see for example Staton 1980; Wilson 1990; Coster 1990; Thomas 1991; McMurray Gibson 1996; Knodel 1997; Lee 1998; Roll 2003) agree that the rite in the Anglican Communion, which emerged from the Latin pre-Reformation Roman Catholic purification rite, is constructed around or elaborated from the Old Testament in the eight short verses of the Book of Leviticus, Chapter 12. The next section of the chapter examines the text of the Old Testament Book of Leviticus 12: 1–8.

A strange text

The Levitical text below is selected from the King James Authorized Version of the Bible,[1] because it is linguistically closest to the English Prayer Book text:

1. And the LORD spake unto Moses, saying
2. Speak unto the children of Israel, saying, if a woman have conceived seed, and born a man child: then she shall be unclean seven days; according to the days of separation [*menstruation*] for her infirmity shall she be unclean.
3. And in the eighth day the flesh of his foreskin shall be circumcised.
4. And she shall then continue in the blood of her purifying three and thirty days; she shall touch no hallowed thing, nor come into the sanctuary, until the days of her purifying be fulfilled.
5. But if she bear a maid child, then she shall be unclean two weeks, as in her separation: and she shall continue in the blood of her purifying threescore and six days.
6. And when the days of her purifying are fulfilled, for a son, or for a daughter, she shall bring a lamb of the first year for a burnt offering, and a young pigeon, or a turtle dove, for a sin offering, unto the door of the tabernacle of the congregation, unto the priest.
7. Who shall offer it before the LORD, and make an atonement for her; and she shall be cleansed from the issue of her blood. This is the law for her that hath born a male or a female.
8. And if she be not able to bring a lamb, then she shall bring two turtledoves, or two young pigeons; the one for the burnt offering, and the other for a sin offering; and the priest shall make an atonement for her, and she shall be clean.

(Book of Leviticus 12: 1–8)

The uncleanness of childbirth to which Leviticus is referring is the discharge of lochia. The lochia (Marchmant *et al.* 1999) is the discharge from the uterus emerging from the vaginal introitus after the completion of labour, consisting of decidua (tissue debris, blood and mucous). Lochia appears in three observable and emerging stages. First, *lochia rubra* is markedly stained with blood for the first four days after birth, while the change to *lochia serosa* occurs from five to fourteen days after childbirth and is brownish pink in appearance. Lastly, *lochia alba* appears, which is pale and creamy, free from red blood cells and may last on average some thirty-two to thirty-six days after birth. For a few women the discharges may continue for as long as six weeks.[2] Thus the law of purification of women as given in Leviticus covers the maximum amount of time that the lochia may appear and continue. The first two stages of red and brownish pink discharge in which red blood cells are apparent coincide with the seven- or fourteen-day period requirement for the parturient's body in Levitical law to be 'unclean' as at the time of her menstruation (Leviticus 12: 2–5). In both instances women are considered to be the defilers of anything with which they may come in contact. During the subsequent thirty-three days, that is, leaking *lochia alba per vaginam*, the maternal body continues in 'the blood of her purifying'. But, and this is important to the discussion in the chapter, the parturient's body is in Levitical law doubly unclean for a further sixty-six days if delivered of a girl. Yet the lochia alba normally ceases by thirty-six days irrespective of the sex of the baby. During the time of her lochia alba, the woman may not enter the sanctuary of the tabernacle. That the postnatal woman underwent a 'ritual cleansing' or 'blessing' in temple or church that symbolically brought her back into the 'community of faith' does not mean that she was not mobilized by degrees before the time of the ritual. Despite the maternal body's implied and considered impurity, nowhere in the Hebraic Old Testament is the process of childbirth considered symbolically unclean. The process of labour involves bodily discharges from the vagina which inevitably smear the neonatal body. Yet the newborn is not considered unclean. Only the post-birth lochia from the vagina renders the woman as 'unclean'. This begs the question: why is the lochia held to be unclean?

Returning to Mary Douglas's (1966) critique of Leviticus, 'defilement' occurs within a system or order of ideas and these ideas are held in relation by rituals of separation. Douglas argues that the organic system of the body provides an analogy of the social system. The more bodily systems are ignored the more likely are they to be set outside, and the more important they become. She proposes that a natural way of investing a social occasion with dignity is to hide organic processes, that is, the dirty, polluting, defiling, unclean processes. My contention is that these organic processes have emerged as rites of the Christian church and as social or celebratory occasions. For example, in live birth, the body of the baby emerges in the symbolism of the infant baptism rite with its subsequent christening party. With the birth of the placenta and membranes and the living mother leaking lochia, the maternal body emerges in the churching rite which in the Christian medieval period was followed by a churching party (Cressy 1993; McMurray Gibson 1996; Cressy 1997; Knodel 1997; Lee 1998). Heterosexual activity (the transmission of semen from penis to vagina which is not perceived as dirty) emerges as the marriage rite followed by the wedding celebration. The dead body or corpse emerges in the burial rite followed by a 'wake'. Douglas writes:

> Matter issuing from them [the orifices of the body] is marginal stuff of the most obvious kind. Spittle, blood, milk, urine, faeces or tears simply issuing forth have traversed the boundary of the body. . . . The mistake is to treat bodily margins in isolation from all other margins.
>
> (Douglas 1966: 121)

The power of defilement is not innate. Defilement's power is in relationship to the power of the forbidden from which it originates: 'it follows from this that pollution is a type of danger which is unlikely to occur except where the lines of structure, cosmic or social are clearly defined' (Douglas 1966: 121).

Douglas's analysis claims that all bodily emissions are viewed as polluting, but Frymer-Kensky takes a different view: 'The only bodily emissions that pollute are those involved with sex' (Frymer-Kensky 1983: 401). I suggest that the bodily emissions that pollute or render unclean are those involved with the risk to life that bring about death of the body.

While I do not disagree with Mary Douglas (1966), I do diverge some-what by seeking to relate physiology to symbolism while trying to avoid collapsing symbolism into physiological pragmatism.

Every childbirth is normally associated with two elements: birth of a live baby, followed by the 'dead' placenta, membranes and cord. The sub-sequent leakage of uterine blood is thus related to birth and death simul-taneously. It is not the leakage of uterine blood which is the pollutant, but what the leakage symbolizes. Unique to women following childbirth is the physiological fact that the empty, firmly contracting, uninjured, non-infected postpartum uterus will naturally reduce its blood loss over a given period of time. But if the body continues to lose blood uncontrollably it will eventually die. The dead body becomes the 'vile body' (Murray 1850: 358).[3] All of the time that a parturient bleeds *per vaginam* in the Levitical context, she is at risk of dying. It is the threat of maternal death, the threat of becoming the 'vile body' which is the pollutant, not the leaking uterine discharges *per se*. I agree with Douglas (1966) that this pollutant is 'a type of danger', because the pollutant may lead potentially to maternal death which is the greatest danger. The living mother at forty days postpartum is the survivor of the pollutant. The language of impurity, uncleanness and pollution in relation to the postpartum woman is, I venture to suggest, a metaphor for the risk of maternal death. Once the lochia ceases, the mater-nal body is no longer in a state of perceived risk. No longer in a state of perceived risk of becoming the 'vile body' is a metaphor for 'purified'.

I am of the view that the separation or seclusion of the parturient from the Hebraic community at large was both symbolic and pragmatic. The isola-tion or segregation most likely became a social mechanism devised by women together with the people as a pragmatic exercise.[4] The segregation of the puerperium was a social mechanism which probably brought health benefits to women. Because of the success of the health benefits to women and by extension to men (success as breeding women), the form of segrega-tion became a social exercise which gained the approval of the people. The postpartum social isolation exercise eventually emerged as a purification ritual. In the ritual of purification, the Hebrew priests found the means to establish a power over women that controlled their reproductive processes, because they conceived the 'leakage of vaginal blood' as something suspi-cious. I concur with Douglas's point, that the Hebrew priests' power over the organic processes of childbirth and the puerperium is disguised by investing the process with the dignity of a social occasion and celebration.

Julia Kristeva (1982) has made a significant contribution to the debate on purity, the unclean and the Biblical narrative of Leviticus. Kristeva's critique is grounded in Lacanian psychoanalytic theory. Because of the provision of the burnt and sin[5] offerings in order to purify the body, Kristeva (1982: 99) demonstrates that there is on the mother's part an acknowledgement of her 'impurity, defilement, blood and purifying sacrifice'. Kristeva moves her argument to include a commentary on the third verse of the chapter relating to the birth of a son and the necessity for his circumcision. She views circumcision as a rite of separation from the maternal, as a separation from women's impurity and defilement, and aligns the meaning of circumcision as a sign of men's alliance with the God of the chosen people:

> that evocation of defiled maternality, in Leviticus 12 inscribes the logic of . . . abominations within that of a limit, a boundary, a border between the sexes, a separation between feminine and masculine as a foundation for the organization that is 'clean and proper' 'individual' and . . . signifiable, legislatable, subject to law and morality.
>
> (Kristeva 1982: 100)

But the text of the Book of Leviticus 12: 1–8 is essentially a protocol designed for postnatal women. Kristeva (1982: 101) asks the question 'by means of what turn-about is the mother's interior associated with decay?' Crucial to the development of an argument related to the notion of 'decay' is the placenta and membranes which have separated from and been expelled by the 'interior', the uterus. And this remarkable and significant 'other' part of the feto-placental unit (which sustained the intrauterine life of the baby) is now dead, and will decay. In childbirth, life and death coalesce. The 'placental body' is always 'stillborn'. The 'placental corpse' is the disposable body organ of the immediate post-birth maternal body. Expelled from that body it is in Kristevian terms a form of 'sanitary effectiveness'. The 'natural wound' left interiorly, Kristeva claims, leaves no trace of its presence. I disagree. Despite the hidden, interior, natural placental-site wound, the fact of its healing is indicated by the leaking, smelling presence and observation of the changing lochia over the ensuing days. The 'natural wound' does leave a trace, if not 'trail', of its presence.

The maternal body may be wounded from the spontaneously occurring rupture(s) of the vagina and perineum at the time of expulsion of the baby from the birth canal. The 'traces or marks of childbirth' will not disappear for some thirty-two to thirty-six days. Thus the maternal body bears the Kristevian hallmark of 'unclean, the impure, the separated, the non symbolic and the non holy'. The postnatal woman in the context of the Levitical narrative becomes an *agent provocateur* in an ordered society:

For whatsoever man be he that hath a blemish, he shall not approach; a blind man, or a lame or he that hath a flat nose or anything super-fluous . . . he shall not come nigh to offer the bread of his God.

(Leviticus 21: 18–21)

But the Levitical text increases in its significance when the parturient is delivered of a daughter. Verse 5 of the Levitical chapter is examined in the next section.

'Doubly unclean': baby girls and baby boys

A woman having given birth to a daughter is considered doubly unclean (Leviticus 8: 5). A 'doubled time of defilement' for the body of a woman delivered of a woman, because both are women? Jacobus de Voragine (1230–1298),[6] a Dominican friar writing in the thirteenth century, asked the question: why had the Levitical law proscribed a doubled time of defile-ment for mothers of daughters? And he replied:

Since the female body requires twice as much time to complete itself in the mother's womb, the soul is not infused into it on the fortieth day as with male infants but only on the eightieth day.

(De Voragine 1969: 150)

Milgrom (1991) and Noth (1977) are puzzled at the increased length of defilement time. Milgrom cites a Rabbi Ishmael who claimed that complete formation of the male embryo occurs at forty-one days and the female embryo at eighty-one days. Milgrom, citing the Greek philosopher Aristotle, claims that the male foetus is formed in forty days and the female in three months. Milgrom refers to Hippocrates the Greek physician as claiming a thirty-day period for male embryonic development and forty-two days for the female. It is likely that de Voragine's medieval thinking emerged from and was informed by similar Greek source material. The Greeks and de Voragine were writing embryology without the benefits of the scien-tific developments of future history. The evidence demonstrated by late twentieth- and twenty-first-century embryologists related to genital devel-opment in the human foetus would more or less concur with the time limitations contained in the old source materials. William Larsen, an embry-ologist, states:

At the end of the sixth week, male and female genital systems are indis-tinguishable in appearance. In both sexes germ cells and sex cords are present in both the cortical and medullary regions of the presumptive gonads and complete mesonephric and paramesonephric ducts lie side by side. The ambisexual or indifferent phase of genital development ends at this point and from the seventh week on the male and female systems pursue diverging pathways . . . maleness is actively induced by a sex determining transcription factor encoded on the sex determining region of the Y chromosome (SRY). If the factor is absent or defective, female development occurs.

(Larsen 1993: 249)

Moore and Persaud (1998) showed that female genital development is slower (there is no testis-determining factor on the X chromosome to act on the 'indifferent gonad'). It is around the twelfth week of gestation that the ovary is identifiable histologically. Carlson (1999) also agrees with this timing and indicates that the testis develops more rapidly than the ovary. In 2004 Jan Jirasek wrote: 'In males, related to primary genetic sex determination (SRY gene) primordial germ cells and coelomic cells constitute testicular cords between 42 and 45 days after fertilization' (Jirasek 2004: 44).

The impossible-to-answer question: how was it possible for ancient sources to have arrived at such authoritative statements related to the Levitical chapter? Even more puzzling is the speculative possibility as to how the Levitical priesthood arrived at such a time limitation upon male and female embryonic development if that is the explanation for the doubled time of defilement. The issue of the defilement effect whether eighty or forty days postpartum remains an enigma. Milgrom says that many would agree with the view that: 'The cultic inferiority of the female sex is expressed in giving the female such a double uncleanness effect' (Milgrom 1991: 2). Milgrom is unable to explain the difference in length of period following the birth of a girl or boy. He also cites other religions in which the disparity in gender-related purification time periods after childbirth is similar to that in Leviticus. The period following a girl's birth is nearly always longer. Levine's (1989) explanation is equally lacking.

If conception and birth are the intersections at which life and death coalesce, then according to Milgrom (1991: 750) 'the nexus points are those in which there appears to be a departure or a transfer of vital force'. Rachel Adler (1976) has claimed that it is the birthing woman who transfers the vital force, but De Troyer *et al.* (2003) counter and maintain that that is the real problem. For De Troyer *et al.* the issue is the life-giving capacity of a 'female grown-up newborn'. In childbirth women not only give life and live while shedding blood, but the birth of a girl means that in time she too will give life in like manner. My understanding is that De Troyer *et al.* see the female neonate as representative of a 'doubled anti-power to the masculine part of the sacred'. In trying to tease out this notion of 'doubled anti-power', let us consider the observable physiological evidence that many girl babies during their adaptation to extra-uterine life demonstrate a 'pseudo-menstruation'. Pseudo-menstruation may appear from the second to fifth day of life: a part of a girl baby's normal adaptive extra-uterine physiology (Avery 1981; Vulliamy 1982; Sweet 1997: 798). To the observer, neonatal pseudo-menstruation contains small streaks of blood mixed with mucous exiting from the baby's vagina and easily seen on the napkin. Neonatal pseudo-menstruation makes it possible to offer an algebraic equation for De Troyer *et al.*'s 'doubled anti-power':

1 postnatal woman + 1 man baby = 1 'leaky' woman = 40 days
1 postnatal woman + 1 woman baby = 2 'leaky' women = 80 days

De Troyer *et al.* hypothesize that such a long transition for the woman delivered of a daughter reflects a threat or dread related to the female neonate's future fertility. They conclude that the Levitical chapter is the result of a reinterpretation of previous translations. As a result of such changes in vocabulary they reflect:

> Far from being in a state of blood purification, parturients have become unclean, as in the days of her menstruation. Literally, the days of secretion of her menstruation have become days of isolation. . . . The Septuagint, however, opened the way for identifying blood of purification with unclean blood and hence uncleanness.
>
> (De Troyer *et al.* 2003: 63)

Brenton (1978) points out that it was in the Septuagint[7] that the notion of unclean blood as a translation of the Hebrew purifying blood first arose.

Returning to where I started, the Hebrew priests were confronted by the fact that postnatal women leaked blood, the cessation of which was outside male control. Thus it was necessary to control and disempower women symbolically 'by means of a filthy defiling element' (Kristeva 1982). The continuity of the postnatal Hebraic legislation remained intact at the time of the birth of Jesus. In the New Testament Book of Luke, the text reads:

> When the time of her purification according to the law of Moses had been completed, Joseph and Mary took him [Jesus] to Jerusalem to present him to the Lord. (As it is written in the Law of the Lord, Every firstborn male is to be consecrated to the Lord.) And to offer a sacrifice in keeping with what is said in the Law of the Lord, a pair of turtle doves or two young pigeons.
>
> (St Luke 2: 22–24)

Two thousand years later, notions of purity and pollution in relation to postnatal women remain.

Churching in the twentieth and twenty-first centuries

The practice of churching has survived (Hancock 2004, personal communication). Michael Staton (1980) carried out a sociological qualitative study related to churching in an urban context. He showed that notions of 'unclean' and 'impure' were passed on by oral tradition. He claims that the churching ceremony helped convey information to those who participated in the rite as a symbol of social action and communication. Among the information conveyed was the notion of uncleanness and sin associated with childbirth. From a transcribed taped interview excerpt he states:

> This gave me the opportunity to ask if any of these women believed that a woman who had had a baby was in any way unclean. They both replied 'Yes' and they both agreed that it was 'because you bleed a lot after you have had a baby'.
>
> (Staton 1980: 263)

Staton (1980: 263) makes the point about this being 'the clue that he had been waiting for to try to explain the mystery that attaches itself to the mother'; the subject that the other women had, as he stated, 'been too embarrassed to mention'. Perhaps he had not recognized the shift that had already begun to take place. The shift from, on the one hand, women's bodies (in his study context) perceived as objects of pastoral and sacramental care, to women as real people, women who were grounded in their church liturgy trying to affirm the goodness and holiness of their bodies in the late twentieth century. Staton takes the view that the two women above clearly viewed churching as a purification rite. It is also clear that for some women 'having babies is a sin': 'It is a sin to have a baby. It is unlucky not to be churched. You don't have any luck if you don't get churched. My mother would shut the door on you' (Staton 1980: 264).

The evidence provided by this late twentieth-century study sheds light on a number of ways in which women's bodies, women's relationships within their urban community and their childbirths were perceived. Postnatal women were regarded with suspicion until they had participated in the rite. Staton makes the point that churching may have value in helping the woman through the emotional crisis of childbirth. Similar claims have been made by Stern and Kruckman (1983) and Cheung (1997).

This chapter is representative of work in progress. Potential conclusions arising from this work are that medieval midwives licensed by the church were a part of an overall elaborate surveillance or audit mechanism. Within this mechanism the medieval churching ritual completed the process of legitimation (or illegitimation) of the birth at six weeks postpartum by the presence of the midwife at the churching ceremony. In this way midwives assisted in securing the legitimacy of the blood line of the family, and by extension property and lands. In a twenty-first-century secularized state, midwifery services provision conveys not dissimilar messages through the Notification of Births mechanism (normally written by midwives) which is confirmed by parental registration of birth at the local Registrar's Office of Births, Marriages and Deaths. In Levitical and Christian 'churching' the maternal body is rendered symbolically clean, or pure. Within a secularized National Health Service maternity system, postnatal women undergo the ritual practice of the 'six-week postnatal examination'. The actual maternal body and its emotional state are assessed in order to identify normal functioning. The maternal body is given 'a clean bill of health'. In this way the present-day maternal body is rendered symbolically clean in a secularized context. The secularized ritual is of significance for midwifery practice when it is set within the threatening context of the risk of 'dirt and pollution' from antibiotic-resistant bacteria, viruses, postnatal depression and suicide as a significant cause of maternal death. The practice of churching with its concepts of dirt, uncleanness and pollution as once sought and practised is not obsolete. It has emerged disguised within a secular health service. Notions of uncleanness, dirt and pollution remain and government has taken cognizance of such notions. As Douglas (1966: 113) comments, 'the power which presents danger for careless humans is very evidently a power inhering in the structure of ideas, a power by which the structure is expected to protect itself'.

Conclusion

Rituals such as those detailed in Leviticus 12: 1–8 concerning postnatal women and the subsequent emergence of churching in the Christian faith have a physiological dimension to them. However, that alone does not explain why the midwife was also held to be affected by association. It is the physiological dimension which takes us to the symbolic dimension, although the former is not necessarily sufficient to account for the latter *in toto* in some kind of universal sense, or as a 'constant'. Where body and ritual meet, as it were, takes us to the epistemic dimension. The epistemic dimension refers to what, at any given period in history, it is possible to think or say and the meaning that envelops and legitimates it. Hence the episteme at the time of Leviticus would be somewhat different from the medieval or pre-Renaissance epistemes, which are different again from the classical and modern epistemes. The meaning ascribed to the ritual surrounding postnatal women will keep changing, even though the ritual itself (in western Christianity) appears much the same. The meaning of the physiological dimension also changes, while also retaining symbolic significance – for example, the current practices in maternity care where 'filth' or 'impurity' becomes 'infection' or normal functioning, and a 'clean bill of health' is granted after the final postnatal visit. When the midwife ceased to be 'affected' by association (whenever that happened?), then it is clear that the epistemic dimension of what is going on in the 'assemblage of the multiple' changed.

Acknowledgements

The foregoing represents part of 'work in progress' of a doctoral thesis. My grateful thanks are extended to Dr J. Drummond, Senior Lecturer, Nursing, University of Dundee School of Nursing and Midwifery, and to Dr H. Walton, Senior Lecturer, Theology, University of Glasgow School of Religious Studies.

Notes

1　My study uses the excerpt from the King James Authorised Version of the Bible because it relates to the language of the Book of Common Prayer. I am aware of more recent and purportedly accurate modern translations, in particular the New Revised Standard Version of the Bible.
2　Further and varied physiological explanations about lochia are to be found in the many textbooks available to students of midwifery and obstetrics. The list that would arise if all were to be cited would be too long for this work. For a recent evidence-based research publication on the topic of vaginal blood loss following childbirth, see Marchmant *et al.* (1999). However there is a facsimile edition of much older evidence, edited by the historian Elaine Hobby (1999) in the Women Writers in English Series 1350–1850: Jane Sharp (an unknown woman but clearly a midwife) is the author of the book *The Midwives Book or The Whole Art of Midwifery Discovered*. The book provides the reader with access to ways in which Sharp's culture understood the maternal body.
3　The term 'vile body' is used in the rubric or text of 'At the Burial of the Dead' in the 1662 version of the Anglican Prayer Book. The term refers to the body of the deceased at the point in the burial service 'while the earth shall be cast upon the Body by some one standing by'. See Murray (1850: 358). In the 1929 reprinted edition of the Prayer Book 'vile body' becomes the 'body of low estate'. The change was related to the meanings of certain words in the English language in the early twentieth century. Changed meanings of words are no less problematic today.
4　It is Michel Foucault who suggests that 'ordinary people have knowledge of their circumstances and are able to express themselves independently of the universal theorizing intellectual'. See Smart (2002: 67).
5　The word 'sin' does not appear in the Anglican rubric or text in the churching rite.
6　Jacobus de Voragine became a Dominican friar in 1244 at the age of 14. He taught theology and bible study. He became Prior of Genoa of the Provincial of Lombardy from 1267 to 1286 and latterly Archbishop of Genoa. He is the author of *The Golden Legend* (1969).
7　According to Clow (1977: 384), the Greek language became the language of scholars and as a result Hebrew ceased to be the spoken language among the Jews. The change led to a Greek version of the Jewish scriptures which became known as the Septuagint or LXX. The Septuagint was used in the early Christian church and all the quotations from the Old Testament are taken from the Septuagint version.

References

Adler, R. (1976) 'Tumah and Taharah: Ends and Beginnings'. In R. Kolton (ed.) *The Jewish Woman: New Perspectives*. New York: Schocken.

Avery, G.B. (1981) *Neonatology, Pathophysiology and the Management of the Newborn*, 2nd edn. Philadelphia: J.B. Lipincott.

Barkley, G.W. (1990) *Origen: Homilies on Leviticus 1–16*, English translation. Washington DC: Catholic University Press.

Barrow, H. (1966) 'The Writings of Henry Barrow 1590–1591'. In C. Leland (ed.) *Elizabethan Nonconformists*. Texts: 5. London: Allen & Unwin, pp. 72–463.

Bradshaw, P. (ed.) (1987) *The Canons of Hippolytus*. Bramcote, England: Grove Books. Trans. C. Bebawi; Alcium/Grove Liturgical Study 2; Grove Liturgical Study 50.

Brenton, L.C.L. (1978) *The Septuagint Version of the Old Testament*, trans. London Bagster (1851). Grand Rapids: Zondervan.

Buckley, T. and Gottlieb, A. (1988) *Blood Magic: The Anthropology of Menstruation*. London: University of California Press.

Carlson, B.M. (1999) *Human Embryology and Developmental Biology*. London: Mosby.

Carlson Leland, H. (1966) *Elizabethan Non Conformist Texts*, 5. London: Allen & Unwin.

Carrette, J. (ed.) (1999) *Religion and Culture by Michel Foucault*. Manchester: Manchester University Press.

Cheung, N.F. (1997) 'Chinese Zuo Yuezi (sitting in the first month of the postnatal period) in Scotland'. *Midwifery* 13: 55–65.

Clow, W.M. (ed.) (1977) *Bible Reader's Encyclopaedia and Concordance*, rev. edn. Glasgow: Collins.

Coster, W. (1990) 'Purity, Profanity and Puritanism: The Churching of Women 1500–1700'. In W.J. Shiels and D. Wood (eds) *Women in the Church*. Studies in Church History, 27. Cambridge, M.A.: Basil Blackwood, pp. 377–387.

Cressy, D. (1993) 'Purification, Thanksgiving and the Churching of Women in Post Reformation England'. *Past and Present* 141: 106–146.

Cressy, D. (1997) *Birth Marriage and Death: Ritual Religion and the Life Cycle in Tudor and Stuart England*. Oxford: Oxford University Press.

Davis, N.A.Z. (1975) *Society and Culture in Early Modern France: Eight Essays*. Stanford, Calif.: Stanford University Press.

De Troyer, C., Herbert, A., Johnson, J.A. and Korte, A. (eds) (2003) *Wholly Woman Holy Blood: A Feminist Critique of Purity and Impurity*. London: Trinity Press International.

De Voragine, J. (1969) *The Golden Legend*, English translation by Granger Ryan and Helmut Ripperger. London: Longmans Green; reprint New York.

Diamont, A. (2002) *The Red Tent*. Oxford: Pan Macmillan.

Donnison, J. (1988) *Midwives and Medical Men: A History of the Struggle for the Control of Childbirth*. Hong Kong: Historical Publications.

Douglas, M. (1966) *Purity and Danger: An Analysis of Concepts of Pollution and Taboo*. London: Routledge & Kegan Paul.

Dresen, G. (2003) 'The Better Blood: On Sacrifice and the Churching of New Mothers in the Roman Catholic Tradition'. In K. De Troyer, J.A. Herbert, J.A. Johnson and A. Korte (eds) *Wholly Woman Holy Blood: A Feminist Critique of Purity and Impurity*. London: Trinity Press International, pp. 143–164.

Eilberg-Schwartz, H. (1990) *The Savage in Judaism. An Anthropology of Israelite Religion and Ancient Judaism*. Indianapolis: Indiana University Press.

Fitzgerald, M.J.T. and Fitzgerald, M. (1994) *Human Embryology*. London: Baillière Tindall.

Forbes, T.R. (1964) 'The Regulation of English Midwives in the 16th and 17th Centuries'. *Medical History* 8: 235–244.

Foucault, M. (1969) *The Archaeology of Knowledge*, trans. Alan Sheridan. London: Routledge.

Foucault, M. (1977) *Discipline and Punish: The Birth of the Prison*, trans. Alan Sheridan. London: Penguin.

Frymer-Kensky, T. (1983). 'Pollution, Purification and Purgation in Biblical Israel'. In C.L. Myers and M.O. O'Connor (eds) (1983). *The Word of the Lord Shall Go Forth: Essays in Honor of David Noel Freedman in Celebration of his Sixtieth Birthday*. Winona Lake, Ind.: Eisenbraums.

Gelis, J. (1991) *History of Childbirth: Fertility, Pregnancy and Birth in Modern Europe*. Cambridge: Polity Press.

Habiger, P. (1998) *Menstruation, Menstrual Hygiene and Women's Health in Ancient Egypt*. Museum of Menstruation and Women's Health: www.mum.org/germnt5.htm

Hancock, Reverend R. (2004) pesonal communication.

Henerey, A. (2005) 'Evolution of Male Circumcision as Normative Control'. *Journal of Men's Studies* 12(3): 265–276.

Jirasek, J.E. (2004) *An Atlas of Human Prenatal Developmental Mechanisms: Anatomy and Staging*. London: Taylor and Francis.

Johnson, J.A. (2003) 'Shedding Blood: The Sanctifying Rite of Heroes'. In K. De Troyer, J.A. Herbert, J.A. Johnshon and A. Korte (eds) *Wholly Woman Holy Blood: A Feminist Critique of Purity and Impurity*. London: Trinity Press International, pp. 189–222.

Knodel, N. (1997) 'Reconsidering an Obsolete Rite: The Churching of Women and Feminist Liturgical Theology'. *Feminist Theology* 14: 106–125.

Korte, A.M. (2003) 'Female Blood Rituals: Cultural Anthropological Findings and Feminist Theological Reflections'. In K. De Troyer, J.A. Herbert, J.A. Johnson and A. Korte (eds) *Wholly Woman Holy Blood: A Feminist Critique of Purity and Impurity*. London: Trinity Press International, pp. 165–188.

Kristeva, J. (1982) *Powers of Horror: An Essay on Abjection*. New York: Columbia University Press.

Larsen, W.J. (1993) *Human Embryology*. Edinburgh: Churchill Livingstone.

Lee, B.R. (1996) 'The Purification of Women after Childbirth: A Window onto Medieval Perceptions of Women'. *Florigelum* 14: 50–61.

Lee, B.R. (1998) 'Women Ben Purifyd of her Childeryn: The Purification of Women after Childbirth in Medieval England'. Unpublished PhD thesis, University of Toronto.

Levine, B.A. (1989) *Leviticus JPS Torah Commentary*. Philadelphia: Jewish Publication Society.

McCulloch, D. (1997) *Cranmer*. London and New Haven: Yale University Press.

McMurray Gibson, G. (1996) 'Blessings from Sun and Moon: Churching as Women's Theater'. In B.A. Hanawalt and D. Wallace (eds) *Bodies and Disciplines: Intersections of Literature and History in Fifteenth Century England*. Minneapolis: University of Minnesota Press, pp.139–154.

Maltby, J. (1998) *Prayer Book and People in Elizabethan and Early Stuart England*. Cambridge: Cambridge University Press.

Marchmant, S., Alexander, J., Garcia, J., Ashurst, H., Alderdice, F. and Keene, J. (1999) 'A Survey of Women's Experiences of Vaginal Loss from 24 Hours to Three Months after Childbirth (The BLiPP Study)'. *Midwifery* 15: 72–81.

Milgrom, J. (1991) *Leviticus 1–16: A New Translation with Introduction and Commentary*. London: Doubleday.

Moore, K.L. and Persaud, T.V.N. (1998) *The Developing Human: Clinically Oriented Embryology*. London: W.B. Saunders.

Murray, J. (1850) *The Book of Common Prayer*. London: Vijitelly Brothers and Co.

Neusner, J. (1975) 'The Idea of Purity in Ancient Judaism'. *Journal of the American Academy of Religion* 43(1): 15–26.

Noth, M. (1977) *Leviticus; a Commentary*, translated from the German by J.E. Anderson. London: SCM Press.

Porter, J.R. (1976) *The Book of Leviticus: Commentary*. Cambridge: Cambridge University Press.

Razi, Z. (1980) *Life, Marriage and Death in a Medieval Pairsh; Economy, Society and Demography in Halesowen 1270–1400*. Cambridge: Cambridge University Press.

Roberton, N.C.R. (1981) *Neonatal Intensive Care*. London: Edward Arnold. 2nd edn 1987.

Roll, S. (2003) 'The Old Rite of the Churching of Women after Childbirth'. In K. De Troyer, J.A. Herbert, J.A. Johnson and A. Korte (eds) *Wholly Woman Holy Blood: A Feminist Critique of Purity and Impurity*. London: Trinity Press International, pp. 117–142.

Sadler, T.I.W. (2000) *Longman's Medical Embryology*, 8th edn. London: Lippincott, Williams and Wilkins.

Sered, S. (1994) *Priestess–Mother–Sacred Sister: Religions Dominated by Women*. New York: Oxford University Press.

Sharp, Jane *The Midwives Book or The Whole Art of Midwifery Discovered* (a facsimile presentation) ed. E. Hobby (1999) Women Writers in English Series 1350–1850. Oxford: Oxford University Press.

Smart, B. (2002 [1985]) *Michel Foucault*, rev, edn. London: Routledge.

Staton, M.W. (1980) 'The Rite of Churching: A Sociological Analysis with Special Reference to an Urban Area in Newcastle upon Tyne', unpublished M.Theol. thesis, University Library, Newcastle upon Tyne.

Stern, G. and Kruckman, L. (1983) 'Multidisciplinary Perspectives on Postpartum Depression: An Anthropological Critique'. *Social Science and Medicine* 17(15): 1027–1041.

Sweet, B.R. (1997) *Mayes' Midwifery: A Textbook for Midwives*. 12th edn. London: Baillière Tindall.

Thomas, K. (1991) *Religion and the Decline of Magic*. London: Penguin Books.

Vulliamy, D.G. (1982) *The Newborn Child*, 5th edn. Edinburgh: Churchill Livingstone.

Walker, S.S. (1973) 'Proof of Age of Feudal Heirs in Medieval England'. *Mediaeval Studies* 35: 306–323.

Wenham, G. (1979) *The Book of Leviticus*. London: Hodder and Stoughton.

Wilson, A. (1990) 'The ceremony of childbirth and its interpretation'. In V. Fildes (ed.) (1990) *Women as Mothers in Pre-industrial England: Essays in Memory of Dorothy McLaren*. London.

4　Pollution: midwives defiling South Asian women

Kuldip Bharj

Introduction

> 'Only paper and wood are safe from a menstruating woman's touch. So they built this room for us, next to the cowshed. Here, we're permitted to write letters, to read, and it gives a chance for our kitchen-scarred fingers to heal . . .'
>
> (Bhatt 1998: 191)

In contemporary health services words such as uncleanness, contamination, contagion, dirt, exclusion and segregation epitomise the culture of everyday life; however, synonymous words such as defilement and pollution have a different meaning. It is these that I want to focus on. The notion of 'pollution' is not new; it has been central to theoretical discourses since the time of the Book of Leviticus. Within the anthropological literature it was as far back as 1966 that authors such as Mary Douglas examined the concept. These discussions have essentially been within the context of primitive or developing societies and in essence concerned with the links between pollution and religion and the sacred. However, the issue of pollution and rites of purification within British maternity services requires a dialogue and this chapter will provide a platform for such a discourse.

The concept of pollution is not new to me, either, though I had given little thought to the practices and indeed accepted many without question. I had personally come across the concept of pollution in many walks of my life – for example, pollution in terms of ritual cleanliness, secular defilement (this was particularly evident when going to the Gurdwara or when praying) – and indeed I personally experienced 'ritualistic purification' after the birth of my two children. My interest around the notion of childbirth pollution, however, was heightened by a comment made by one of the participants in a research study I conducted as part of my doctoral studies. Parveen (to preserve her identity a pseudonym has been used) was employed as an interpreter in one of the NHS Trusts in the north of England. She stated that some of the Pakistani Muslim women for whom she had interpreted reported that during the course of receiving midwifery care, midwives had defiled and polluted them.

This was the first time I had come across the notion of pollution expressed in this context, and if it is an issue for Pakistani Muslim women then midwifery needs to respond to this. I therefore set out to explore this notion with the women who were participating in my study. Concomitant with this I located literature which attempted to examine the notion of childbirth pollution. There were myriad cross-cultural essays on pollution, which linked mainly to 'blood pollution' and 'childbirth pollution', and indeed it is from this literature that I have drawn the framework and evidence. My attempts to explore the literature which examined childbirth pollution in respect of Pakistani Muslim women were largely unsuccessful – no citations were found during my literature search, although there was a body of knowledge concerning women of South Asian background. I have therefore focused in this chapter on South Asian women and their experiences of pollution during childbirth.

The purpose of this chapter is to explore the notion of pollution and its relationship with childbirth within British midwifery, and debate the issues for maternity service provision and delivery for women from South Asian backgrounds. I will set the scene by exploring the notion of pollution and its related concepts. I will then analyse the statement made by Parveen in order to identify the issues which are perceived to pollute women. Finally, I will examine the emerging issues and their implications for delivery of maternity services for women from South Asian backgrounds.

Pollution: a theoretical explanation

In 1966 Mary Douglas, a British anthropologist, in her book *Purity and Danger* attempted to explain societies' beliefs in ritual pollution. In her analysis pollution ideas work in two ways. First, pollution ideas work instrumentally (Douglas 2002: 3), for example the socially powerful use ideas of contamination to uphold social rules and the moral order. Moreover, those who break these rules are threatened by 'danger-beliefs'. Second, Douglas asserts that pollution ideas relate to social life as symbols where 'some pollutions are used as analogies for expressing a general view of the social order' (2002: 4). She emphasises that some things that are thought to have special religious significance are seen as sacred whilst others are seen as polluted, and pollution is a result of a symbolic system. Thus sacred things, considered as 'pure', are merely a vision of 'order'. So, in practice, when considering purity there is an image of order where things are assigned to their naturally occurring position, and each thing is in its rightful place. However, when things are 'out of order' and 'out of place' they become 'filth', 'dirt' and 'pollution'. This suggests that concepts of dirt and its façade, purity, are strongly related to the cultural ordering of societies.

It is in this sense that sacred things are to be protected from defilement. Therefore, prohibitions, sacred rules, may apply to only some things and actions and not to others. There are many rules within cultures to maintain a state of purity and rules that prevent defilement. Pollutions are perceived, Douglas argues, when a sense of coherence in our thought is threatened. At that point, we may avoid confusion by declaring that the thing which confused us is evil, and to be avoided. Prohibitions on touching, using or even seeing certain foods, objects, animals, plants or people may be embedded in a belief that such things are too 'good' for humans to have contact with or that they are 'dirty' or 'polluting'. According to Douglas, when things do not fit neatly into a society's classification of the world, they are likely to be seen as 'taboo' or 'danger'. Taboo 'is concerned with all the social mechanisms of obedience which have ritual significance and with specific and restrictive behaviour in dangerous situations' (Steiner 1956: 20). Douglas (2002) asserts that things which exist at the borders of society, or on the boundaries between categories, are perceived as possessing both power and danger and in both circumstances there is likely to be a rule against contact with the marginal person or thing. Pollution avoidance is therefore seen essentially as fear of danger. Some ritual taboos apply to a whole community at all times – for example, the rule against Muslims eating pork, Hindus eating beef and so on – and others only to part of a community at set periods – for example, in many cultures certain foods are taboo to pregnant women, or the isolation of menstruating women, or isolation of women from the rest of the community during childbirth.

Whilst the analysis of dirt is based on hygiene, like ritual pollution it is also expressed within symbolic systems. Douglas's thesis about dirt suggests that it is merely a matter of being out of place and 'there is no such thing as absolute dirt: it exists in the eye of the beholder'; dirt is thus 'essentially disorder' (2002: 2). This means that it is not the quality of things that is considered as dirty, but it is where they stand in the order of things as determined by that society's system of symbols. Things which are 'dirt' in one context may become pure just by being put in another place – and vice versa. For example, walking with bare feet in a street is viewed as unclean and shoes are worn to prevent feet getting dirty and getting infected. However, those very shoes are not worn in the Gurdwara as they are seen to pollute the sacred place. Likewise, handling of blood coming from a wound on a hand is seen completely differently from that of blood from the vagina. Dirt, defilement and pollution are concepts concerned with ideologies within society and it is about how the environment is reordered in order for it to fit in with the ideology. However, ideologies change over time and are governed by the state of knowledge. Indeed, states of cleanliness and uncleanliness can be relative categories where something can be clean in relation to one thing yet unclean in relation to another. Douglas (1966) argues that pollution beliefs should be viewed as a continuum covering both danger beliefs relating to religious thinking and the ideas about dirt which are usually taken for granted.

From the above explanation it is apparent that rules about touching or not touching certain people (castes) or people at certain times (during menstruation for example) and eating some foods and not others are not related to ideas about hygiene only but they emerge from the society. One such example is the belief that the upper part of the body is clean and the lower half is polluted. There are thus many rules which are based on this belief – for example, having a shower with free flowing water from the upper part of the body, which is cleaner, to the lower part of the body, which is unclean. Likewise, bodily secretions and excretions, for example blood, pus, urine and faeces, are sources of impurity and are seen as defilement, but the bodily fluids closer to the head are less polluting than those from the lower body. However, the degree to which these substances are considered dangerous differs from culture to culture around the world. These perceptions of bodily pollution are often a reflection of the dangers perceived by the society in question. Dirt relates to the boundaries and to objects that are not within the boundaries but are at the margins. Douglas argues,

> any structure of ideas is vulnerable at its margins. We should expect the orifices of the body to symbolise its especially vulnerable points. Matter issuing from them is marginal stuff of the most obvious kind. Spittle, blood, milk, urine, faeces or tears by simply issuing forth have transversed the boundary of the body.
>
> (2002: 150)

She asserts that things which exist at the boundaries are perceived as possessing both power and danger. Whilst for some purposes this may be seen as power, for others it is danger. In both circumstances there is likely to be a rule against contact with the marginal person or thing. It is this which is a likely explanation of the variation in what is perceived as 'purity', 'dirt', 'pollution' and 'taboo' from culture to culture.

Death, birth and pregnancy exist at the border between different stages of life, and are frequently surrounded by taboos, for example corpses may be seen as polluting and blood may be seen as polluting. So when people are exposed to pollution, such as coming into contact with corpses or with blood either during menstruation or childbirth, they are defiled. Mary Douglas asserts that these people must be moved to new statuses through rituals (rites of passage) to 'purify' them to correct such confusion.

Pollution and childbirth

In many cultures, childbirth is seen as a highly contagious and polluting situation. In this section, I will explore cultural practices and ceremonies around childbirth in relation to South Asian women which focus on the idea of holiness and views that women must be purified after childbirth. I will begin by deconstructing an excerpt from an interview which I conducted with Parveen which essentially led me to examine this issue.

My purpose in interviewing Parveen was to explore interpreters' perspectives on Pakistani Muslim women's experiences of British maternity services. It was when she was explaining some of the encounters reported by Pakistani Muslim women as in-patients on the antenatal wards that she stated that some women indicated that:

> I need to be clean I need to be . . . they [midwives] should not be touching me, they have not had a 'woo zoo', they don't clean themselves when they have been to toilet or whatever, they might not have a bath every time whatever . . . Oh they [midwives] just delivered a baby and they got a 'shetta' – splash [of blood] on them . . . on their . . . they are not 'paleth' [clean] enough and then they are sort of touching me and touching my tummy and now I can't say my prayer and I have to have a bath now . . .
>
> (Interview with Parveen, 2002)

'Woo zoo', also referred to as 'Wudzû', 'wudu' or 'ablutions', is ritual washing with clean water of mouth, nostrils, face, hands and forearms, the wiping of the head and ears, and washing of the feet (Winter 2000: 20).

From the analysis of this excerpt, categories such as 'personal belief about purity', 'perception of defilement', 'midwives as agents of defilement' and 'blood as defilement' were identified. Table 4.1 demonstrates these.

I found Parveen's statement fascinating. It suggests that the two main issues which lead to defilement are the midwives (birth attenders) and the blood. When I followed this concept through with the future participants,

Table 4.1 Identification of categories from an interview excerpt

Excerpt from the interview	*Category*
'I need to be clean I need to be . . .'	Personal belief about purity
'they [midwives] should not be touching me . . .'	Perception of defilement
'they have not had a "woo zoo", they don't clean themselves when they have been to toilet or whatever, they might not have a bath every time whatever . . .'	Midwives as agents of defilement as they do not observe ritual cleanliness
'Oh they [midwives] just delivered a baby and they got a "shetta" – splash [of blood] on them . . . on their . . . they are not "paleth" [clean] enough and then they are sort of touching me and touching my tummy and now I can't say my prayer and I have to have a bath now . . .'	Blood as defilement

both the interpreters and the women, insufficient data emerged to validate this category. However there is sufficient published literature which suggests that for South Asian women there are two main events that are seen as polluting. One is menstruation and the second is childbirth. A common factor in both these events is 'blood', which is seen as a pollutant.

Pollution: blood as agent

The event of menstruation is universal and many ethnic groups – 'in particular those socially organised around religious taboos – ascribe diverse symbolic meaning to this regular biological event' (Yanay and Rapoport 1997: 652). The women are perceived to be in a state of pollution during this period and prohibitions and taboos to prevent the dangers of this impurity are observed. For example in Judaism menstruating women are bounded by laws of '*niddah*' (laws of impurity concerning menstruation) (Yanay and Rapoport 1997: 651) and are forbidden to enter the temple and have to observe sexual prohibition. In Hinduism and Sikhism women are also perceived to be polluting during menstruation. Thompson's (1985) study, which was conducted in central India, found that during the menstruation period Hindu women are considered 'caukkebãhar', which means 'outside the kitchen' (1985: 702), and as such are not expected to enter the kitchen. In addition they are prohibited from sexual intercourse during this period. Thompson also reported that during menstruation women were prohibited from participating in the 'benevolent deities' such as practices of worshipping gods and taking part in weddings or funerals (1985: 702).

In Islam menstrual blood is referred to as 'Haid blood' and this blood is perceived as defiling and women are considered to be temporarily impure. During menstrual periods the women are required to observe a number of rules which prohibit them from saying prayers, fasting during the month of Ramadan, entering the mosque and engaging in sexual intercourse until the women have been purified. Once the Haid blood flow has stopped it is obligatory for women to observe the practice of 'ghusl' (Winter 2000: 20), which is pouring clean running water over the whole body. Women pass into a pure state and resumption of normal life can begin.

As seen from the model offered by Douglas (1966, 2002), menstrual blood exhibits the phenomenon of crossing the boundary and renders the woman temporarily 'impure' and as such a threat to the order valued by the South Asian societies. Douglas argues that rituals preoccupied with the body represent social contradictions, and that the private body and the social collective mirror one another in the symbolic domain. Here menstrual blood, like pus, semen and excreta and other bodily issues, is a polluting social marker.

The danger of impurity is expressed and institutionalised in practices – menstrual taboos – which may cause domestic upheaval, for example the women have to abstain from the kitchen. In traditional situations this domestic upheaval can be overcome in many ways particularly when there are other women within the extended family unit. However this may not be the case in many cultures in present-day society and it is likely that there are variations in the way women observe these taboos.

Pollution: birth attenders as agent

In South Asian societies childbirth is seen as a 'highly polluting event' (Thompson 1985: 704). The state of being pregnant is not polluting but it is the period after the birth of the baby; it is the blood loss during delivery and the postnatal period which is most polluting. The period of pollution lasts for around forty days after birth (Jeffery *et al.* 1989). Douglas's theoretical explanation would suggest that the conception material which was within the boundary of the body for the nine months has come out of the mother and it is this material which is 'dirt' and seen as 'pollution'. In Hindu society the nine months' dirt is known as 'narak' (Thompson 1985: 704; Chawla and Ramanujam 2004: 15) and the women are perceived to be highly polluting for one and a quarter months after birth. Thus they occupy the position of untouchables (referred to as 'achut') during this period and essentially observe the same taboos and prohibitions as they would if they were menstruating. In addition to this, because the period around birthing is seen as polluting, the physical process of giving birth is denigrated (Thompson 1985). However many authors highlight that there is great regional variation among Hindu societies in India in the way in which birth pollution is experienced and expressed (Jeffery *et al.* 1989; Van Hollen 2003).

There are some pollutions which are permanent, for example having membership of a particular caste or sect, and irreversible. Unlike this, childbirth pollution and menstrual pollution are considered temporary. As these pollutions are associated with women's bodily state the women are considered to be in a polluting state during the period when they have vaginal blood loss. They have to observe taboos and prohibitions during periods of menstruation and childbirth pollution so that they do not place their menfolk, children or other women in danger. They are also excluded from worshipping, for example Muslim women refrain from reading the Quran and Hindu women are not permitted in the temple. Many observers have also noted cultural ceremonies at the end of forty days to mark the 'passing off' or removal of 'defilement' when the polluting period ends, for example the ceremony of 'tiddukkarital' in Hinduism (Van Hollen 2003: 196).

Given that childbirth pollution is considered to be highly defiling it is not surprising that in South Asian societies the dais' (traditional birth attendant) work, which is predominantly around the birth of the baby, is seen as most defiling. Cecilia Van Hollen (2003: 200) cites an excerpt from the 1918 report of the Victorian Memorial Scholarship Fund which highlights the views held of dais at the time 'as low caste, filthy, "vermin-ridden" woman whose main function was to deal with the "pollution" of childbirth rather than to impart specialised knowledge of the reproductive body'. Disappointingly, though unsurprisingly, this view of the dais changed little over time. For example, a birth study conducted in Uttar Pradesh (a state in north India) in the 1980s by Jeffery *et al.* indicates that 'most Hindu dais are Harijans (formerly untouchables), who often also perform other forms of defiling-work and whose presence is generally anathema to Caste Hindus (and many Muslims as well)' (1989: 108); and furthermore, 'village dais are not considered to have esoteric knowledge or specialised techniques; their distinctiveness rests on their willingness to accept payment for cutting umbilical cords, unpalatable defiling-work that no ordinary woman values or wishes to perform' (1989: 67).

However, more recent work from India (Chawla 2000; Van Hollen 2003; Chawla and Ramanujam 2004) and Pakistan (Chesney 2003) indicates that there have been some positive developments in the way the work of the dais is becoming valued as their skills and knowledge in assisting women with their birthing are being recognised. Nevertheless Janet Chawla, Renuka Ramanujam and Margaret Chesney acknowledge that cutting of the cord and handling of the placenta is carried out by the dais and it remains the most defiling aspect of their work. Chawla and her colleague have noted that 'sometimes dais, family and neighbourhood women will manage the birth itself and call a low or outcaste woman only to cut the cord and handle the afterbirth' (Chawla and Ramanujam 2004: 16).

The literature therefore suggests that birth attendants are seen as agents of pollution for two reasons. The first reason is that the majority of them are from poor backgrounds and from lower castes and many are likely to have to do this work out of necessity. As one of the respondents in Jeffery *et al.*'s study stated, 'I used to go out very little and I never liked to take food and water in other people's houses. I used to be very careful about cleanliness. But when my husband died – so, out of necessity, I became a dai' (1989: 66). Similarly Chawla and Ramanujam (2004: 63) cite a dai in Pubjabi: 'I was poor and took up Dai work for economic reasons. My husband lost his eyesight and I had small children.' The women during their birthing are attended by low caste birth attenders who are likely to be from poor backgrounds. The Hindu caste system denotes that 'the lower castes are the most impure and it is they whose humble services enable the higher castes to be free of bodily impurities' (Douglas 2002: 152). So in normal circumstances the women would avoid contact with such birth attenders for fear of becoming polluted. The second reason is that the dais' work is intrinsically linked with childbirth pollution and carrying out work which is labelled as 'defiling', for example clearing the vomit, urine and faeces. In addition to this the 'touching of the amniotic sac, placenta and umbilical cord', assert Jeffery *et al.* (1989: 106), is considered as the most dirty task.

In Islam, vaginal bleeding, which may start with the commencement of contractions, during labour and post-delivery, is referred to as 'Nifass' and prohibitions similar to menstruation pollution apply.

I have attempted to explain that for women from South Asia, menstruation and childbirth may be considered to be states of pollution; they are temporary and childbirth pollution is the more 'dangerous' of the two pollutions. There are of course many practices which are concerned with avoiding pollution and maintaining purity. As these pollutions are temporary, then impurity has to be eliminated and this is achieved by specific ceremonies which 'cleanse' the woman by getting rid of the impurities and returning the woman to her 'pure', 'non-polluting' state.

Pollution: issues for service provision and delivery

A review of the literature has highlighted that there is a wealth of literature concerning 'purity and pollution' globally, for example the work of Mary Douglas (1966), Charles Hudson (1976) and Julia Kristeva (1982) in which ideas about menstruation and childbirth pollution have been incorporated. In addition, there is literature around menstruation and childbirth pollution (Thompson 1985; Jeffery *et al.* 1989; Van Hollen 2003). The latter literature, though it discussed the polluting nature of the birth attendants, did not investigate the implication of childbirth pollution on birth attendants working within institutions. Therefore there is little to be drawn from the literature which can be extrapolated to the role of British midwives, and hence in this final section I pose some questions for the profession to consider.

Similarities and dissimilarities between Indian subcontinent midwifery and British practice

Evidence appears to suggest that one of the key differences in the practice of midwifery in the Indian subcontinent and Britain is the place of care. The above studies from the Indian subcontinent involving South Asian women appear to suggest that the place of birth is predominantly the home, as opposed to the majority of births in Britain which take place in hospital. The birth culture in British midwifery is based on the technocratic model, whereas the birth culture in South Asian societies is based on a cultural, non-interventionist model. Recent work in the United Kingdom suggests that South Asian women are strongly committed to western maternity care and perceive western obstetric and midwifery care as being superior (Woollett *et al.* 1995; Watson 1984; Bahl 1987).

During labour and in the postnatal period the women in the Indian subcontinent are cared for largely by other women in the household – for example, mothers-in-law and older sisters-in-law – and the dais are only called to attend the birth and in some instances only to cut the cord and clear the defiling material. In contrast, in Britain midwives are the main providers of care to the women during labour and the postnatal period, the majority of births take place in hospital and women are required to comply with the care and behave like patients (Kirkham 1983; Hunt and Symonds

1995). Interestingly, in both the Indian subcontinent and Britain labouring women are passive partners – in the Indian subcontinent the mothers-in-law take control of the birth and in Britain midwives. By implication, therefore, the labouring women perceive that the expert knowledge about birth lies with others – mothers-in-law and midwives.

The majority of birth attendants in the Indian subcontinent are dais, who may be trained or untrained, and in Britain they are midwives who are trained. It is possible that women place British midwives on a high pedestal because of their expert knowledge gained through education and training and because the British midwives are 'conductors of the orchestra' with knowledge and authority invested in them. It is possible that women perceive that midwifery in South Asian societies is 'primitive' when compared to British midwifery. By not criticising British midwifery, women from South Asian backgrounds may wish to demonstrate that they are 'moving on'.

Are midwives polluting?

As stated above, the notion of midwives polluting women was raised in the qualitative data I collected for my doctoral studies.

Interestingly, the childbearing Pakistani Muslim women did not validate the notion that midwives were defiling them and were agents of pollution. However, during the interviews when older women (either mothers or mothers-in-law) were present they reported that although midwives do undertake 'dirty' work in the course of caring during labour and the postnatal period, they are not perceived as 'polluting' in the same way as the dais. The main reason given was that the dais were mainly women from a lower caste. It is likely that birthing women see British midwives as of a higher status than South Asian dais and this does not violate their notion of purity. It is also likely that with the belief that western midwifery is superior women's pollution beliefs may change in respect of the defiling nature of the midwives' work.

It is possible that some women see midwives as carrying pollution, especially when there are visible stains on their clothing, but they feel they cannot express this from their position as patient. Interpreters are in a more secure and professional position and hear the views of many mothers. Should the women from South Asian backgrounds perceive that the midwives are agents of 'defilement' and are of low status then it is likely that they will not comply with care and the influence of the midwives will be limited.

Is ritual cleansing practical?

The earlier excerpt from the interview with Parveen suggested that it is possible that women see midwives as ritually unclean as they have not observed the practice of 'woo zoo'. Clearly it is not a practical solution for midwives to ritually clean themselves between providing care to different patients. It is likely that the measures taken to prevent infection and cross-infection – for example, washing of hands, wearing of gloves and changing uniform if it is contaminated with blood – are adequate and acceptable measures.

Conclusion

Investigating the concept of 'purity' and 'defilement' has been an interesting learning experience for me. In my quest to examine the implications of 'pollution' for maternity service provision and delivery there are many unanswered questions and this subject warrants further examination.

References

Bahl, V. (1987) Results of the Asian mother and baby campaign. *Midwife Health Visiting and Community Nurse* 23(2): 60–62.

Bhatt, S. (1998). Udaylee. In K. McCarthy *Bittersweet: Contemporary Black Women's Party*. London: Women's Press.

Chawla, J. (2000) *Crossing Boundaries and Listening Carefully*. MATRIKA – Motherhood and traditional resources, information, knowledge and action. Final report January 1997–March 2000. Pakistan.

Chawla, J. and Ramanujam, R. (2004) *Hearing Dais' Voices: Learning about Traditional Birth Knowledge and Practice*. New Delhi: MATRIKA.

Chesney, M. (2003) Birth for some women in Pakistan: defining and defiling. Unpublished PhD thesis, University of Sheffieldd.

Douglas, M. (1966) *Purity and Danger: An Analysis of the Concepts of Pollution and Taboo*. London: Routledge & Kegan Paul.

Douglas, M. (2002) *Purity and Danger: An Analysis of Concepts of Pollution and Taboo*, reissue. London: Routledge.

Hudson, C. (1976) *The Southeastern Indians*. Knoxville: University of Tennessee Press.

Hunt, S. and Symonds, A. (1995) *The Social Meaning of Midwifery*. Basingstoke: Macmillan.

Jeffery, P., Jeffery, R. and Lyon, A. (1989) *Labour Pains and Labour Power*. London: Zed Books.

Kirkham, M. (1983) Admission in labour: teaching the patient to be patient? *Midwives Chronicle*, February: 44–45.

Kristeva, J. (1982) *Powers of Horror: An Essay on Abjection*. Translated by Leon S. Roudiez. New York: Columbia University Press.

Steiner, F. (1956) *Taboo*. New York: Philosophical Library.

Thompson, C. (1985) The power to pollute and the power to preserve: perceptions of female power in a Hindu village. *Social Science and Medicine* 21(6): 701–711.

Van Hollen, C. (2003) *Birth on the Threshold: Childbirth and Modernity in South India*. Berkeley, Calif.: University of California Press.

Watson, E. (1984) Health of infants and use of health services by mothers of different ethnic groups in East London. *Community Medicine* 6(2): 127–135.

Winter, T.J. (2000) 'The Muslim grand narrative'. In A. Sheikh and A.R. Gatrad (eds) *Caring for Muslim Patients*. Oxford: Radcliffe Medical Press, pp. 17–28.

Woollett, A., Dosanjh, N., Nicolson, P., Marshall, H., Djhanbakhch, O. and Hadlow, J. (1995) The ideas and experiences of pregnancy and childbirth of Asian and non-Asian women in east London. *British Journal of Medical Psychology* 68(1): 65–84.

Yanay, N. and Rapoport, T. (1997) Ritual impurity and religious discourse on women and nationality. *Women's Studies International Forum* 20(5/6): 651–663.

5   Drained and dumped on: the generation and accumulation of emotional toxic waste in community midwifery

Ruth Deery and Mavis Kirkham

Introduction and context

When I (RD) was a community midwife I used to describe to my colleagues feeling 'worn out' and 'psychologically drained' and that I needed to 'recharge'. Similar feelings had occurred as a hospital-based midwife but I became more aware of my emotions during community midwifery. Listening compassionately to women, empathising with them, protecting them and often absorbing their 'feelings' was beginning to pay its price. It came as no surprise to me when my PhD work revealed a group of community midwives whose emotional well-being had become compromised. This chapter reports some of the findings from an action research study and how emotion work (Hochschild 1983) was experienced by a team of National Health Service (NHS) community midwives. The study comprised three phases. Phase one involved individual in-depth interviews with the midwives. Phase two involved focus groups, workshops and the introduction of clinical supervision so that the 'emotional disturbance' of caring work could 'be felt within the safer setting of the supervisory relationship, where it can be survived, reflected upon and learnt from' (Hawkins and Shohet 1989: 3). Phase three comprised final individual interviews with the midwives. Although the midwives were community-based the organisational culture of the hospital, and changes happening within it, had had a major impact, often to their detriment.

Working in an 'emotional minefield'

At its inception the National Health Service was an inventive public service idea. Since then it has become a large, extremely complex organisation with a strong, well-developed culture (Walter 2001) that appears to have changed very little over the years. Yet within this culture, the demands upon midwives have changed greatly, as have ways of organising the service, so that midwives now find themselves working within contexts that are extremely uncertain and changeable. Massive large-scale change is happening as a result of varying policy directives and local, regional and national reconfiguration (DOH 2004). Without the mediation of a supportive organisational culture, this has led to competing organisational and client demands and midwives have learnt to cope by regulating and controlling their midwifery work in ways that entail considerable emotional energy (Deery 2003; Hunter and Deery 2005). This particular climate has become a potential health hazard for midwives in terms of stress-related disease (Mackin and Sinclair 1998; Sandall 1997, 1998, 1999) and is further complicated by the inherent uncertainties of birth and of relationships with women and their families. In this context midwives can become susceptible to a particular type of occupational stress known as 'burnout syndrome' (Sandall 1995, 1997). Constant scrutiny from the users of the service exacerbates the situation further, as well as a culture of risk management that produces endless streams of rules and regulations that stifle the practice of any midwife who wants to 'think' or practise differently.

Emotions can only contribute to healthy interpersonal growth in an individual if they can be mobilised appropriately. Emotions become unhealthy, or toxic, if they reappear unconsciously in ways which are destructive and unhelpful (Bond and Holland 1998; see also Hunter and Deery 2005). Emotion work was experienced by these midwives as a hindrance, and detrimental, to midwifery work in the bureaucratic context of the NHS. Pressure to meet organisational demands meant the midwives had to regulate and control their emotional engagement, since the revelation of emotions had become 'matter out of place' (Douglas 1966: 44), which consumed their time and emotional energy with unhealthy and unpredictable results for themselves. Their negative experience of emotion work could be considered a 'by-product of a systematic ordering and classification of matter' (Douglas 1966: 44), that is, the organisational demands of the NHS far outweighed their own emotional needs.

> I don't think you include yourself in women's needs . . . I think we see ourselves as . . . I try to respond to the needs of the service if you like . . . so we make ourselves available . . . we give everyone the mobile phone number . . . and we've got four hundred women between us . . . we have to give a time when we visit and we have to go within two hours of this time and if not we ring the person and give a reasonable excuse as to why not . . .
>
> (Stella)

The high value placed on technical competence and efficiency in the NHS leaves little space for the emotion work of midwives in relationships, with toxic effects upon the midwives themselves. As Frost and Robinson state, 'emotional competence is irrelevant; it doesn't show up on the bottom line, or so the thinking goes . . . they [managers] still consider the job to be the corporate version of society's "women's work" – the stuff of daily life that must be done but is thankless' (1999: 102). Unfortunately when organisations have become chronically toxic they can also generate cultures of toughness and blame. Frost and Robinson describe toxic handlers 'who voluntarily shoulder the sadness and the anger that are endemic to organizational life' (1999: 98). This 'shouldering' is strategically important work because toxic handlers can be powerful sources of organisational effectiveness, helping to listen empathetically, work behind the scenes, suggest solutions and reframe difficult messages (Frost and Robinson 1999). The midwives reported in this chapter, however, found toxic handling physically, psychologically and professionally detrimental to their well-being.

Midwives as 'toxic handlers'

It was not surprising to find the midwives experiencing toxic handling as negative when their emotional needs were not regarded as a fundamental part of their work (Kirkham and Stapleton 2000; Hunter 2002; Deery 2003). This is unfortunate because dealing with emotions is an important and demanding component of working with people, entailing the management of feelings and the expression of emotion (Hochschild 1983). This often requires the use of acting techniques or 'impression management' (Goffman 1990). Unless the midwives managed to maintain face and status with peers, clients and managers they ran the risk of allowing their 'mask to slip' (Fineman 2003: 37). Positive emotional energy was experienced by these midwives as a finite resource. Competing organisational and client demands led them to regulate and control their midwifery work which required considerable emotional energy. They reported reaching the limit of their capacity to deal with clients emotionally.

> I feel wrung out . . . they [the women] drain you . . . I feel wrung out by them . . . I feel as if there is nothing else I can give them . . . and yet they expect more . . .
>
> (Eileen)

> . . . some of the postnatal visits are like that . . . you come out feeling like a wet rag . . . they've absolutely wrung every ounce out of you and you've tried to give everything . . .
>
> (Maureen)

> I just feel empty . . . I feel like they've just absorbed every bit of energy . . . my duracells are flat when I come out . . .
>
> (Amy)

Relationships with clients were depicted as a one-way draining of emotional energy, leaving the midwives feeling 'empty' and at the end of their emotional resources. Acting as 'protective buffers or sponges, absorbing and deflecting the worst of the organizational fear or pain for the good of others' (Fineman 2003: 88) meant that the midwives suppressed their emotions and suffered the 'negative repercussions of toxic handling' (Frost and Robinson 1999: 100).

Midwives as 'toxic handlers' for their peers

Emotions were viewed as 'interferences' (Fineman 2003: 114) with the smooth running of the service, and emotional distress was experienced by these midwives as toxic waste accumulated in their interactions with colleagues as well as clients. This was often attributed to interpersonal problems within the team. There seemed to be a fear in the work team of hurting a colleague by relating clumsily or communicating inappropriately. In order to save each other from emotional discomfort the midwives dealt with work-related issues superficially, sometimes manipulatively, often destructively, and in a manner that often sabotaged their good intentions. This is behaviour akin to ladylike saboteurs as identified in Deery's 2003 action research. These midwives avoided dealing with difficult issues which later surfaced to disrupt their presentation of themselves as a team. Thus by avoiding and denying the consequences of what they perceived as bumbling and inept communication, they prevented themselves from learning from difficult experiences (Deery 2003).

> [. . .] we bury a lot because we don't want to fall out as a team [. . .] we all recognise the value of having this gelled team and we all swallow bits and pieces that we are maybe not happy with and then we don't act on things that we think should be acted on because we don't want to destroy the team [. . .]

> [. . .] one of us is very emotional at the moment [. . .] I remember coming in [. . .] I'd been to a home birth and I was hoping I could just hand over and go to bed [. . .] I just wanted to say 'here have the work' and then go to bed [. . .] and she was in pieces [. . .] so then it was a question of looking at the work [. . .] I took visits [. . .] I said 'I've got to go home and get some sleep now' – so I had a few hours in the morning and then did eight visits in the afternoon [. . .] I got her clinic covered [. . .] I was out of my brains [. . .] I keep saying to myself 'I'm eating, drinking, sleeping so I can't be that bad' [. . .] and I just keep pushing myself [. . .] I find I'm going from one crisis to the next [. . .] I spent three days of my holidays doing booking letters [. . .] sorting out my cards [. . .] I'm just not organised . . .
>
> (Amy)

Such self-blame is common in NHS midwifery (Kirkham 1999).

Midwives as 'toxic handlers' for clients

In a similar vein, toxic handling meant that Amy and Sarah were only able to depict relationships with clients as a one-way draining of emotional energy where it was impossible to feel energised by relationships with women.

> [. . .] there's often comments about 'my women' or 'your women have been ringing again' . . . the demands are different . . . I get 'can you tell me how to perform neonatal resuscitation on my baby' from my women – not, 'how do I change a nappy?'
>
> (Amy)

> I think the further you come up the social class [. . .] then the more demands they [the women] make on you [. . .] the demands they make are emotionally draining [. . .] they've got two sides of A4 paper of questions . . .
>
> (Sarah)

> . . . particularly people who have got problems . . . you listen . . . you are sympathetic . . . but then you can get over-reliance . . . and I think it's difficult where you cut off because I have had episodes in the past where it had been difficult to dissolve the relationship . . .
>
> (Susan)

The midwives reach the limit of their capacity for dealing with clients emotionally, with Susan identifying a difficulty with dissolving relationships. Thus setting boundaries within relationships caused even more emotional distress.

Managers as 'toxic bosses'

The midwives perceived that the distress of clients and colleagues was 'dumped' upon them and often made worse by their managers who unloaded their own distress and frustrations onto the work team. They described themselves as a 'big dumping ground' for the problems of the organisation as well as those of their clients. The midwives sought opportunities to 'offload' this accumulated burden but found little opportunity for this within the service. This burden was experienced as both heavy and toxic, damaging the practice and the stamina of the midwives concerned. The managers were perceived as 'toxic bosses', with the midwives having yet another area within their midwifery work where they acted as 'toxic handlers'.

> . . . people [the managers] think that you can cope and think that you are alright . . . this is something you often perpetuate because you wouldn't have them know anything else . . .
>
> (Amy)

> I went home and I sat in the chair for about an hour and a half . . . just like zombified . . . thinking about what had gone on . . . and if I had done everything . . .
>
> (Joan)

> . . . we were so badly off for staff . . . I worked my days off . . . two out of three weeks . . . because we were so short-staffed . . .
>
> (Susan)

Thus, the midwives' only response to mounting demands upon them was to endlessly endeavour to meet, or appear to meet, those demands until they exhausted their personal capacity.

Midwives who did not fit into the organisation were placed within this work team of midwives because they were seen as a team that could cope emotionally with the distress of others. Dumping distress (Orbach 1994: 31) in this manner exacerbated the difficulties that were already present within the work team.

> . . . it just felt like a dumping ground because we were getting people that had problems of their own, dumping them on us . . . we already had our own problems and it just felt like a big dumping ground at one point.
>
> (Kathy)

The midwives wanted to put a hold on containing others' distress so that their own team could sort out its difficulties. The midwives sought opportunities to 'offload' this accumulated burden but found little opportunity for this within the service.

'Healthy toxic handling' through clinical supervision

Clinical supervision offered a means of examining and learning from the toxic effects of emotional distress to the benefit of the midwives, their clients and the organisation. The study introduced clinical supervision with the aim of creating the opportunity to develop skills in reflecting upon, and learning skills to deal with, emotional distress. Despite some success, the main response was resistance to change. The midwives felt too bogged down and burdened to make full use of this opportunity. Neither they nor the organisation recognised the positive effects of toxic handling. Instead this was seen as burdensome and damaging and the midwives were left to 'toil in danger zones completely exposed' (Frost and Robinson 1999). As these authors go on further to state:

> Organizations must recognize the toxic handlers in their midst so that their important work can be supported before a crisis strikes . . .

although toxic handlers save organizations from self-destructing, they often pay a steep price professionally, psychologically, and sometimes physically. Some toxic handlers experience burnout; others suffer from far worse . . .

(Frost and Robinson 1999: 98)

Dumping distress and maintaining order

Throughout this study positive emotional energy was seen as a finite resource, which was 'drained' from midwives by the attention they gave to demands of their clients, colleagues and managers. The emotional distress of others was seen as toxic waste, which was 'dumped' upon midwives. The burden thus created became increasingly heavy and they in their turn needed to 'dump' it elsewhere. Nowhere in this study did midwives speak of the emotional distress of those they dealt with as something from which they could learn or gain in experience or insight. In dealing with distress, midwives demonstrated two separate categorisations, both of which can be seen as attempts to control uncertainty and achieve order by limiting emotional engagement. First, a 'spontaneous coding practice' (Douglas 1966: pxiii) sets up what is taboo: the things that midwives do not attempt to deal with, the relationships that are not challenged and the discomforts that are not revealed. Second, in the relationships with clients which form the centre of midwives' work, stereotyping is widespread (Kirkham *et al.* 2002). This can be seen as a manifestation of the 'yearning for rigidity which is in us all' (Douglas 1966: 200): a way of dealing with uncertainty and establishing order in the face of uncertainty and change. Linguistic techniques are used to pre-empt conversation which may be painful or organisationally disruptive for the midwife (Stapleton *et al.* 2002; Kirkham 1983). As Mary Douglas stated, 'dirt offends against order' (1966: 2) and distress offends against an orderly model of birth, particularly against an industrial model of birth. In avoiding or 'dumping' emotional distress, the accumulation of which is experienced as burdensome and toxic, midwives seek to make their working environment orderly and maintain control. Where maternity services are experienced as a production line (e.g. Dykes 2006) and run according to an industrial model, this aids the smooth running of the service. However, midwives and mothers can pay a high price for the maintenance of such order. Many studies have shown midwives' unmet support needs (e.g. Stapleton *et al.* 1998; Kirkham and Stapleton 2001), though support, where experienced, can have very positive outcomes, as has been shown for childbearing women (Hodnett *et al.* 2003). Yet this model, where attention to emotional distress is experienced by the midwife as draining and being dumped upon, may enable she who dumps her distress upon the midwife to feel heard, but does not go beyond this to the actual provision of support. It may also make her feel guilty for taking up the midwife's time (Kirkham and Stapleton 2001).

Is it possible to recycle emotional toxic waste?

Since the model of draining and dumping has a negative effect upon mid-wives and limits their relationships with clients, we are led to ask whether there are better ways of dealing with emotional distress. Within this project, midwives were experiencing such stress and alienation in their work that, even when clinical supervision, designed to their own model, was made available to them, they resisted the opportunity to examine and learn from difficult emotional experiences in their work. Nevertheless, examples of learning from difficult emotional experiences, rather than just dumping them on someone else, can be found in the midwifery literature.

Examples of such recycling

There are various processes by which difficult emotional experiences can be used as learning opportunities. Within NHS midwifery they are, however, often resisted, as was the case in this study. This makes successful cases parti-cularly valuable.

Structured reflection upon clinical experience is important here. Olive Jones set up a process of guided reflection for midwives, facilitated by a supervisor of midwives, as a fundamental practice in a new birth centre.

> At first some midwives tended to continue with practices rooted in hospital consultant unit experience with which they felt comfort-able but did not necessarily reflect the philosophy of the birth centre. Following discussion of one birth, it was encouraging when a midwife commented, 'I didn't know that before, I think I would manage the situation differently next time.'
>
> (Jones 2000: 161)

This process was experienced as empowering, providing opportunities for debriefing and learning together 'as the story of a birth unfolds' (2000: 162).

> It took time for midwives to become confident in group reflection, to accept critical enquiry as non-judgemental and to trust each other in terms of confidentiality and support.
>
> *It would be unrealistic to say that nobody's feelings are ever hurt because some-times this causes inevitable pain. We all care deeply that what we do is right, so realising that there could be a better way causes us discomfort . . . these are growing pains and far preferable to the anaesthetised routine that has always been good enough. (Midwife)*
>
> (Jones 2000: 162)

Trust was crucial here. Once trust was established, the midwives in Jones's study valued reflective sessions. The midwives in our study did not reach that level of trust and expended considerable energy upon protecting themselves from knowing and understanding each other at a level where such trust could develop.

The neonatal unit in Exeter provides clinical supervision for its staff, including midwives. Group supervision was set up because it 'allows for the exploration of issues, problem solving, recognition of others' knowledge and skills and shared learning' (Derbyshire 2000: 171).

> Outcomes have been audited and there have been many changes in practice as a result. The groups enable staff to reflect on their professional activity and structures within their working environment. Problems in the work area are addressed and solutions found. Thinking and learning processes have been enhanced.
>
> (Derbyshire 2000: 172)

Frances Derbyshire gives useful insight into the philosophy underpinning this unusual development in midwifery.

> Quality in patient care is not achieved by decree, nor by striving to reach standards set by others. Rather, it is achieved by the endless pursuit, by each individual practitioner, of greater understanding and better practice. Clinical supervision is central to this. In the Exeter neonatal unit we are fortunate to have had the vision to develop the unit to meet our needs.
>
> (Derbyshire 2000: 172)

Others achieve similar results by reflecting upon their experience in writing.

> We go to school to a complex, demanding art so that we may learn a device for discharging tensions and apprehensions which we might otherwise not have strength to bear, and which as it is, become simply transposable *energy*. So grief itself is transposed into a curious joy.
>
> (Sarton 1980: 21; emphasis in the original)

To write thus requires 'transference from feeling to thinking, a conscious exploration and manipulation of what the subconscious brings'. This is seen to require 'unremitting ruthless analysis' (Sarton 1980: 43).

Skills and prerequisites for recycling emotional distress

In order to reflect upon emotional distress and painful clinical and personal experience, considerable skill is needed. Some learn these skills and practise them as individuals, as May Sarton describes above, but most of us learn these skills from and with others. In the examples given by Jones and Derbyshire, skilled facilitators demonstrate and model such skills, as well as enabling midwives to learn from each other. Skills in analysis and deconstruction of experiences make it possible to see in a new light, to learn from experience and re-align our view of negative experience as valuable learning material. Such skills also enable us to recognise and use other resources in our learning.

In order to learn such skills, midwives have to feel safe enough to open themselves to the possibilities of change with all its 'growing pains'. In our study, the midwives did not feel safe enough with each other, even in clinical supervision, to move from self-protection to self-analysis. Trust is of key importance here. The culture within which midwives practise in the NHS is one of blame and self-blame, not trust (Kirkham 1999; Kirkham and Stapleton 2004). The midwives described by Jones and Derbyshire were able to move beyond this because they worked within a small, contained setting with the appropriate philosophy: a free-standing birth centre in one instance and a relatively small neonatal unit in the other. This provided a safe space, or 'creative compartment' (Fairtlough 1994), within which openness and trust could develop and creativity was fostered. In such a context, midwives' skills can develop greatly (Hunter 2000), not least their skills in relationships and dealing with emotions.

Context and the potential for creative recycling

In a large-scale, industrial model of maternity care, distressing emotions can only be experienced as matter which is out of place, impeding the smooth running of the 'conveyor belt' of the service. Such dirt is burdensome and corrosive for those who carry it. The draining of resources and the dumping of toxic emotional waste are damaging for all concerned, not least in inhibiting change and learning.

In small, safe settings without much of the rigidity of the industrial model, more flexible responses are possible. The safety of mutual trust and the potential for flexible responses are both essential for midwives to re-classify and break down 'dirt' into nutrient learning material, which can feed professional growth. Working in small groups with appropriate philosophy and facilitation can enable midwives to learn from their experience, to recycle as useful that which was previously perceived as toxic matter which could only be dumped on someone else. It is significant that the small, flexible and emotionally safe settings in which this is possible also have a positive impact upon the experience of childbearing women and their families and are marked by generosity in professional relationships (Kirkham 2003).

Sadly, though we studied community midwives, their situation within the wider context of local maternity services prevented them from 'feeling safe enough to let go' (Anderson 2000) of their defences against the system in which they worked. Those defences included the definition and wasting of emotional experience through dumping, as well as rigid personal barriers to change.

References

Anderson, T. (2000) Feeling safe enough to let go: the relationship between a woman and her midwife during the second stage of labour. In M. Kirkham (ed.) *The Midwife–Mother Relationship*. Basingstoke: Palgrave Macmillan.

Bond, M. and Holland, S. (1998) *Skills of Clinical Supervision for Nurses: A Practical Guide for Supervisees, Clinical Supervisors and Managers*. Buckingham: Open University Press.

Deery, R. (2003) Engaging with clinical supervision in a community midwifery setting: an action research study. Unpublished PhD thesis, University of Sheffield.

Deery, R. (2005) An action research study exploring midwives' support needs and the effect of group clinical supervision. *Midwifery* 21(2): 161–176.

Derbyshire, F. (2000) Clinical supervision within midwifery. In M. Kirkham (ed.) *Developments in the Supervision of Midwives*. Manchester: Books for Midwives Press.

DOH (2004) *National Service Framework for Children, Young People and Maternity Services*. London: Department of Health.

Douglas, M. (1966) *Purity and Danger*. London: Routledge.

Dykes, F. (2006) *Breastfeeding in Hospital: Mothers, Midwives and the Production Line*. Oxford: Routledge.

Fairtlough, G. (1994) *Creative Compartments: A Design for Future Organisation*. London: Adamantine Press.

Fineman, S. (2003) *Understanding Emotion at Work*. London: Sage.

Frost, P. and Robinson, S. (1999) The toxic handler; organizational hero – and casualty. *Harvard Business Review* 77(4): 96–107.

Goffman, E. (1990) *The Presentation of Self in Everyday Life*. Harmondsworth: Penguin. First published in 1959.

Hawkins, P. and Shohetm, R. (1989) *Supervision in the Helping Professions*. Milton Keynes: Open University Press.

Hochschild, A.R. (1983) *The Managed Heart: Commercialization of Human Feeling*. Berkeley, Calif.: University of California Press.

Hodnett, E.D., Gates, S., Hofmeyr, G.J., Sakala, C. (2003) Continuous support for women during childbirth. *The Cochrane Database of Systematic Reviews*, Issue 3, art. no.: CD003766. DOI: 10.1002/14651858.CD003766.

Hunter, B. (2001) Emotion work in midwifery: a review of current knowledge. *Journal of Advanced Nursing* 34(4): 436–444.

Hunter, B. (2002) Emotion work in midwifery: an ethnographic study of the emotional work undertaken by a sample of student and qualified midwives in Wales. Unpublished PhD thesis, University of Wales Swansea.

Hunter, B. and Deery, R. (2005) Building our knowledge about emotion work in midwifery: combining and comparing findings from two different research studies. *Evidence Based Midwifery* 3(1): 10–15.

Hunter, M. (2000) Autonomy, clinical freedom and responsibility: the paradoxes of providing intrapartum midwifery care in a small maternity unit as compared with a large obstetric hospital. Unpublished MA thesis, Massey University, Palmerston North, New Zealand.

Jones, O. (2000) Supervision in a midwife managed birth centre. In M. Kirkham (ed.) *Developments in the Supervision of Midwives*. Manchester: Books for Midwives Press.

Kirkham, M. (1983) Labouring in the dark; limitations on the giving of information to enable patients to orientate themselves to the likely events and timescale of labour. In J. Wilson-Barnett (ed.) *Nursing Research: Ten Studies in Patient Care*. Chichester: John Wiley, pp. 81–100.

Kirkham, M. (1999) The culture of midwifery in the NHS in England. *Journal of Advanced Nursing* 30(3): 732–739.

Kirkham, M. (ed.) (2003) *Birth Centres: A Social Model for Maternity Care*. Oxford: Elsevier Science.

Kirkham, M. and Stapleton, H. (2000) Midwives' support needs as childbirth changes. *Journal of Advanced Nursing* 32(2): 465–472.

Kirkham, M. and Stapleton, H. (eds) (2001) *Informed Choice in Maternity Care: An Evaluation of Evidence Based Leaflets*. York: NHS Centre for Reviews and Dissemination.

Kirkham, M. and Stapleton, H. (2004) The culture of maternity services in Wales and England as a barrier to informed choice. In M. Kirkham (ed.) *Informed Choice in Maternity Care*. Basingstoke: Palgrave Macmillan.

Kirkham, M., Stapleton, H., Curtis, P. and Thomas, G. (2002) Stereotyping as a professional defence mechanism. *British Journal of Midwifery* 10(9): 509–513.

Mackin, P. and Sinclair, M. (1998) Labour ward midwives' perceptions of stress. *Journal of Advanced Nursing* 27: 986–991.

Orbach, S. (1994) *What's Really Going on Here? Making Sense of Our Emotional Lives*. London: Virago Press.

Orbach, S. (1999) *Towards Emotional Literacy*. London: Virago Press.

Orbach, S. and Eichenbaum, L. (1987) *Between Women. Love, Envy and Competition in Women's Friendships*. London: Arrow Books.

Sandall, J. (1995) Burnout and midwifery: an occupational hazard? *British Journal of Midwifery* 3(5): 246–248.

Sandall, J. (1997) Midwives' burnout and continuity of care. *British Journal of Midwifery* 5(2): 106–111.

Sandall, J. (1998) Occupational burnout in midwives: new ways of working and the relationship between organisational factors and psychological health and well being. *Risk Decision and Policy* 3(3): 213–232.

Sandall, J. (1999) Team midwifery and burnout in midwives in the UK: practical lessons from a national study. *MIDIRS Midwifery Digest* 9(2): 147–152.

Sarton, M. (1980) *Writings on Writing*. London: Women's Press.

Stapleton, H., Duerden, J. and Kirkham, M. (1998) *Evaluation of the Impact of the Supervision of Midwives on Professional Practice and the Quality of Midwifery Care*. London: English National Board.

Stapleton, H., Kirkham, M., Thomas, G. and Curtis, P. (2002) Language use in antenatal consultations. *British Journal of Midwifery* 10(5): 273–277.

Walter, M. (2001) Organisation and management. In J. Naidoo and J. Wills (eds) *Health Studies: An Introduction*. Basingstoke: Palgrave.

Section 2

Breastfeeding as pollution

6 Resisting the gaze:
the subversive nature of
breastfeeding

Fiona Dykes

Introduction

In this chapter I focus upon the dissonance experienced by women related to juxtaposing competing notions of breastfeeding, that is, 'natural' and 'subversive'. To illuminate this issue I draw upon a recently conducted critical ethnographic study within a hospital setting, the maternity ward, in the north of England. Within this highly public place and space women are encouraged to breastfeed as a sign of natural and self-sacrificing motherhood and yet within their local community breastfeeding is rarely carried out in open spaces and carefully hidden from the public gaze. Within some northern English communities, despite the increasingly pervasive public health messages that 'breast is best' and 'breastfeeding is natural', the act of breastfeeding is often seen and indeed experienced as a subversive manifestation of women's sexuality. The hospital culture reflects and indeed potentiates the public–private dilemmas for women who have little autonomy over their space and the 'gaze' of their neighbours, visitors and hospital staff. Women's accounts are analysed with regard to the ways in which women negotiate the 'natural'–'subversive', 'private–public' dilemmas and resist the 'gaze' in hospital by, for example, using their curtains to create a 'safe place'.

To contextualise the dilemmas for breastfeeding women it is useful to highlight some relatively recent historical changes. During the seventeenth to nineteenth centuries, in Europe, there was a massive proliferation in industrialisation. During this era, as factories sought labourers and the age of rationalistic science developed, there were accompanying changes that affected women. There was an increasing demarcation of public and private spheres for women, growing medical involvement in infant feeding and, more latterly, a media-based sexualisation of women's breasts. I will now refer to each of these areas of change for women.

Separating spheres

While men and women have always adopted different roles, the development of industrialised societies in Europe contributed to a very defined separation of roles. Males became increasingly associated with 'culture' and women with 'nature'. Martin (1987) refers to this doctrine of two spheres by first connecting the development of industrialised and capitalist societies with displacement of production from the home to the factory. This contributed to the construction of public and private domains. The public world of paid work, that is, work involved in the production process, came to be seen as separate from the private world centred in the home. Previously, within agricultural communities, work had been located in and around the home, with the extended family being seen as united in an endeavour to make provision for their own needs. The private world came to be associated with the 'natural', that is, bodily functions, sexuality, intimate relationships, morality, kinship and expression of emotions. Women, who were seen as 'natural', increasingly came to be seen as located within the private world of the home, as wives and mothers. Their role was one of reproduction rather than production in the industrial and economic sense. The public world, on the other hand, was seen as related to the impersonal process of efficient, goal-oriented competitive production. It was not only seen as breaking away from nature, but indeed dominating and controlling it. This was the world of the wage-earning male who came to be seen as cultural, in contrast to and in a superior position to the feminine and natural (Martin 1987). During the era of growing industrialisation, breastfeeding was seen as part of the natural role of women, although women from wealthy families commonly employed wet nurses. Women from poor families were less bounded by the public–private divide in that they were forced into the ambiguous position of juggling paid employment and home responsibilities (Doyal and Pennell 1981).

Growing medical imperative to control women's activities

Towards the end of the nineteenth century and into the twentieth century there was growing scientific, medical and governmental interest and involvement in infant feeding practices. Prior to this era infant feeding had been largely the domain of women. Both public policy and medical recommendations were related to concerns regarding high rates of infant mortality and the quality of the population (Doyal and Pennell 1981; Lewis 1980; Carter 1995). As Doyal and Pennell (1981) note, this agenda was driven by the need for the nation to provide plentiful 'fit' individuals to engage in the various forms of production. The behaviour of the mother was consequently scrutinised and called into question at all stages of the ongoing policy decision-making (Fildes 1989; Carter 1995).

One of the first major areas of medical debate and subsequent influence appears to be the practice of wet nursing, a key way in which women engaged either significant others or paid employees to nurture their babies when they were unavailable or indisposed (Fildes 1989). The medical profession increasingly discredited this practice during the nineteenth century. They expressed concerns about its biological, social and moral shortcomings, so that by the twentieth century wet nursing was virtually non-existent in western culture (Apple 1987; Fildes 1989; Ebrahim 1991; Palmer 1993). During the same period the quality of the mother's milk and her infant feeding practices came to be scientifically scrutinised and questioned. Although breast milk was considered to be natural and ideal it was proclaimed that not all women could produce enough or adequate milk, with a growing list of medical reasons being put forward (Apple 1987; Wolf 2000). Thus there was a growing and persisting western cultural belief that human lactation was an inherently unreliable bodily function (Dykes and Williams 1999; Wolf 2000; Dykes 2002, 2005a, 2005b, 2006). Given these 'problems', while breastfeeding was portrayed as the natural ideal, the alternative of feeding with infant formula became an increasingly acceptable option as the twentieth century progressed.

The scientific discourses around infant feeding at the turn of the twentieth century (Rotch 1890; Budin 1907; Vincent 1910; King 1913) reflected the mechanistic, dualistic and reductionist assumptions of that era. They also reflected the growing medical imperative to supervise and regulate women's bodies and minimise the threat of chaos (Palmer 1993; Carter 1995; Blum 1999). Breastfeeding was increasingly seen as potentially 'dirty', contaminating and representative of the body being out of control (Bramwell 2001; Bartlett 2002). On the other hand, there was a persisting discursive connection being made between mothering, breastfeeding and naturalness (Apple 1987; Leff *et al.* 1994; Carter 1995; Schmied and Barclay 1999; Shaw 2003). This connection in itself created many difficulties for women as notions of natural as a cultural construction were and are ever changing, as Franklin argues:

> Not only are constructions of the natural culturally and historically specific; they are also shifting and contradictory. As is the case in the analysis of science, a cultural domain to which ideas of the natural are central, it is important not to overstate the discursive or cultural determinism operative in the 'naturalising' process.
>
> (1997: 97)

Equally, as Shaw argues:

> The relation between maternal desires, one's identification as a 'good mother' and actual experiences of breastfeeding are not so straightforward. Bad experiences of breastfeeding – for whatever reason – may in fact induce or motivate women to distance themselves from disciplinary technologies and social norms and expectations they regard at odds with their own sensory understandings and dispositions.
>
> (2003: 64)

This complex combination of medical interference, growing concern regarding the efficacy of breastfeeding, essentialist messages that breastfeeding was the natural option and yet increasing acceptability, availability and marketing of breast milk substitutes set the scene for the dramatic decline in breastfeeding that swept across many parts of western Europe in the 1960s and early 1970s.

Sexualisation of women's breasts

To add to the challenges for women, as the twentieth century unfolded there was an increasing trend towards the sexual portrayal of women's breasts through the growing media channels. As Palmer (1993) asserts, our era is the first in recorded history in which the breast has become a mass fetish for male sexual stimulation while simultaneously its primary function has diminished on a massive scale. This, Palmer observes, has led to the seemingly legitimate use of women's bodies, and in particular breasts, to sell commodities such as peanuts, newspapers and cars. McConville sums up the issues around display of women and their breasts:

> Bare breasts aren't confined to the tabloids. They turn up everywhere from clubs to pubs to workshops. And because the models either have that soppy 'come-hither' message in their eyes, or the corny 'dying for it' look, the topless image constantly promotes a phoney male fantasy of relationships with women. Perhaps it wouldn't be so bad if we saw topless women with expressions of irony, of intelligence – even of boredom – on their faces. At least we would know they had some identity, some individuality . . . The bare breasts themselves are often beautiful: it's the paid-for, male-adoring expressions on the faces which are so dishonest.
>
> (1994: 41)

The marginalisation of breastfeeding in the UK was illustrated by Henderson *et al.* (2000) in a study that elicited ways in which breastfeeding and bottle feeding were portrayed in newspapers and on television. Breastfeeding was rarely shown and this contrasted with bottle feeding which was almost invariably presented as the norm. When breastfeeding was shown it tended to be associated with the 'out of control body, sexuality and embarrassment' (2000: 1197). For example, in the famous British television soap *Coronation Street*, humour was invoked when a breastfeeding woman, working in a bar, approached a stunned male and asked him if he could see that her bra was stuffed with toilet paper. This media research and other related studies and commentaries provide reasons why breastfeeding, although commonly referred to as 'natural', has become far from natural as a public activity, creating dissonance, embarrassment and anxiety to women from all social groupings (McConville 1994; Rodriguez-Frazier and Frazier 1995; Nadesan and Sotorin 1998; Blum 1999; Dykes 2003; Dykes *et al.* 2003).

Breaching boundaries

The combination of the public–private divide that developed with growing industrialisation and increasing sexualisation of women's breasts during the twentieth century led to breastfeeding becoming increasingly seen as a private activity to be conducted away from the public gaze (Maher 1992; Carter 1995). As Stearns argues, breastfeeding in public was and is seen and experienced as 'transgressing the boundaries of both the good maternal body and woman as (hetero)sexual object', with the sexual breast and maternal breast being required to be independent of each other as the 'meaning and place of women's breasts is contested' in western culture (1999: 310). The dissonance created for women by this blurring of boundaries between breastfeeding as a maternal activity and display of sexual breasts is repeatedly highlighted (Young 1990; Carter 1995; Rodriguez-Frazier and Frazier 1995; Blum 1999; Murphy 1999; Stearns 1999; Pain *et al.* 2001; Mahon-Daly and Andrews 2002; Dykes 2003; Dykes *et al.* 2003).

The discord felt may be increased by the embodied experience of breastfeeding as intimate, sensuous and erotic (Odent 1992; Rodriguez-Frazier and Frazier 1995; Shaw 2003). The leakiness of the body may further potentiate dissonance as women contend with the additional dualism between breast milk being portrayed as a natural, pure and life-giving fluid and yet on the other hand being seen as a secretion and, as such, a subversive corporeal manifestation of unboundedness (Britton 1997; Shildrick 1997; Bramwell 2001; Bartlett 2002; Spiro 2006). In its subversive state breast milk may be seen as akin to other body secretions and as representative of the uncontrolled, chaotic, dangerous and polluting female body (Douglas 1966; Kristeva 1982; Young 1990; Grosz 1994; Bramwell 2001).

As breastfeeding became less visible due to its general decline and to women's ambivalence about feeding in public during the twentieth century, bottle feeding became more visible. This was an activity on the increase but also its acceptability in public meant that it became the visual norm within many western communities. This served as a marker of and trigger to the further marginalisation of breastfeeding. We therefore now have a situation in some communities in England in which breastfeeding has been rarely practised, seen or even spoken about for several generations.

While notions of public and private are spoken about, it also needs to be remembered that there is considerable blurring between these spaces. Even private places such as one's home cannot be assumed to be truly private. As Carter notes, even in the 'privacy' of the woman's own home breastfeeding is not a neutral activity. Women wherever they are still have to negotiate 'what to do, where to do it, in whose presence, and with whose approval it can be done' (1995: 107). Carter further argues that what remains consistent is 'women's responsibility for being modest and discreet and checking out the implications of breastfeeding in each particular setting' (1995: 114). To illustrate some of the dilemmas and ambiguities for women between breast-feeding in specific places and spaces in the public domain I turn to a recent critical ethnographic study that I conducted within maternity units in the north of England.

Critical ethnography

The study explored the influences upon women's experiences of breast-feeding within postnatal ward settings (Dykes 2004, 2005a, 2005b, 2006). Ethnography involves participating in people's lives, including watching what happens, listening to what is said and asking questions (Hammersley and Atkinson 1995). It uncovers two types of cultural knowledge, tacit knowledge, a knowledge that remains largely outside our immediate aware-ness, and explicit knowledge, a form of knowledge that people may com-municate about with relative ease (Spradley 1980). Critical ethnography places additional emphasis upon ideology, power and control in the research process, analysis and theoretical conceptualisations. As Thomas argues, it involves a:

> Type of reflection that examines culture, knowledge and action. It expands our horizons for choice and widens our experiential capacity to see, hear and feel. It deepens and sharpens ethical commitments by forcing us to develop and act upon value commitments in the context of political agendas. Critical ethnographers describe, analyze, and open to scrutiny otherwise hidden agendas, power centres, and assumptions that inhibit, repress, and constrain.
>
> (1993: 3)

The study was adopted in two maternity hospitals in the north of England, with sixty-one postnatal women and thirty-nine midwives participating. The ethnographic study involved long periods of observation of activities on the maternity wards and interactions between midwives and breastfeeding women. The observations were supplemented by interviews with both mid-wives and breastfeeding women. Ethical approval for the study was gained through the relevant local research ethics committees. At all stages partici-pant autonomy and confidentiality were protected (ASA 1999). Pseudonyms are used throughout. This chapter refers to women's experiences related to being under the public gaze while breastfeeding in hospital.

Magnifying dilemmas

Women's experiences of breastfeeding in hospital provided a striking representation and indeed magnification of the ambiguous positions women are faced with when breastfeeding in western communities. The typical English maternity ward now consists of several rooms leading off a central corridor. The rooms, commonly referred to as bays, usually open out into the corridor so that women may be observed by health workers. They form an attenuated version of the traditional wards that were based on the principles of Bentham's panopticon (Foucault 1977), in which women were placed in rows either side of a completely open central aisle so that surveillance of both staff and 'patients' could be maximised. Each person's bed has a set of curtains that may be drawn around the woman either by a member of staff or the woman herself.

While maternity wards tend to be seen as women's areas, in reality they are highly public places. They often have a mixture of antenatal women with obstetric problems, some of whom may be in early labour, and post-natal women including post-operative women following Caesarean section. There is a constant stream of people moving in and out of the bays including physiotherapists, midwives, health care assistants, doctors and women's family members and friends. Women are surrounded by relative strangers and commonly bombarded with noise from passing people, buzzers, foetal heart monitoring machinery and babies crying. Consequently, while efforts may be made to make the area as private as possible, maternity wards are indeed public places.

Women's use of curtains in such a place illuminates some of their dilemmas. Burden (1998) observed the range of uses of curtains in a UK postnatal ward and reported that the primary reason for curtain closing was a desire for privacy. She found that women used curtains to secure privacy or to send signals to other room occupants, visitors and midwives. They completely closed the curtains for total withdrawal, semi-closed their curtains as a signal that they wanted information or support, and partly closed them across, that is, just pulled one curtain across, for periods of solitude or rest. In this way women created boundaries and barriers when they felt they needed them.

In my study, women tended to close their curtains either fully or partially to breastfeed. The closed curtains symbolically represented the dilemmas around the maternal versus sexual breast and public–private places for women. Women tended to constantly monitor and resist the male gaze, as illustrated by Corinne: 'I like the privacy, while I'm feeding . . . you don't want an audience do you [laughs] and there's husbands and that [laughs]'. Young (1990) refers to this ambivalence for women as stemming from the objectification of the female breast within a male-dominated society and under the male gaze.

Corinne was also concerned about how the visitors would feel: 'I mean I don't want to feed in front of visitors, like I'm not bothered, but it puts them in an awkward position.' Stella referred to a similar concern about others viewing her body:

> Well, I just leave them [curtains] round cos I'm feeding all day. Like if any of my own relatives come and that like . . . that doesn't bother me but um . . . and like trying to get out of bed it's not very ladylike really.

This concern of women about others' reactions to them and their bodies is referred to by Stearns (1999). When the women I interviewed spoke about privacy issues they often related breastfeeding in a hospital to dilemmas regarding breastfeeding in external public places. This was illustrated by Selina who was surrounded by three bottle-feeding mothers who had their curtains open. This left her as the only person with curtains closed, making her feel awkward. After a postnatal examination by the midwife she declined to have her curtains opened:

Felix (midwife):	How do you want the curtains?
Selina:	I'd rather have them left closed because the visitors will be here soon.
Felix:	You don't want everyone watching you?
Selina:	I don't [laughs]

Selina expressed antipathy towards breastfeeding in public places. This related in part to her feelings of inexperience and lack of confidence but her feelings were also influenced by attitudes to breastfeeding in the public domain:

Selina:	I'd prefer to have them [curtains] around, because I'm recovering from the birth and also when I'm breastfeeding, until I get used to it, I'd feel better having them around . . . Yeah, I think it'll be a while before I'm confident to do it in front of people. I mean when you go out you can express and give it in a bottle, can't you?
Fiona:	Would it bother you to breastfeed in public?
Selina:	It's the attitudes of people that would bother me really. I mean they may think ooh, she shouldn't do that here . . . and I don't think shops and places of leisure have anywhere near what they should have, and the shop changing rooms; I've seen them and they're not very nice really. So, I'd have to express and put it in a bottle, but you don't really want them to use a teat too early do you?

Clearly, Selina was thinking through the ways in which she would negotiate breastfeeding in public, by giving expressed milk by bottle, but was also concerned about jeopardising breastfeeding by introducing a teat too early. The feeling that to breastfeed in public was problematic was reiterated by Jasmin who had breastfed her last baby:

'I do think there's a certain attitude to breastfeeding, particularly when you're round and about, there's an awful lot of negativity around and that's a pressure for people who want to breastfeed. I mean I wanted to do it . . . but, I'm sure it could put people off. It certainly colours things for me, you know, I have to stick my head down and get on with it.'

Women still tended to feel under surveillance even behind the curtains, as Chloe illustrated:

'The thing about hospitals is that you feel as though. . .um, you're a bit on display and even with the curtain round you, there isn't a lot of sanctuary, and um I find that quite hard because you can't just shut yourself off from people, or sort of go and be a part of it if you want to . . . I find it quite difficult not being able to just close the doors and say that's it now. You generally feel that people can hear your conversations and I think you feel . . . you know . . . when you sort of come into hospital that your body is not your own, then when you go home again, you're sort of back in your own safe place.'

Chloe's comments illustrate the blurring of boundaries between public and private spaces and places and the ways in which, even if conditions are created to improve privacy, there are still restrictions on the ways in which women may feel that they have a safe space. These feelings of not having a safe space were reinforced for women by repeated invasions by health staff, as illustrated in the following interaction:

Shannon (midwife): Right are you ready for feeding love? [The baby was crying and Jackie, the mother, was sitting in her bedside chair preparing to feed.]

Jackie: Yes

Shannon: Right, I need you to get some of these teddies and things taken home because we need some space, all right love?

Jackie: Yes, all right, I'll tell my husband this afternoon

Shannon: Let's get baby feeding under your arm. [The midwife then moved forward and grasped the woman's breast and baby and put them together.] All right, love, we'll leave you to it.

The baby came off in a couple of minutes and Jackie, looking tearful, carried on trying.

This midwife first asserted her territorial power in terms of what was 'allowed' in the space, and then invaded Jackie's bodily boundaries in her handling of her breast, as if it was a disembodied receptacle, without permission or discussion.

I only found one discrepant 'case', a woman who appeared to be un-inhibited about breastfeeding in front of male visitors. Denise, a multiparous woman, appeared to reject and personally resist all social imperatives for being 'discrete'. She sat with both breasts fully exposed while vigorously hand expressing into a cup in front of a male visitor sitting with the woman opposite. The health care assistant came along and, looking rather embar-rassed, asked her if she would like the curtains closed. She said 'no – I'm past bothering now' and laughed. The male visitor carefully avoided looking at her! This situation also illustrates that it was not only the women who saw closing curtains for breastfeeding as the preferred option but also some of the staff on the wards. Staff attitudes therefore tended to reinforce feeding in private as a cultural norm during the first few days of a woman feeding her baby.

The interactions and narratives above illustrate that breastfeeding on maternity wards in northern England presented and indeed magnified dilemmas for women at the very heart of dualistic discourses around public versus private and maternal versus sexual. The notion of 'natural', as Blum asserts, usually signals what is 'good, authentic, and untainted by social or human manipulation, and thus "natural" motherhood seems to belong out-side the public realm' (1999: 13). However, as Martin states, 'women's bodily processes go with them everywhere, forcing them to juxtapose biology and culture' (1987: 200).

Foucault's (1977) reference to the 'productive' yet 'subjected' body seems to be very appropriate to breastfeeding mothers in England who are expected to be productive – producing breast milk – but their bodies are also sub-jected to forms of surveillance which Foucault describes as the 'gaze'. This 'gaze' may be public, medical, or both. Indeed Foucault refers to breast-feeding as a 'dangerous period . . . saturated with prescriptions' (1981: 37). Foucault's concept of the gaze upon individual bodies and its self-regulating potential is highly relevant to the female body. As Shildrick argues:

> The gaze now cast over the subject body is that of the subject herself. What is demanded of her is that she should police her own body, and report in intricate detail its failure to meet standards of normalcy; that she should render herself, in effect transparent. At the same time the capillary processes of power reach even deeper into the body, multiply-ing here not desire but the norms of function/dysfunction. As with con-fession, everything must be told, not by coercive extraction, but 'freely' offered up to scrutiny.
>
> (1997: 49)

The careful negotiation of space and place in relation to breastfeeding that I have illustrated has become a feature of women's breastfeeding experiences in England and other western cultures (Stearns 1999; Pain *et al.* 2001; Mahon-Daly 2002). As Stearns states, 'women accomplish the breastfeeding

of their children with constant vigilance to location, situation, and observer'
(1999: 322). As stated earlier, negotiation does not simply occur in public
places such as shopping areas, but may occur in so-called private places,
even within the home.

Accepting leaky distinctions

Is there a way out of this complex maze of dualisms and associated dissonances? It seems unlikely that the prolific sexualisation, in the media, of
women's breasts will stop, neither will medical interference in infant feeding
practices. Indeed both appear to be on the increase in a range of insidious
ways. So how can breastfeeding be normalised as an activity in public
domains? Perhaps this requires a reconceptualisation of breastfeeding that
takes us away from dualistic representations of breastfeeding as purely
maternal, on the one hand, and women's breasts as sexual on the other. The
time has come for us to accept what Haraway refers to as 'leaky distinctions',
'transgressed boundaries' and 'potent fusions' (1991: 154). This requires us
to acknowledge complexity, difference and diversity in the way women
breastfeed while avoiding disembodiment. I believe that women could come
to recognise and celebrate a unique blend of embodiment, relationality,
caring/nurturance and sexuality, whilst avoiding a return to essentialism
that simply binds women to reproduction. This requires a collective effort
by us, as women, to erode the dominant metaphors applied to our bodies
and to theorise new forms of embodiment, as suggested by Shildrick:

> What a feminist project might aim to do is to uncover the mechanisms
> of construction, flaunt the contradictions and transgressions which
> destabilise the binaries, and insist on a diversity of provisional bodily
> identifications. The move towards embodied selves need not entail a
> new form of essentialism nor a covert recuperation of biological deter-
> minism. Rather it celebrates embodiment as process, and speaks both to
> the refusal to split body and mind, and to the refusal to allow ourselves
> to be either normalised or pathologised. At the same time to stress both
> particularity and substantiality for the female body challenges the uni-
> versalised male standard and opens up for us new possibilities of (well)
> being-in-the-world.
>
> (1997: 61)

A key to disrupting dualisms around breastfeeding centres upon seeing
breastfeeding in relational terms rather than simply nutritional and health-
related terms. When breastfeeding is conceptualised as a relational activity
then varying constructions may co-exist. After all, relationships are dynamic,
highly complex and many-faceted. There are times of distance, closeness,
sensuality, sexuality, dialogue, silence, sharing, independence, interdepen-
dence, pleasure, partiality, exclusivity, mutuality, interaction, distraction

and interrelatedness. By accepting complexity, diversity and leaky distinctions we can celebrate breastfeeding and, at the same time, collectively disrupt and divert the range of penetrating 'gazes' upon our bodies, our being and our activities.

References

Apple, R. (1987) *Mothers and Medicine: A Social History of Infant Feeding 1890–1950.* London: University of Wisconsin Press.

Association of Social Anthropologists of the UK and the Commonwealth (ASA) (1999) *Ethical Guidelines for Good Research Practice.* www.asa.anthropology.ac.uk/ethics2.html

Bartlett, A. (2002) Breastfeeding as headwork: corporeal feminism and meaning for breastfeeding. *Women's Studies International Forum* 885(1): 1–10.

Blum, L.M. (1999) *At the Breast: Ideologies of Breastfeeding and Motherhood in the Contemporary United States.* Boston, Mass.: Beacon Press.

Bramwell, R. (2001) Blood and milk: constructions of female bodily fluids in western society. *Women and Health* 34(4): 85–96.

Britton, C. (1997) 'Letting it go, letting it flow': women's experiential accounts of the letdown reflex. *Social Sciences in Health* 3(3): 176–187.

Budin, P. (1907) *The Nursling.* London: The Caxton Publishing Co.

Burden, B. (1998) Privacy or help? The use of curtain positioning strategies within the maternity ward environment as a means of achieving and maintaining privacy, or as a form of signalling to peers and professionals in an attempt to seek information or support. *Journal of Advanced Nursing* 27: 15–23.

Carter, P. (1995) *Feminism, Breasts and Breastfeeding.* London: Macmillan.

Douglas, M. (1966) *Purity and Danger: An Analysis of the Concepts of Pollution and Taboo.* London: Routledge & Kegan Paul.

Doyal, L. and Pennell, I. (1981) *The Political Economy of Health.* London: Pluto Press.

Dykes, F. (2002) Western marketing and medicine – construction of an insufficient milk syndrome. *Health Care for Women International* 23(5): 492–502.

Dykes, F. (2003) *Infant Feeding Initiative: A Report Evaluating the Breastfeeding Practice Projects 1999–2002.* London: Department of Health. http://www.dh.gov.uk/assetRoot/04/08/44/59/04084459.pdf

Dykes, F. (2004) 'Feeling the pressure, coping with chaos': breastfeeding at the end of the medical production line. Unpublished PhD thesis, University of Sheffield.

Dykes, F. (2005a) 'Supply' and 'demand': breastfeeding as labour. *Social Science and Medicine* 60(10): 2283–2293.

Dykes, F. (2005b) A critical ethnographic study of encounters between midwives and breastfeeding women on postnatal wards. *Midwifery* 21: 241–252.

Dykes, F. (2006) *Breastfeeding in Hospital: Midwives, Mothers and the Production Line.* Oxon: Routledge.

Dykes, F. and Williams, C. (1999) 'Falling by the wayside': a phenomenological exploration of perceived breast milk inadequacy in lactating women. *Midwifery* 15: 232–246.

Dykes, F., Hall Moran, V., Burt, S. and Edwards, J. (2003) Adolescent mothers and breastfeeding: experiences and support needs. *Journal of Human Lactation* 19(4): 391–401.

Ebrahim, G.L. (1991) *Breastfeeding: The Biological Option*. London: Macmillan.

Fildes, V. (1989) *Breasts, Bottles and Babies: A History of Infant Feeding*. Edinburgh: Edinburgh University Press.

Foucault, M. (1977) *Discipline and Punish: The Birth of the Prison*. Harmondsworth: Penguin Books.

Foucault, M. (1981) *The History of Sexuality: An Introduction*. London: Tavistock.

Franklin, S. (1997) *Embodied Progress: A Cultural Account of Assisted Conception*. London: Routledge.

Grosz, E. (1994) *Volatile Bodies: Towards a Corporeal Feminism*. London: Allen & Unwin.

Hammersley, M. and Atkinson, P. (1995) *Ethnography: Principles in Practice*, 2nd edn. London: Routledge.

Haraway, D.J. (1991) *Simians, Cyborgs, and Women: The Reinvention of Nature*. London: Free Association Books.

Henderson, L., Kitzinger, J. and Green, J. (2000) Representing infant feeding: content analysis of British media portrayals of bottle feeding and breast feeding. *British Medical Journal* 321: 1196–1198.

King, F.T. (1913) *Feeding and Care of the Baby*. London: Macmillan & Co.

Kristeva, J. (1982) *Power of Horror: An Essay on Abjection*. New York: Columbia University Press.

Leff, E., Gagne, M. and Jefferis, S. (1994) Maternal perceptions of successful breast-feeding. *Journal of Human Lactation* 10(2): 99–104.

Lewis, J. (1980) *The Politics of Motherhood: Child and Maternal Welfare in England 1890–1939*. London: Croom Helm.

McConville, B. (1994) *Mixed Messages: Our Breasts in Our Lives*. London: Penguin Books.

Maher, V. (1992) Breast-feeding in cross-cultural perspective: paradoxes and pro-posals. In V. Maher (ed.) *The Anthropology of Breastfeeding: Natural Law or Social Construct*. Oxford: Berg, pp. 1–36.

Mahon-Daly, P. and Andrews, G.J. (2002) Liminality and breastfeeding: women negotiating space and two bodies. *Health and Place* 8: 61–76.

Martin, E. (1987) *The Woman in the Body: A Cultural Analysis of Reproduction*. Milton Keynes: Open University Press.

Murphy, E. (1999) 'Breast is best': infant feeding decisions and maternal deviance. *Sociology of Health and Illness* 21(2): 187–208.

Nadesan, M.H. and Sotorin, P. (1998) The romance and science of 'breast is best': discursive contradictions and contexts of breastfeeding choices. *Text and Performance Quarterly* 18: 217–232.

Odent, M. (1992) *The Nature of Birth and Breastfeeding*. Westport, Conn.: Bergin & Garvey.

Pain, R., Bailey, C. and Mowl, G. (2001) Infant feeding in North East England: contested spaces of reproduction. *Area* 33.3: 261–272.

Palmer, G. (1993) *The Politics of Breastfeeding*. London: Pandora.

Rodriguez-Frazier, R. and Frazier, L. (1995) Cultural paradoxes relating to sexuality and breastfeeding. *Journal of Human Lactation* 11(2): 111–115.

Rotch, T.M. (1890) The management of human breast milk in cases of difficult infantile digestion. *American Pediatric Society* 2: 88–101.

Schmied, V. and Barclay, L. (1999) Connection and pleasure, disruption and distress: women's experience of breastfeeding. *Journal of Human Lactation* 15(4): 325–334.

Shaw, R. (2003) Theorizing breastfeeding: body ethics, maternal generosity and the gift relation. *Body and Society* 9(2): 55–73.

Shildrick, M. (1997) *Leaky Bodies and Boundaries: Feminism, Postmodernism and (Bio) Ethics*. London: Routledge.

Spiro, A. (2006) Gujarati women and infant feeding decisions. In V. Hall Moran and F. Dykes (eds) *Maternal and Infant Nutrition and Nurture: Controversies and Challenges*. London: Quay Books.

Spradley, J.P. (1980) *Participant Observation*. New York: Holt, Rinehart & Winston.

Stearns, C.A. (1999) Breastfeeding and the good maternal body. *Gender and Society* 13(3): 308–325.

Thomas, J. (1993) *Doing Critical Ethnography. Qualitative Research Methods Vol. 26*. London: Sage.

Vincent, R. (1910) *The Nutrition of the Infant*. London: Baillière, Tindall & Cox.

Wolf, J.H. (2000) The social and medical construction of lactation pathology. *Women and Health* 30(3): 93–109.

Young, I.M. (1990) *Throwing Like a Girl and Other Essays in Feminist Philosophy and Social Theory*. Bloomington: Indiana University Press.

7 Not in public please: breastfeeding as dirty work in the UK

Susan Battersby

Although breastfeeding has been increasingly promoted as important to the health of both the infant and the mother there are still many in the UK who object to it being undertaken in the public arena. Recently, a mother was told to stop breastfeeding in Hampton Court Palace (Narain 2005) and mothers are also asked to leave restaurants (Narain 2005) and deserted bars (Sears 2000). Breastfeeding is perceived as primitive and crude by many men and women. It is the cause of embarrassment, and the butt of smutty jokes and innuendoes. It arouses feelings of disgust and disdain. Bottle feeding is seen as sterile and clean whilst breast milk is considered a pollutant, a bodily fluid that should be contained. There are limited facilities available for mothers to feed their infants outside of the home; they either breastfeed openly to the disdain of those around them or alternatively are pointed towards mother and baby rooms, which are either attached to the public toilets or within the public toilet. Why is there this objection to mothers breastfeeding in public? And is it just in public? Do mothers also encounter difficulties with breastfeeding within the private domain? The aim of this chapter is to explore the issues and feelings associated with breastfeeding under the public gaze. The basis for this study is drawn from a review of the pertinent literature and also from data collected for my PhD research. This entailed data collected during interviews of 39 breastfeeding mothers and 10 midwives, and a survey of 291 midwives who had personal experience of breastfeeding in the north of England (Battersby 2006). Within the text these will be referred to as midwife-mothers.

Sanctions by society

In 1993 the Royal College of Midwives conducted a survey which demonstrated that 93 per cent of the respondents disagreed with women breastfeeding anywhere they choose (Modern Midwife 1993). There have been many campaigns to try to increase awareness of the importance of breastfeeding but these do not appear to have removed the stigma that is associated with breastfeeding in the presence of others in the public domain and even within the private domain. As identified above, there have been recent cases where mothers have been asked to leave public places because of the need of their child for food. Mothers are frequently asked to leave shops, restaurants, shopping malls, museums and many other public places if they attempt to breastfeed their child, however discreetly. This is not the case if a mother wishes to bottle feed her infant. Although breastfeeding is perceived as better and is as natural as breathing, it is also perceived by some as dirty, unclean or even obscene. The reasons for sanctions are therefore twofold: for some, breastfeeding and breast milk are seen as dirty and polluted, whilst for others it is the sexual connotations associated with the breast. Whatever the cause, the reaction of others to breastfeeding may cause distress to mothers and in some instances can be a reason why mothers do not commence breastfeeding in the first instance (Fitzpatrick and Fitzpatrick 1994). In the study by Scott and Mostyn (2003) women reported how they would confine themselves to home or restrict their movement whilst breastfeeding in order to avoid the need to breastfeed in public.

Breast milk as polluted and dirty

Although breastfeeding is a natural and biological act it has also taken on an enormous and sometimes irrational emotional significance which has resulted in some people perceiving breastfeeding as indecent, disgusting, animalistic, sexual and even, for some, a perverse act (Yalom 1997). Breast-feeding can arouse feelings of disgust and disdain and one reason for this is associated with the connotations of breast milk as dirty or polluted. Forbes *et al.* (2003) highlight how shame and guilt are associated with both bodily functions and bodily fluids and this is particularly significant with fluids and functions associated with reproduction. Bramwell (2001) explores how breast milk and menstrual blood are constructed within western society and highlights how negative constructions of women's bodily fluids may undermine breastfeeding. Breast milk, menstrual blood and lochia (the vaginal discharge following childbirth) are all products resulting from bodily functions that are only experienced by women. Menstrual blood and lochia are considered as polluted by many cultures and strict codes of conduct are established relating to cleansing processes once the discharge has ceased (Schott and Henley 1996). Even in cultures where these rituals are not observed there is still a perception that bodily secretions are more or less disgusting, although to varying degrees. Menstrual blood and lochia are viewed as waste products and aligned with faeces and urine.

Morse (1989) believes that the fact that women are often asked to go to a toilet to breastfeed or to express breast milk suggests that breast milk and breastfeeding are also perceived as dirty and disgusting. Fluids that are escaping from the female body are expected to be contained or controlled by women. Breastfeeding is under neuro-hormonal control and the letdown reflex which is responsible for the ejection of the milk from the breast is unconditional initially and requires physical stimulus by the baby before becoming effective. This alters and eventually becomes a conditional reflex so that even thinking about the baby can result in ejection and leaking of milk from the breasts. Even when a mother is not breastfeeding her baby publicly, she can still be distressed and embarrassed by the unpredictability of the letdown process and the appearance of damp patches on her clothing.

> 'I had an embarrassing situation. Suddenly, that was it, I felt it and I thought, "Oh my God" and there it was, leaked all over the place. My breast pads had failed me. I had two great big wet patches . . . I didn't want it to happen but it did, typical.'
>
> (Britton 1997: 181)

This situation may cause distress and embarrassment to the woman because she and others may perceive her body as out of control, and observers may feel disgusted by the visible evidence. Women are provided with information within health education discourses which encourages them to exercise rational, individual and instrumental control of bodily processes (Lupton 1995). The media have also taken up this theme, particularly television adverts, which encourage women to control extraneous bodily fluids by wearing the appropriate sanitary protection or incontinence pads. Recently there has been an increasing consumerism around products related to breastfeeding which include breast pads to absorb leakage of breast milk. Unfortunately, as can be seen from the quote above, these are not always as good as they are advertised to be. At the same time as health education discourses encourage women to control bodily fluids, medical discourses portray the letdown reflex as one that is determined by stimulus/response linkages and one that will operate within the autonomic nervous system over which the woman has no control.

In many traditional societies, colostrum is perceived as dirty or unhealthy because it has been stored in the breast for a long time (Tran 1999). Colostrum may also be seen as polluted in some cultures because it is perceived as being similar to 'pus' because of its colour and texture and because of this may cause diarrhoea or other ill health (Rice 1999). Consequently, some women may worry about the effects that colostrum could have on their child and either express colostrum and discard it before breastfeeding or feed the baby with formula milk until the milk comes in at around three days after birth.

Breastfeeding and sexual connotations

Dykes and Williams (1999) argue that within the UK societal approval for breastfeeding in public is unfortunately lacking, and consequently Stewart-Knox *et al.* (2003) believe that breastfeeding in public is seen as taboo. This is because in some people's minds the physical and emotional intimacy of breastfeeding is connected with sexual activity. As a result, Pugliese (2000) believes that when a woman uses her breasts for their natural function, in an intimate relationship with her baby, she may consciously or unconsciously mistake it as something that is sexual which should be done in privacy. This is understandable as Li *et al.* (2002) highlight that the sexuality of the female breasts is a common image in the mass media whilst visual images of breast-feeding are rare. Ida May Gaskin (2003) has diagnosed our society as suffering from 'nipplephobia' and she sees the issue of women breastfeeding in public as symptomatic of a social epidemic. Wickham (2004) also believes that the veneration of breasts as sexual objects has not helped the cause of breastfeeding as a sacred pursuit, and as a consequence the issue of sexuality and breastfeeding has become very muddled and has resulted in many men and women being uncomfortable with the dual role of the breasts.

The cultural concept of the female breast

Dykes and Griffiths (1998) highlighted that conflicting cultural beliefs about women's breasts can undermine a woman's desire to breastfeed and also create problems for those who do breastfeed. Although this is not a new phenomenon, it is one that is constructed in a particular social and historical context (Stephen 2002). The increasing intrusion of the media into the home and everyday aspects of life has hastened the sexualisation of women's breasts through their increased display and objectification (Shilling 1993). Within western society, there has also been the construction of language specific to the sexuality of breasts. Within the UK, breasts are now viewed primarily as sexual objects and both men and women see breastfeeding as primitive and crude, especially if undertaken for more than the first few months. Sadly, an association between breastfeeding and indecent exposure has developed (Rodriguez-Garcia and Frazier 1995). This was highlighted recently when a person reported a mother to the police for breastfeeding in public. The police responded by sending an officer out to ask her to refrain from breastfeeding in public (Blacklock 2005). It appears that it is more acceptable in society to expose breasts within the tabloid press or through wearing transparent clothing for erotic purposes than for breasts to be exposed for the natural biological purpose of feeding an infant.

Baumslag and Michels (1995) highlighted the fact that if women are self-conscious about baring their breasts they will seek alternative ways of infant feeding. Foucault (1978) highlighted that sexuality is not a natural quality of the body, but rather the effect of historically specific power relationships. Feminists have used this concept to explain how women's experiences are controlled by culturally determined images of feminine sexuality. Palmer (1993) develops this further by stating that the sexualisation of the female breast has led to the breasts being appropriated by men, which has resulted in some men discouraging their partners from breastfeeding.

The cultural identity of the breast has seen a marked shift in the last thirty years and the breast has become an icon of sexuality. Along with this have come potential conflicts between the sexual and the mothering/nurturing role of the breast (Mahon-Daly and Andrews 2002). This has led to confusion for women who have been taught through socialisation that the sexual aspects of women and the maternal aspects should be independent of each other (Stearns 1999). For those who choose to breastfeed the conflict may cause embarrassment when breastfeeding within the public domain (Pugliese 2000).

Embarrassment

Embarrassment belongs to the general class of self-conscious emotions and is the emotion of self-exposure (Lewis 1995). Many women are not ashamed of breastfeeding but are shy of exposing themselves in public in order to undertake the process. It is the feeling of exposing oneself to others when breastfeeding that elicits the feeling of embarrassment. Lewis reiterates that embarrassment due to exposure is more similar to shyness rather than shame. This is not always the case because Stewart-Knox *et al.* (2003) in their qualitative analysis of infant-feeding perceptions found that women were embarrassed by the thought of breastfeeding, embarrassed to be seen with breastfeeding women and thought of women feeding publicly as breaching a cultural taboo.

Mothers' embarrassment

When I interviewed breastfeeding mothers the issue of feeding in public and embarrassment arose for all except five of the mothers (Battersby 2006). There were fourteen mothers who found breastfeeding natural and would feed the baby where and when it was necessary and did not get embarrassed feeding in public or in front of men; many of these were aware of the people about them being embarrassed but for them the baby's needs came first, as one mother explains:

> 'I'm not bothered any more. If some people, I can tell if they are uncomfortable, I'll just cover myself with a shawl. But other than that I'm OK. You know we went to the cinema yesterday, Crystal Peaks [a local shopping mall], so I breastfed him on the tram, because I had no choice. Well I was waiting for the tram, they don't have any benches anymore, so you can't sit down, can you? So as soon as I got on, I think the conductor was a bit, you know at first he didn't know what was going on, I had them covered, but I was more worried about him crying, I wasn't bothered about what was happening around me. You know for my first baby I kept looking for where you could go and sit down and breastfeed children, now I do it anywhere, I'm more worried about the baby than I'm worried about people.'

This was the mother's third child and she had worked through the issues of embarrassment during previous episodes of breastfeeding. The mother was also very confident of her role and had an outgoing personality. These are factors which were highlighted in Mahon-Daly and Andrews's (2002) study where they noted that the mothers' ability to 'feed the baby anywhere' was usually related to the more confident and outgoing mothers.

For the other mothers there was a range of feelings about breastfeeding publicly and the embarrassment it caused. Two mothers had found that they had not been embarrassed, although they had thought they would be embarrassed prior to giving birth. Two had been embarrassed about feeding their first baby but not their subsequent babies. Some mothers felt able to feed in front of friends and family but not publicly. Conversely, one mother would feed publicly but would not do it in front of some relatives. Two mothers found that their own fathers were embarrassed and four stated that they did not like the thought of feeding in front of any man.

For women, breastfeeding raises many possibilities for public performance (Stearns 1999) as on average a newborn baby will nurse about every two hours. As a consequence, most women will have to think about how they will go about breastfeeding in public, that is unless a woman decides to stay at home for several months following the birth and is able to only breastfeed at home, and in private. Although Stearns's study (1999) was conducted in the United States of America, the findings are reminiscent of the situations that women in England find themselves in when breastfeeding. Many women in her study reported instances when they received direct or indirect feedback from family, friends and others about the appropriateness of breastfeeding in front of others. Therefore, many women in the study proceeded with breastfeeding as though it was a deviant behaviour, occurring in a hostile environment. This would not be conducive to successful breastfeeding.

Embarrassment at breastfeeding can become a cause of social isolation for breastfeeding women and can be a cause of women discontinuing breastfeeding earlier than they had anticipated (Heath *et al.* 2002) or even not commencing breastfeeding in the first instance (Hoddinott and Pill 1999). Stearns (1999) found that women in her study often felt intimidated and embarrassed when breastfeeding their first baby but became more liberated with subsequent children. Stearns found that many women will try to plan their breastfeeding experiences when in the public domain; whilst Pugliese (2000) states that how a woman reacts to objections will vary depending upon her relationship with the objectors, her personality and the support she has. Some countries are now supporting women in their breastfeeding, and countries such as Scotland have brought in legislation to enable women to breastfeed in public without fear of complaint. England has yet to establish the right of mothers to breastfeed in public.

Midwife-mothers and embarrassment

The issue of embarrassment was raised by some of the midwife-mothers I interviewed (Battersby 2006). Midwife 4 raised the issue when relating how she had difficulty recalling her first exposure to breastfeeding. None of her family had breastfed and she thought this was due to embarrassment. Within the questionnaire there was a direct question asking the midwives if they would be embarrassed to feed in front of male relatives and friends, and another asking them if they would breastfeed in public. Embarrassment did not appear to be a major issue for many of the midwives because although the midwives talked about embarrassment it was more to state that they would not be embarrassed rather than to state that they would be embarrassed. The comments showed that the majority of midwives believed that they would not be embarrassed to breastfeed in public (68 per cent) or in front of male relatives (69.8 per cent). This, however, still leaves over 30 per cent who would feel embarrassed or were unsure. A midwife who had breastfed three children for nine months each 'still found it embarrassing and very personal'.

Kitzinger (2000) describes embarrassment as 'an expression of social interchange between the observed and the observer in an act considered shameful or immodest'. The fact that most midwives do not believe that breastfeeding is shameful or immodest may be the crux of why they state that they would not be embarrassed. This may be because midwives are generally confident and outgoing because of their chosen role in life, but also because of their profession they are more likely to view the function of the breasts as providing nutrition for the infant rather than endowing them with sexual connotations.

Embarrassment of others

Breastfeeding can be a major source of embarrassment not only for the mother who is breastfeeding but also for those who are witnessing the act. Earle (2000) reports that there is no dedicated research around the topic although the issue of breastfeeding and embarrassment has been introduced into breastfeeding literature. Edelmann (1987) identified embarrassment as an unpleasant feeling having to do with some form of discrediting of one's own image, either through the loss of self-esteem, the esteem of others, or both. In order for embarrassment to occur, three factors need to be present. These are the presence of another person, the person becoming aware that she is the centre of attention, and that person feeling that she is being judged.

The embarrassment of others was an area that was considered by a number of the mothers but the way they handled it varied. In one instance the mother would take a bottle to church to prevent embarrassment; in other instances those who were embarrassed were asked to leave the room or given the option to do so. In several instances, where the mothers knew breastfeeding their baby would cause embarrassment they prevented the embarrassment by opting to feed in a different room.

There were instances where the midwife-mothers were not embarrassed but others around them were. One midwife recalled how male relatives 'have been embarrassed and did not like me to do it', and another told how 'my parents asked me not to'. One midwife 'did not find it necessary to breastfeed in front of male relatives or friends. They always chose to keep a low profile whilst I fed.' Several midwives felt feeding in front of men was dependent upon 'the person, some I would feel comfortable with, others not', whilst another found it 'easier to feed with strangers than males in the family'. Therefore, embarrassment may not only be felt by the breastfeeding women themselves but breastfeeding women were aware of possible embarrassment of others and would initiate strategies to try to avoid embarrassment in others.

Breastfeeding and modesty

Davis-Floyd and Sargent (1997) believe that the modesty norm is still a significant factor in our culture. Moran (1999), however, identifies that modesty may be a significant variable impacting upon breastfeeding outcomes in western cultures. She conceptually defines modesty and places it in a cultural context. Kitzinger (2000), however, criticises Moran for using dictionary definitions for modesty and for failing to sufficiently explore the relation between linguistic meanings and social interaction. Moran's real failure is to link the concepts of modesty and embarrassment, which are very closely interlinked, with modesty being a personal attribute whilst embarrassment is a more active component where there is interaction between the observer and the observed in an act considered shameful or immodest. Although this may still be a factor for the older generation, still enshrined in Victorian values, it is difficult to believe that it is a factor for the younger generation who willingly expose vast expanses of their bodies on a daily basis.

Kitzinger (2000) explains that being immodest always involves an audience but being embarrassed can be unilateral. This means that although a woman may not be embarrassed when breastfeeding publicly, those around her may be, or vice versa. Therefore, the construction of the good maternal body involves constant vigilance to how breastfeeding is viewed by others (Stearns 1999). Many women find it difficult to breastfeed publicly but many also find it difficult to breastfeed in front of family and friends, particularly if they are male.

The need for discretion

Many see breastfeeding in front of others as exhibitionism. Women, however, in everyday life are constantly invading someone's territory, whether it is in the public domain or within their own domestic territory. Britton (2003) believes that many women will either give up breastfeeding or quickly develop an awareness of where they can breastfeed away from the public gaze. In an observational study undertaken by Mahon-Daly and Andrews (2002) this was done by the women deliberately seeking out mother-and-baby facilities, or by sitting in a position that removed them from the direct line of vision, or by wearing clothing that helped maintain modesty whilst breastfeeding.

A recurrent theme in many of the midwife-mothers' comments (Battersby 2006) was the necessity to be discreet when breastfeeding and to use supportive companions and concealing clothes to provide insulation from the disapproval of others. One stressed, 'It is important to breastfeed discreetly in company so as not to embarrass others.' Another told how, 'I breastfed my children discreetly in public places and in the company of male friends.' MW482 highlighted that it 'is possible to breastfeed discreetly without exposing yourself'. In order to be discreet some midwife-mothers wore 'clothes which enabled me to breastfeed without drawing attention to the fact'.

The size of their breasts caused embarrassment for some midwife-mothers, as MW368 explained, 'I only find breastfeeding in public embarrassing as I have large breasts and therefore difficult to be discreet.' Thus when many women speak of breastfeeding publicly they highlight the need for discretion.

Noisy breastfeeding as pollution

There were two mothers in my study who were not so much embarrassed at exposing themselves but were embarrassed because the babies were very noisy feeders and therefore drew attention to the act of breastfeeding (Battersby 2006). One mother explained:

> 'Yes because she makes a right noise. My friend came one day, and my boyfriend was here and she was crying. I said "I'll feed her and go upstairs". He said "do her here, you're all right". There was no telly on and no radio on and all you could hear was her. I said "can we please turn the telly on" because I felt really embarrassed. Some people can just get their boob out and do it wherever but I'm not one of them.'

If a baby feeds noisily and is demonstrative whilst feeding this may be perceived as breaching the normal bounds of modesty and may attract critical attention. Kitzinger (2000) argues that it is not only the exhibition of the breasts that causes embarrassment but also the fact that the baby may actually be enjoying being breastfed. Pugliese (2000) also believes that physical contact between mother and baby, which results in the mother and baby responding to each other both physically and emotionally, is the source of embarrassment. This close contact does not occur with bottle feeding. Smale (2001) extends this notion by considering the psychodynamic under-standings of breastfeeding as a relationship. Onlookers may perceive the baby as an impossible problem because it is seen as insatiable. Others may see a baby being instantly gratified whilst their own needs are not being met, therefore generating anger. Consequently, mothers are expected to breastfeed their infants in a quiet and detached manner, with any emotional display being regarded as taboo. This will be particularly evident if the mother is nursing an older child. Consequently, to avoid embarrassment for themselves and others many mothers will opt to breastfeed away from the public gaze.

Mother-and-baby facilities

Many women will seek out mother-and-baby facilities as places of privacy, but the use of these facilities is not without problems. Many are attached to or are part of public toilets which compounds the view of breastfeeding as dirty or polluted, whilst for other mothers they feel as if they are being segre-gated from society. A midwife recalled how she made her sister feed in public because she 'was sick of sitting in the toilet at the Early Learning Centre whilst she breastfed' (Battersby 2006).

The facilities themselves are often dirty and lack equipment, and some are available to men as well. Therefore women who have strived to reduce per-sonal embarrassment may still be confronted by it. In my study (Battersby 2006) a mother went to breastfeed her baby in the mother-and-baby room and was distressed because there was a man sitting with his partner who was bottle feeding the baby; this resulted in her getting the assistant to ask him to leave.

> 'The "Mothercare" facilities are brilliant but I went into town a few weeks ago and he was really hungry and I walked into "Mothercare" and there was a man sat in with his wife and she was just bottle feeding. There's benches outside to bottle feed, outside where you go to breast-feed. It said "Mother and Baby" room and then there's a place where dads feed and this man was sat in with his wife while she was bottle feed-ing her baby. I went in to breastfeed him and it just put me off. I went and saw one of the sales assistants and she said "Leave it with me" and I said "oh don't let him know it was me" but he must have known it was me. I walked in and walked back out and went and told them, and they went in and sent him out.'

Many of the midwife-mothers who had breastfed their own children told of how they had breastfed 'anytime, anywhere, in front of anyone' and 'found it easy to feed anywhere and rarely used special facilities'. Others did feed in public but felt they 'would rather find somewhere private'.

Breastfeeding as a private act

Breastfeeding, for many, is perceived as a private domestic event and this was reinforced by the midwives and mothers who opted out of the 'visual' environment in order to afford privacy for themselves and/or prevention of embarrassment for themselves or others (Battersby 2006). Four mothers stated that they would not feed in front of anyone, one because she believed it was personal and she explained that part of the reason for this was that she had large breasts and felt that she could not do it discreetly. Another mother felt very self-conscious, whilst the next mother was embarrassed herself when watching other mothers breastfeeding. The last mother stated that she did not like feeding in front of people; she said that her partner did not mind her doing it but she just could not relax. She went on to say:

> 'I breastfeed in private really. If someone came, well I just wouldn't do it. I would think that the person would be embarrassed anyway, if it was a man or whatever. I think they'd be embarrassed if you just started feeding your baby. I think they'd be a bit surprised really.'

The issues of embarrassment and mothers' desire for privacy are areas that have been touched on within much of the breastfeeding literature, but they are areas that have not been subjected to dedicated research. As already stated, breasts have acquired a sexual connotation and Shilling (1993) argues that partly due to the role of the media women's bodies are more displayed, objectified and sexualised. This arouses conflicts between the breasts as sexual objects and their role in mothering and nurturing the infant. The issue of exposing one's breasts in order to feed a baby could be argued to contravene known and accepted social and cultural boundaries. Accordingly, some women may feel that they need to negotiate space within their own domestic domain, especially if there are males present or in a crowded home.

Conclusion

Breastfeeding in public, and even at times in the private domain, remains a controversial issue. Although breastfeeding is readily accepted as the 'gold star' of infant feeding, breastfeeding in public is still seen as wrong and inappropriate. Sanctions on feeding in public arise from women as well as men. They arise because of breast milk being perceived as unclean and because of sexual connotations placed on the breasts. These sanctions cause anxiety and embarrassment for mothers wishing to breastfeed and for those who witness the act. The embarrassment is not always linked to exposure of the breasts and can also result from the baby feeding noisily and drawing attention to the act. Mothers may confine themselves to their homes to avoid the public gaze, whilst the fear of breastfeeding publicly may inhibit a mother from initiating breastfeeding. Mothers who breastfeed publicly often seek ways of being discreet and thus try to prevent embarrassment for themselves and others. Midwife-mothers do not appear to be as embarrassed about breastfeeding in public as non-midwife mothers but this is understandable because of their profession. The use of mother-and-baby facilities for breastfeeding can compound the view of breastfeeding as dirty and can cause social isolation for mothers. There needs to be designated research looking at breastfeeding in the public domain alongside a strong public awareness campaign by the government to highlight the natural function of breastfeeding, which should be reinforced by legislation to prevent discrimination of mothers who 'dare' to breastfeed publicly.

References

Battersby, S. (2006). 'Work in progress.'

Baumslag, N. and Michels, D. (1995). *Milk, Money and Madness: The Culture and Politics of Breastfeeding*. Westport, Conn.: Bergin and Garvey.

Blacklock, M. (2005). 'Police treat mother "like a criminal" for breast-feeding baby.' *Daily Express*, 22 November, p. 15.

Bramwell, R. (2001). 'Blood and milk: constructions of female bodily fluids in Western society.' *Women and Health* 34(4): 85–96.

Britton, C. (1997). 'Letting it go, letting it flow: women's experiential accounts of the letdown reflex.' *Social Science in Health* 3: 176–187.

Britton, C. (2003). 'Breastfeeding: a natural phenomena or a cultural construct?' In C. Squire (ed.) *The Social Context of Birth*. Oxon: Radcliffe Medical Press.

Davis-Floyd, R. and Sargent, C. (1997). *Childbirth and Authoritative Knowledge*. Berkeley: University of California Press.

Dykes, F. and Griffiths, H. (1998). 'Societal influences upon initiation and continuation of breastfeeding.' *British Journal of Midwifery* 6(2): 76–80.

Dykes, F. and Williams, C. (1999). 'Falling by the wayside: a phenomenological exploration of perceived breast-milk inadequacy in lactating women.' *Midwifery* 15(4): 232–246.

Earle, S. (2000). 'Why some women do not breastfeed: bottle feeding and the father's role.' *Midwifery* 16(4): 323–330.

Edelmann, R. (1987). *The Psychology of Embarrassment*. Chichester: Wiley.

Fitzpatrick, C. and Fitzpatrick, P. (1994). 'Factors associated with the decision to breastfeed among Irish women.' *Irish Medical Journal* 87: 145–146.

Forbes, G. and Adams-Curtis, L. *et al.* (2003). 'Perceptions of the woman who breast-feeds: the role of erotophobia, sexism and attitudinal variables.' *Sex Roles* 49 (7/8): 379–388.

Foucault, M. (1978). *The History of Sexuality, Volume 1*. London: Penguin.

Gaskin, I. (2003). *Ida May's Guide to Childbirth*. New York: Bantam.

Heath, A., Tuttle, C. *et al.* (2002). 'A longitudinal study of breastfeeding and weaning practices during the first year of life in Dunedin, New Zealand.' *Journal of American Dietetic Association* 102: 943–957.

Hoddinott, P. and Pill, R. (1999). 'Qualitative study of decisions about infant feeding among women in the east end of London.' *British Medical Journal* 318: 30–34.

Kitzinger, S. (2000). 'Comments on: analysis and application of the concept of modesty to breastfeeding.' *MIDIRS Midwifery Digest* 10(3): 370–371.

Lewis, M. (1995). 'Embarrassment: the emotion of self-exposure and evaluation.' In J. Tangney and K. Fischer (eds). *Self-conscious Emotions: The Psychology of Shame, Guilt, Embarrassment, and Pride.* New York: Guilford Press.

Li, R., Fridinger, F. *et al.* (2002). 'Public perceptions on breastfeeding constraints.' *Journal of Human Lactation* 18(3): 227–235.

Lupton, D. (1995). *The Imperative of Health: Public Health and the Regulated Body.* London: Sage.

Mahon-Daly, P. and Andrews, G.J. (2002). 'Liminality and breastfeeding: women negotiating space and two bodies.' *Health and Place* 8: 61–76.

Modern Midwife (1993). 'Men's attitudes to breastfeeding.' *Modern Midwife* 3(6): 7.

Moran, M. (1999). 'Analysis and application of the concept of modesty on breastfeeding.' *Journal of Perinatal Education* 8(4): 19–26.

Morse, J. (1989). 'Euch, those are for your husband! Examination of cultural values and assumptions about breast feeding.' *Health Care for Women International* 11: 223–232.

Narain, J. (2003). 'Restaurant orders out mum who breastfed baby.' *Daily Mail*, 20 November. London.

Narain, J. (2005). 'Mother told breast is not best at the palace.' *Daily Mail*, 10 August. London.

Palmer, G. (1993). *The Politics of Breastfeeding.* London: Pandora Press.

Pugliese, A. (2000). ' Breastfeeding in public.' *New Beginnings.* November/December: 196–200.

Rice, P.L. (1999). 'Child health and childbearing: traditional and changed patterns among Hmong women.' In P.L. Rice (ed.) *Asian Mothers, Western Birth.* Melbourne: Ausmed Publications.

Rodriguez-Garcia, R. and Frazier, L. (1995). 'Cultural paradoxes relating to sexuality and breastfeeding.' *Journal of Human Lactation* 11(2): 111–115.

Schott, J. and Henley, A. (1996). *Culture, Religion and Childbearing in a Multiracial Society: A Handbook for Health Professionals.* Oxford: Butterworth-Heinemann.

Scott, J. and Mostyn, T. (2003). 'Women's experiences of breastfeeding in a bottle-feeding culture.' *Journal of Human Lactation* 19(3): 270–277.

Sears, N. (2000). 'No room at the inn: mother turned away after she tries to breast-feed her baby son in a deserted bar.' *Daily Mail*, 18 July. London.

Shilling, C. (1993). *The Body and Social Theory.* London: Sage.

Smale, M. (2001). 'The stigmatisation of breastfeeding.' In T. Mason, C. Carlisle, C. Watkins and E. Whitehead (eds) *Stigma and Social Exclusion in Healthcare.* London: Routledge.

Stearns, C. (1999). 'Breastfeeding and the good maternal body.' *Gender and Society* 13(3): 308–325.

Stephen, K. (2002). 'Sexualized bodies.' In M. Evans and E. Lee (eds) *Real Bodies: A Sociological Introduction.* Basingstoke: Palgrave.

Stewart-Knox, B., Gardiner, K. *et al.* (2003). 'What is the problem with breastfeeding? A qualitative analysis of infant feeding perceptions.' *Journal of Human Nutrition and Dietetics* 16: 265–273.

Tran, H. (1999). 'Antenatal and postnatal maternity care for Vietnamese women.' In P.L. Rice (ed.) *Asian Mothers, Western Birth*. Melbourne: Ausmed Publications.

Wickham, S. (2004). *Sacred Cycles: The Spiral of Women's Well-Being*. London: Free Association Books.

Yalom, M. (1997). *A History of the Breast*. New York: Ballantine.

8 'Milk for Africa' and 'the neighbourhood' but socially isolated

Cheryl Benn and Suzanne Phibbs

Introduction

The issue of having an excessive breast milk supply appears to have been overlooked since research into breastfeeding began. It is complex and confusing as babies fight at the breast in the same way babies do when there is insufficient milk to satisfy their needs. Studies such as those by Schmied and Barclay (1999) and Schmied and Lupton (2001) indicate that some of the women had experiences similar to those in the current study but there was no identification of the problem as being one of an excessive milk supply and the overwhelming focus was on the negativity of the experiences of the participating Australian woman. In contrast, the majority of women in our research, while acknowledging difficulties and problems, talked positively about managing their excessive breast milk supply.

In this chapter use is made of two scenarios to illustrate the clinical situation and experience that led to the research study titled 'Too much milk'. The study design is described briefly while the main focus of the chapter is on two themes that were identified from the transcripts of interviews conducted with the first twelve women who volunteered to participate in the study. The themes, *having milk for Africa and the neighbourhood*, and *social isolation*, are illustrated using verbatim quotes from some of the women's transcripts. We discuss how the women were influenced by the masculine body politic, which underpins cultural expectations about bodily autonomy, containment and control, using a range of strategies to positively manage their open and secreting bodies and those of their babies. At the same time, socially isolating themselves and their babies in a way that protected other people from discomfort is indicative of the liminal and potentially polluting activity of breastfeeding and the disruptive potential of the maternal body.

Background and case scenarios

> We cannot possibly interpret rituals concerning excreta, breast milk, saliva and the rest unless we are prepared to see in the body a symbol of

society and to see the powers and dangers credited to social structure
reproduced in small on the human body.

(Douglas 1966: 115)

The title of Douglas's (1966) book *Purity and Danger* seems an apt metaphor
for the contradictory meanings surrounding breastfeeding for women in
general and those who experience an excessive breast milk supply in particular. Discourses about *purity* may be found in literature committed to the
promotion of breastfeeding. International agencies such as the World Health
Organization (WHO 2002), government reports and policies (NZMOH
1996, 1997, 2000, 2002, 2004; UK DoH 2002) and health professionals
currently promote breast milk as the safest, most hygienic and appropriate
source of nutrition for babies (Whit 2004; Murphy 2004), recommending
that women breastfeed exclusively up until 6 months of age (WHO 2002).
Women also draw on moral discourses about being a good mother (Murphy
2004; Schmied and Lupton 2001; Schmied *et al.* 2001) and doing their best
for baby (Murphy 1999; Ertem *et al.* 2001) to describe their decision to
breastfeed, while those who use infant formula are implicitly constructed as
'deviant', neglecting their duty of care and placing their infants in 'moral
danger' (Murphy 1999, 2004; Minchin 1998; Balsamo *et al.* 1992).

The other side of the coin, *danger*, is also represented by breast milk as a
source of pollution – dirty and dirtying. Schmied and Lupton (2001), for
example, reported that women in their study who experienced leaky breasts
described this occurrence as messy, embarrassing and a source of disgust.
Similarly Schmied and Barclay (1999) identified that some of the women
who contributed to their study found the embodied experience of breastfeeding to be disruptive and unpleasant. The women in the Schmied and
Lupton study also talked about the need to manage not only their own
bodies but those of their babies as well in order to minimise public embarrassment and/or revulsion caused by uncontained bodily fluids. Douglas
(1966) argues that the dominant social order is reproduced in ideas about
bodily pollution, which delimits boundaries, symbolising danger to the community, and wider concerns about the maintenance of existing social hierarchies. For Douglas 'all margins are dangerous' (1966: 121) including
those associated with the body; as such their transgression threatens the body
politic.

In her seminal article on the body politic, Moira Gatens (1996) argues
that traditional philosophical accounts of what it means to be human are
governed by understandings of what it means to be male. Within these
accounts woman are constructed as that which is 'not man'. Feminists have
documented the ways in which these male accounts of the human subject
have adversely affected understandings about women and femininity
(Gatens 1996: viii). Breastfeeding is a deeply embodied and 'liminal' activity
(Mahon-Daly and Andrews 2002; Turner 1979) that challenges enlighten-
ment ideas that privilege bodily transcendence, autonomy and separation

(Shildrick 1997). The act of breastfeeding in which milk flows directly from the mother to the baby, and the expression of milk through mechanical means, depends upon an open and secreting rather than an isolated and closed body (Mol and Law 2004: 51), blurring taken-for-granted assumptions about the margins of the body (Mol and Law 2004). At the same time, the extent to which women attempt to manage and present their own bodies as well as those of their babies as contained and discrete is indicative of the power of the masculine body politic which privileges ideas about bodily control and containment (Shildrick 1997). Thus women experience breastfeeding as simultaneously a domain of possibility and a means of constraint. In this way the multiple meanings and contradictory discourses about the body, breastfeeding and mothering shape, and are shaped by, how women understand their embodied experiences of breastfeeding and craft their identities as women and mothers.

Case scenarios

The issue of excessive milk supply caught Cheryl's attention when she was asked to assist some women with breastfeeding issues, as their babies were 'clicking' when feeding and that was thought by their midwife to be a bad sign that needed remedying. When she went to visit the women she decided to just sit and watch them feed in order to find out what was really happening. As she sat observing the baby suckling without much noise being emitted, some time into the feed she noticed the clicking start and that the baby seemed to be swallowing powerfully and noisily. On discussing the issue with the mothers they informed her that their babies tended to choke when the letdown happened and as they took baby off to assist them their milk squirted all over the baby, the room and onto their clothes, the sofa, the carpets. They did not complain of sore nipples and seemed to have the baby well latched. Cheryl deduced that they had a strong letdown reflex and a large milk supply that seemed to affect the babies, who pulled back as a means of protecting themselves from choking. This was when the clicking started.

   Suzanne, a sociologist, became interested in the issue after a close friend had her first baby and asked if the midwives at her work had any advice about breastfeeding. The friend was having ongoing problems with latching baby due to engorged breasts and fast letdown, she also leaked milk constantly – all signs of an excessive breast milk supply. In her search for help, the friend had consulted many sources (her midwife, the doctor, her Plunket (Well Child) nurse, the La Leche League, the internet). She was determined to breastfeed until at least 6 months but had lost confidence in her ability to do so and was at the end of her tether. She was resistant to advice from health professionals to express milk in order to soften the breast so that baby could latch because all the information that she read, and the advice that she was given, confirmed that expressing increased breast milk supply – an outcome that she did not want. Suzanne asked Cheryl, who specialises in breastfeeding support, for any advice that she could pass on to her friend; a conversation ensued that there was very little research about, or information available for, women who experienced excessive breast milk supply and the idea for a joint research project emerged.

Literature review and research context

Schmied and Barclay (1999) identify that there is a paucity of literature on women's experience of breastfeeding. On consulting the literature on the topic of an excessive milk supply, it was found that there is a lot of anecdotal information that seems to be available to health professionals (see Hoover, n.d., for example,[1] and the Australian Breastfeeding Association (ABA) booklet titled *Too Much. Managing an Over-abundant Milk Supply* (2002)). However, there was very little research found on the subject other than a few case studies published on pathological conditions such as pituitary tumours which led to women having an excessive milk supply which was not necessarily related to a recent pregnancy and breastfeeding (Zargar et al. 2005; Theunissen et al. 2005; Kroese *et al.* 2004). Cases of hyperprolacti-naemia with associated galactorrhoea have also been found in those using antipsychotic drugs (Medsafe Editorial Team 2001; Haddad *et al.* 2001; Meaney and O'Keane 2002).

Some information about factors that are associated with excessive breast milk supply may be cobbled together from various sources; however excessive breast milk supply tends not to be the major focus of these articles. Britton (1997, 1998), for example, explored women's experiences of the let-down reflex, but the main focus was not on the letdown reflex in relation to a large milk supply. Humenick *et al.* (1994) measured patterns of breast engorgement in 114 breastfeeding mothers during the first two weeks after delivery, with 20 per cent of the respondents reporting intense engorgement for the entire two-week period. Much of the discussion in this article focuses on the relationship between a lack of engorgement and insufficient milk supply. No mention is made of an excessive breast milk supply. Both Britton in relation to the letdown reflex and Humenick *et al.* in relation to engorge-ment identify the diversity of breastfeeding women's experiences which have not necessarily been supported by knowledge gained from scientific research evidence.

Schmied and Lupton conducted a qualitative study of twenty-five Australian women's experiences of breastfeeding and found that there was a predominant group of women who had difficulty reconciling their breast-feeding relationship with their baby 'with notions of identity that value autonomy, independence and control' (2001: 234). They draw attention to the female body and bodily secretions which are indeterminate and un-controlled and thus 'invested with cultural meanings as dangers, pollutants, dirt or contaminants' (2001: 245). In a qualitative study conducted by Schmied and Barclay eight of the twenty-five Australian women who participated in the study described their embodied experience of breastfeeding as painful or uncomfortable and the changes in their breasts as 'repulsive' (1999: 330). Factors that contributed to the women's distress about their breastfeeding experience included excruciating pain upon letdown, fast letdown and having to constantly attend to their leaking breasts, all possible signs of having had an excessive milk supply.

Many of the women who participated in the current study were keen on finding answers to what seemed to be a very personal and individual problem they were experiencing, but found little information to help or inform them. As an example, Anne, a health professional, who experienced an extreme 'stabbing pain' upon letdown and an excessive breast milk supply and had embarked upon extensive internet searches (including health databases), commented: 'I found there wasn't enough "out there" to help me; especially with the pain of letdown that I dreaded every time I fed my son.' Anne, a first-time mother, actively searched for information that would validate her experience of breastfeeding. Anne's midwife had not been able to reassure her about the 'normality' of her experience of pain upon letdown or to provide advice that Anne found either useful or practical about how to cope with her excessive milk supply.

In New Zealand there are a handful of La Leche League members who are lactation consultants who, either as a result of their own breastfeeding experiences or because they have themselves identified it as an unmet need, have specialised in helping women with excessive breast milk supply. However these women tend to be located in large urban centres and few women know of this aspect of the service. Some of the women whom we interviewed for example were already networked into home birth and La Leche League circles; others said that they stumbled across a specialist La Leche League lactation consultant after weeks of having problems with latching their baby, not coping and feeling inadequate. Few midwives who provided the postnatal care and support knew much about the issue and thus most were unable to provide the information and support the women needed. For these women, having too much milk became one of those 'silent' issues that no one spoke about. Hence the need for this qualitative study.

Research method

A qualitative approach was used as a starting point to find out about women's experiences of having too much milk. After having gained ethics approval for the study, recruitment was initiated using newspaper advertisements, but to no avail; this was followed by contacting women through existing networks such as lactation consultants, La Leche League and midwifery colleagues. While the latter method was of great value it was decided that a more diverse group of women was needed, as most interviewed at that time had been well supported by a lactation consultant and/or contact with La Leche League. One woman's story (used with her permission) and an advertisement calling for participants were inserted into a national mothering magazine, *KiwiParent*, produced by the Parent's Centre of New Zealand. This was the best means of recruitment, as calls and emails were received from women all over the country who told their stories with absolute relief that someone was interested in knowing about their experiences of having too much milk. The following extract is a typical representation of the type of response that we received from women interested in participating in the study (the extract is reproduced with the writer's permission):

> Currently I am breastfeeding my first baby who is 10 weeks old and just like the article in KiwiParent I can totally identify with Rosie. I have also had no answers on how to deal with this situation and have a couple of times thought it would be just easier to give up breastfeeding but I'm determined to see the six months out so have tried different ways of coping with the situation myself with varying degrees of success!

This chapter draws on extracts from the first twelve interviews conducted, which we consider to be largely representative of the qualitative information obtained in the wider and ongoing study. The volunteering women were from rural and urban areas, and were of varying ages and parity, with some now having grown-up children. The face-to-face interviews were audio-taped and transcribed with the women's permission; all names used in the discussion of interview extracts are fictitious. Two of the themes identified from the transcripts are presented and discussed in the following sections – the first, women's experiences of having too much milk, and the second, the issue of social isolation.

Having milk for Africa and the neighbourhood

There is no standard definition by which one may measure whether a woman has an excessive or 'normal' supply of breast milk. As breast milk production works on a supply and demand system, women's supply may vary according to how frequently or infrequently their baby feeds. However, it appears that for women with an excessive milk supply the frequency of feeding may not necessarily influence their supply to the same extent as for a woman who has an insufficient supply due to infrequent suckling. The concept of normal was an enigma to many of these women experiencing a large milk supply, especially if this was their first baby or first experience of breastfeeding a baby:

> 'because you don't know, it's the first time I've ever breastfed, and your boobs feel really full and, were leaky and, so I don't know, what's the

normal, you know you don't know what's normal when you've got nothing to compare it with.'

(Jane)

'Baby wasn't latching because I had so much milk, and on the second day [after the birth], I think, they decided to express and I filled a container full . . . 150 mls off one breast. It was like bloody hell!'

(Rosie)

In these extracts sets of understandings about what is normal are articulated in relational and comparative terms. Rosie, for example, thought that filling a container was normal until she took the milk to the fridge in the hospital for storage and found the other mothers had only managed to express about 25 mls of milk. This was the start of Rosie's recognition that she was different from other mothers – a recognition that influenced her participation in discussions at postnatal teas or gatherings for mothers. Even though all of the women whom we interviewed shared membership with a group of women who participated in what has been termed a liminal and marginal activity (Mahon-Daly and Andrews 2002), namely breastfeeding, women with a large milk supply felt ostracised and isolated as they perceived themselves to be different and abnormally so. Some of the women who participated in this research and did not find the large milk supply overly troublesome still regarded it as a 'problem' and were a little nervous to say anything about their supply in gatherings of young mothers, especially as they were aware that other women did not have the same experience. Thus it became an issue around which silence existed:

'You get quite despondent about it. So if you have, I think someone who's a friend, it would have been nice to just maybe talk to someone else that had the same problem.'

(Anne)

Women who participated in this study self-identified as having an excessive milk supply, as we did not have a definition as such. Their description of their milk supply frequently referred to how many other babies they could feed locally, nationally or internationally as well as to how large their breasts were:

'[I had so much milk it felt] like being able to feed the world'

'I had enough to feed Africa . . .'

'I just had so much and I would've, I would've filled the freezer in a week'

'My breasts were humungous; I had heaps of milk and filled six milk cube trays in three days. I had enough to feed two to three babies'

Having a large supply had obvious benefits for some of the women, such as never being concerned about their supply and being able to express enough so that they could go out and leave an aunt or grandmother to babysit, and having a sense of achievement that they have grown their baby themselves.

'This "excessive" production has made it really easy for the occasions that we have needed babysitters or got "caught short". We do not need to plan going out and could stay out all afternoon and half the night if we needed to. We also know how much she drinks at different times, which is a lot easier for the sitter if she knows this and baby has always taken the bottle, another huge relief for the sitter. We also know baby has been exclusively breastfed to this point and we have done our best for baby's start in the world.'

(Rebecca)

'I actually felt quite proud of my body in a way, there was that, not wanting to have milk squirting everywhere embarrassment side, but then in myself . . . I mean my mother and my midwife said I was a great cow, and I actually sort of took that in as something to be proud of that I was being a really good supplier of milk for my baby and so I actually felt quite proud of that.'

(Sarah)

However, this sense of freedom was counterbalanced in some women's talk about the need to ensure that a private space was available in case they had to use the breast pump. In the following extract, for example, Rosie talks about finding a suitable place to express and having to take both the baby and the breast pump with her when she left home:

'If you had to express finding a place to express . . . I could see that for . . . women who have to go to work definitely [they might give up] because there is no place to express that is private . . . To my own detriment if I did not remember to take the express pump with me . . . We went to the beach [house] one day and she didn't latch that day and I had so much milk and I did not have a pump and so I had to go home . . . as I was having a few pains . . .'

(Rosie)

If breastfeeding is a liminal activity that is marginally acceptable in public (Scott and Mostyn 2003; Mahon-Daly and Andrews 2002; Schmied and Lupton 2001; Hoddinott and Pill 1999), using a breast pump is definitely not acceptable. The use of a breast pump outside of the home requires forward planning to ensure that a suitably private space is available. This need for a private space reflects general cultural understandings about the maintenance of bodily products, particularly those associated with procreation and digestion (Douglas 1966), as belonging solely to the private sphere.

For some women the negative effects associated with having an excessive breast milk supply were overwhelming and these women tended to give up feeding after having exhausted all avenues of help and support, rather than persevering through the difficulties experienced:

> 'I had a horrendous time breastfeeding due to excessive milk supply, and after six weeks of breastfeeding and visiting lactation consultants, I gave up, as it was too much for me. I have to say that bottle feeding has made my life and my daughter's so much easier, and I certainly have bad memories of what breastfeeding, dressing, going to places, were like because of my milk supply.'
>
> (Ngaio)

Some of the women whom we interviewed talked about self-imposed social isolation because it was sometimes too challenging to try to get ready to go out and have to change themselves and their baby numerous times before being able to leave the house. In addition, health challenges such as mastitis made it impossible for them to go out or even want to do so. Many of the women, but not all, suffered from repeated bouts of mastitis. This was identified by the women as being related to whether their very full breasts leaked or did not leak:

> 'But I think, if I did [have leaking breasts] it would be like a release valve, I wouldn't have got the mastitis as often.'
>
> (Jackie)

The participating women described their milk volume in relation to the world around them, coming to recognise that they had a large milk supply through social contact with other women who had different experiences from themselves. Breastfeeding is not simply a mechanical exercise, it is also a relational activity (Dykes 2005; Schmied and Barclay 1999; Leff *et al.* 1994), with women also being concerned about the ways in which having an excessive breast milk supply impacted upon their babies.

Effect of too much milk on the baby

The effect on the babies influenced the women greatly in terms of their acceptance or otherwise of having a large milk supply. Women talked about how their babies seemed to swallow a lot of air and required frequent burping/winding, and spilled a lot:

'[I was always] stopping for winding, in the middle, because she obviously would swallow a lot of air.'

(Christine)

'I had other issues such as drowning my baby with milk. My son had excess wind due to gulping the large quantities of milk and had to be winded a number of times during feeding, severe pain on letdown, embarrassment related to milk spurting all over my son's face and into the air when he came off the breast suddenly, as well as problems with milk leakage. I still wear breast pads, where none of the other mothers in my mothers' group do.'

(Jasmine)

'[My son was] pretty much, blown off [the breast] you know he had to really work to stay latched on . . . [He was] very windy, and he was very spilly right from the beginning. Just really spilly after every feed, numerous clothing changes for him and for me. I went to the doctor and the doctor just said that he was just a happy chucker and that is just the way [he was]. He did not get upset with it, but he was always really, really very spilly.'

(Nancy)

'At first, baby would latch on, but the flow was so fast that she had trouble establishing a rhythm to her sucking and she would choke and splutter her way through a feed, but she quickly learnt to feed little and often and looking back over my postnatal notes she was feeding every 30–40 minutes for 10 minutes from one side only. She has never been able to drain one side and then move onto the other in one sitting. We also learnt to feed with an old pillowcase on top of the feed pillow to mop up spillage, and yes, we often had the experience of squirting milk across the room.'

(Rebecca)

Babies were 'spilly', 'windy' and 'gulped the milk'; they had to 'work to stay latched on' and required 'numerous clothing changes'. Mothers were 'embarrassed' and concerned about their babies 'drowning', 'choking', 'spluttering' and being 'blown off the breast'. 'Squirting milk', 'leakage' and 'pain on letdown' are used to describe the embodied experience of having an excessive breast milk supply. It is the open, secreting, interdependent and relational maternal body that is described in these interview extracts. Thus, bodily margins are blurred in the very talk of women who have an excessive breast milk supply.

Some babies fed less frequently in order to cope with the large milk supply:

'. . . people started to say, you know "she should be feeding more often" . . . and I started to get this so often, that I started to think "ooh" you know "I'm doing something wrong, maybe I should feed her more often, because she's only feeding every six hours that's four times in twenty-four hours". So . . . I started to wake her up four-hourly, 'cos you know of course that's what everyone recommends, you know, if they, don't wake then you should not let them go longer than four hours without a feed. So, I started to wake her and she, would take it, and then she'd just have, awful, awful colic, just scream and scream . . . until the next feed and then the four hours would be up and it'd be time for the next one, it was a total disaster. And I think it took someone like my mother, and I only, only did it for about two or three days, I can't quite remember exactly how long that was, it's probably in my Plunket (Well Child) book. And she said "you know I don't think it was such a good idea, she was very contented before you did that" and I, thought, "you know she was too".'

(Catherine)

Well-meaning health professionals and friends tried to give good advice on how to deal with the baby in terms of its frequency of breastfeeding. While these women responded to their suggestions they found they did not work and thus they tried to avoid the advice that came with some of the social contact. However, self-imposed social isolation was not only due to a wish to avoid advice that on the whole was contradictory and confusing; their bodies, and those of their babies, also made it necessary to impose restrictions.

Social isolation

Some women would not go out at all because of the large milk supply and the flow of milk which occurred at unexpected times and in unexpected places. Catherine described herself as becoming reclusive and making a firm decision in the first six weeks after her baby's birth not to go out.

'If I had missed a feed and I'd brush against somebody, and I didn't have breast pads in there would be milk everywhere . . . So, in the very early days I think, I just gave up getting dressed, I just stayed in, in, in. Well it was summer, 'cos she was a Christmas baby, and I just stayed in [the house], 'cos I had a whole lot of cotton nightgowns, housecoat things . . . and, once it was drenched, then I just, changed to another one. I just didn't put clothes on; because I knew I was gonna have to take them off . . . I remember taking, I remember that if ever we went out to anything, I just insisted on taking the baby with me. Maybe I was a bit, over the top [laughs]. At least until the baby was three months old anyway, if we were invited to a work do I said "well the baby has to come too", which wasn't totally, the accepted thing. And that would of course have solved that, letting down, problem. And I think also I was probably prepared for the first six weeks or something, not to go to things without baby, and I know, for a lot of women they wouldn't want to do that.'

(Catherine)

The only way Catherine found she could cope with an excessive supply and copious milk flowing everywhere when out in public was to take her baby with her so that she could be fed when Catherine demanded or needed her baby to feed. According to Uvnas Moberg (2003) the close relationship that develops between a mother and a baby has a physiological basis in the hormone of oxytocin and is necessary for survival of the species, and for continuing enhancement of the relationship. The presence of the baby promotes touch and thus probably the release of oxytocin, which has been found to be released in animals who are touched. In Catherine's case her baby's presence prevented those unexpected conditioned letdowns of her milk and the resultant flow in public when the baby was mentioned or thought of but was not there as a reassurance for her. Taking the baby with her was not a socially acceptable action as the presence of babies and lactating/breastfeeding women was considered inappropriate at business dinners/luncheons. As a result, Catherine would stay at home and not go out much, and was glad she did not have to go to work. This self-imposed social isolation might be considered to be conducive to the development of postpartum stress and depression, an idea proposed by Thorpe *et al.* (1991) and supported by the work of Macarthur (1991). However, the women who participated in the current study who continued to breastfeed did not mention depression as a consequence of their experience of having too much breast milk, but those who stopped feeding did refer to the bad memories and stress caused by the excessive milk supply. Further research is needed into the calming and connecting effects of oxytocin on postnatal moods.

Other women did go out but experienced some challenges which were often related to the baby not coping with the large supply and the effects of a rapid flow such as 'spilling' large amounts of milk all over themselves. Dirty clothes and the smell of partially digested milk were socially unacceptable and made the women feel dirty and concerned that their babies looked uncared for. Many of these babies gulped the milk, or fought at the breast to protect themselves from the overwhelming supply, thus drawing attention to the breastfeeding mother:

'So if ever I was out and tried to feed her somewhere I often got so covered in vomit, and, you know, she'd have to be completely changed and often I'd have to be completely changed. So it was sort of a bit embarrassing, and it was, quite noisy too, 'cos often you didn't know, you know if she broke away, and your milk was still squirting out, sort of quite embarrassing . . .'

(Jackie)

'The thing about the puking was just, fact of cleaning it up, because you know the navy couch used to look lovely with puke all over it. And going out, and you just get ready to go to work or something and she'd puke all over you and then you'd have to change it again. So I used to, run round in my knickers and bra in the morning, and, put her in her car seat and then get dressed . . .'

(Liz)

'She's never been a great feeder. Sometimes she'd feed here [in the lounge at home] and she would have a, a little spastic and have a scream and, probably feeding in front of people would be a bit embarrassing, you know, then they'd make you more anxious and, it doesn't work, as well.'

(Christine)

'He really struggled to latch and to cope and I found it quite embarrassing. If I would go to mothers' groups and things he was a very noisy drinker and I found that a little bit embarrassing I guess and I ended up getting cracked nipples.'

(Nancy)

'. . . my first day back at work, everyone asked me about [baby] and I had to go home at the end of the day 'cos my top was soaking, I couldn't believe how wet it was [laughs] it was drenched. And I had expressed so much milk off at work that day, 'cos I obviously was just, I dunno if it was related to the anxiety of leaving her for the first time and, I think I walked around the whole day letting down actually.'

(Christine)

In the above interview extracts women talked about their baby's ability to embarrass them in public by puking, being a noisy drinker or screaming while trying to latch on during a feed.

Breastfeeding babies are also embarrassing for other family members. One woman's family tried to 'put' her away at a family wedding so as not to be an embarrassment while feeding:

'Oh I went to my brother's wedding and I wanted to breastfeed him there and they kind of wanted to put me away in a separate room, and I was like "oh I don't know". I suppose I did have a dress on that did make it a bit difficult but it was just a bit like "would you like this room, this separate room?", and I was like "oh I don't know about that". I was a bit surprised that they wanted to just sort of put you away.'

(Sarah)

The women also tended to isolate their babies, especially if they spilled or vomited up large volumes of milk. This was to prevent them messing up visitors' or relatives' clothes and furniture, or their baby receiving a look of disgust from the person holding the baby:

'Yeah so it was probably just the, social thing really about it, that was the most annoying and a couple of people that saw her puking you know, they'd hold her, and you'd see them pick up a baby and instead of, I used to always hold her upright, and or sitting right upright, and I never ever, you know how some people hold babies in their arms, I never held her like that, and she hated it too and I'm sure it had something to do with her neck. She used to always grizzle when she was held like that, and you see people wanna hold the baby and you'd be watching them thinking, I just see she's gonna puke. And a couple of times she did do pukes over them, and they're like "Ohhh", the look on their face as she'd do a huge big puke.'

(Christine)

The passing of stools in public was another factor that influenced one woman to either not go out or delay trips from home when a stool was due:

'No [bowel motions were] about once every five to seven days but when he went . . . And that was an issue as well, like if I knew that he was due to do [a motion] I would not go to a mall or anything like that because it would be just a huge major download. But then when he got onto solids he was far more regular and he goes just sometimes three times a day at the moment. But when it was just breast milk and when it was quite excessive yes, it was about once every five to seven days, major download.'

(Sarah)

Scott and Mostyn suggest that 'many women are reluctant to socialize and go outside the home with their newborn baby until they are feeling confident and in control' (2003: 272). The women who participated in this research struggled to control not only their own maternal bodily fluids but also the excretions and secretions of their babies which they perceived to be excessive due to their milk supply. This resulted in two forms of social isolation. The women experienced geographical isolation because they were unwilling to leave the safety of the home. They were also reluctant to share their 'spilly' babies with extended family and friends, resulting in a type of interpersonal isolation. 'Sharing' in this context was experienced as a stressful event that needed to be carefully managed, requiring vigilant attention to the bodily rhythms of their baby on the part of the mother.

Conclusions

This chapter has examined how the stories of women who experienced an excessive breast milk supply both conform to, and disrupt, understandings about the body politic. The women who participated in this study were implicitly aware of the body politic that underpins sets of understandings about bodily secretions as dirty and polluting, working hard to keep themselves and their babies safe from the adverse comments or actions of those around them. Women talked about the need to manage not only their own bodies but those of their babies as well, in order to minimise embarrassment and/or disgust caused by uncontained bodily fluids. Attention to interpersonal body-space so as to prevent a person accidentally brushing across the breast, controlling their surroundings so that cues such as a crying baby did not trigger the letdown reflex, and managing their leaking breasts in order to minimise their own embarrassment or to prevent others from being embarrassed were recurring themes. Perceptions about excessive burping, vomiting and bowel motions, as a result of their babies gorging themselves on their milk, resulted in the need to manage their babies in ways that they considered to be socially appropriate. As a consequence, some women strategically used forms of geographical and interpersonal isolation to manage and control unruly bodies that were 'leaky', 'spilly' or otherwise 'embarrassing' to themselves and others.

Preliminary results from our research suggest that conventional received knowledge about breastfeeding is challenged by most of the women interviewed who have an excessive breast milk supply. Traditional advice about expressing, spacing of feeds and alternating breasts, for example, may not be appropriate for some women who have too much milk. We have also suggested that contemporary understandings about embodiment are disrupted by the open, secreting, interdependent and relational maternal body. In the quote from *Purity and Danger* reproduced at the beginning of this chapter Douglas writes that the 'social structure [is] reproduced in small on the human body' (1966: 115); through attention to the leaky maternal body it is possible to explore the different ways in which the symbolic order is reproduced in and through the body. Rather than being an exception to forms of embodiment that privilege autonomy and control, the leaky maternal body suggests how general social rules about the management of bodily fluids come to be codified, constructed and crafted in and through the everyday practices of individuals.

Note

1 Kay Hoover (USA IBCLC) has produced information on practical suggestions and strategies regarding an Overabundant Supply and Rapid Milk Ejection Reflex.

References

Australian Breastfeeding Association (2002). *Too Much. Managing an Over-abundant Milk Supply*. Victoria: ABA.

Balsamo, F., De Mari, G., Maher, V. and Serini, R. (1992). Production and pleasure: research on breast-feeding in Turin. In V. Maher (ed.) *The Anthropology of Breast-Feeding: Natural Law or Social Construct*. Oxford: Berg.

Britton, C. (1997). 'Letting it go, letting it flow': women's experiential accounts of the letdown reflex. *Social Sciences in Health: International Journal of Research and Practice* 3(3): 176–187.

Britton, C. (1998). 'Feeling letdown': an exploration of an embodied sensation associated with breastfeeding. In S. Nettleton and J. Watson (eds) *The Body in Everyday Life*. London: Routledge.

Douglas, M. (1966). *Purity and Danger: An Analysis of the Concepts of Pollution and Taboo*. London: Routledge & Kegan Paul.

Dykes, F. (2002). Western medicine and marketing: constructions of an inadequate milk syndrome in lactating women. *Health Care for Women International* 23: 492–502.

Dykes, F. (2005). 'Supply' and 'demand': breastfeeding as labour. *Social Science and Medicine* 60(10): 2283–2293.

Dykes, F. and Williams, C. (1999). Falling by the wayside: a phenomenological exploration of perceived breast-milk inadequacy in lactating women. *Midwifery* 15: 232–246.

Ertem, I.O., Votto, N. and Leventhal, J.M. (2001). The timing and predictors of the early termination of breastfeeding. *Pediatrics* 107(3): 543–548.

Gatens, M. (1996). *Imaginary Bodies: Ethics, Power and Corporeality*. New York: Routledge.

Haddad, P.M., Hellewell, J.S. and Wieck, A. (2001). Antipsychotic induced hyperprolactinaemia: a series of illustrative case reports. *Journal of Psychopharmacology* 15(4): 293–295.

Hill, P.D. and Aldag, J. (1991). Potential indicators of insufficient milk supply syndrome. *Research in Nursing and Health* 14(1): 11–19.

Hoddinott, P. and Pill, R. (1999). Qualitative study of decisions about infant feeding among women in east end of London. *British Medical Journal* 318: 30–34.

Humenick, S., Hill, P. and Anderson, M. (1994). Breast engorgement: patterns and selected outcomes. *Journal of Human Lactation* 10(2): 87–93.

Kroese, J.M., Grootendorst, A.F. and Schelfhout, L.J. (2004). Postpartum amenorrhoea-galactorrhoea associated with hyperprolactinaemia and pituitary enlargement in primary hypothyroidism. *Netherlands Journal of Medicine* 62(1): 28–30.

Leff, E.W., Gagne, M.P. and Jefferis, S.C. (1994). Maternal perceptions of successful breastfeeding. *Journal of Human Lactation* 10(2): 99–104.

Macarthur, P. (1991). *Women's Health after Childbirth*. University of Birmingham: HMSO.

Mahon-Daly, P. and Andrews, G.J. (2002). Liminality and breastfeeding: women negotiating space and two bodies. *Health and Place* 8(2): 61–76.

Meaney, A.M. and O'Keane, V. (2002). Prolactin and schizophrenia: clinical consequences of hyperprolactinaemia. *Life Sciences* 71(9): 979–992.

Medsafe Editorial Team (2001). Hyperprolactinaemia with antipsychotics. Prescriber Update articles downloaded 12/1/06 from http://www.medsafe.govt.nz/Profs/PUarticles/hyperpro.htm

Minchin, M. (1998). *Artificial Feeding: Risky For Any Baby?* St Kilda, Victoria: Alma Publication.

Mol, A. and Law, J. (2004). Embodied action, enacted bodies: the example of hypoglycaemia. *Body and Society* 10(2–3): 43–62.

Murphy, E. (1999). 'Breast is best': infant feeding decisions and maternal deviance. *Sociology of Health and Illness* 21(2): 187–208.

Murphy, E. (2004). Risk, maternal ideologies, and infant feeding. In J. Germov and L. Williams (eds). *A Sociology of Food and Nutrition: The Social Appetite*. Melbourne: Oxford University Press.

NZ Ministry of Health (MOH) (1996). *Food and Nutrition Guidelines for Healthy Breastfeeding Women – A Background Paper*. Wellington: MOH.

NZ Ministry of Health (MOH) (1997). *Infant Feeding – Guidelines for New Zealand Health Workers*. Wellington: MOH.

NZ Ministry of Health (MOH) (2000). *Food and Nutrition Guidelines for Healthy Infants and Toddlers (Aged 0 – 2 years)*. Wellington: MOH.

NZ Ministry of Health (MOH) (2002). *Breastfeeding: A Guide to Action*. Wellington: MOH.

NZ Ministry of Health (MOH) (2004). *Review of the New Zealand Interpretation of the World Health Organization's (WHO) International Code of Marketing of Breast-milk Substitutes (the WHO Code)*. Wellington: MOH.

Schmied, V. and Barclay, L. (1999). Connection and pleasure, disruption and distress: women's experience of breastfeeding. *Journal of Human Lactation* 15(4): 325–333.

Schmied, V. and Lupton, D. (2001). Blurring the boundaries: breastfeeding and maternal subjectivity. *Sociology of Health and Illness* 23(2): 234–250.

Schmied, V., Sheehan, A. and Barclay, L. (2001). Contemporary breast-feeding policy and practice: implications for midwives. *Midwifery* 17(1): 44–54.

Scott, J. and Mostyn, T. (2003). Women's experiences of breastfeeding in a bottle-feeding culture. *Journal of Human Lactation* 19(3): 270–277.

Shildrick, M. (1997). *Leaky Bodies and Boundaries: Feminism, Postmodernism and (Bio)ethics*. London: Routledge.

Theunissen, C., De Schepper, J., Schiettecatte, J., Verdood, P., Hooghe-Peeters, E.L. and Velkeniers, B. (2005). Macroprolactinemia: clinical significance and characterization of the condition. *Acta Clinica Belgica* 60(4): 190–197.

Thorpe, K., Golding, J. and Magillivray, I. (1991). Comparison of the prevalence of depression in mothers of twins and singletons. *British Medical Journal* 302(678): 875–878.

Turner, V.W. (1979). Betwixt and between: the liminal period. In W. Lessa (ed.) *Rites De Passage. Reader in Comparative Religion: An Anthropological Approach*. New York: HarperCollins.

UK Department of Health (2002). *Improvement, Expansion and Reform – the Next 3 Years: Priorities and Planning Framework 2003–2006*. London: DoH.

Uvnas Moberg, K. (2003). *The Oxytocin Factor: Tapping the Hormone of Calm, Love and Healing*. Cambridge, Mass.: De Capo Press.

Whichelow, M.J. (1982). Factors associated with the duration of breast feeding in a privileged society. *Early Human Development* 7(3): 273–280.

Whit, W. (2004). World hunger. In J. Germov and L. Williams (eds) *A Sociology of Food and Nutrition: The Social Appetite*. Melbourne: Oxford University Press.

WHO (2002). *Infant and Young Child Nutrition: Global Strategy on Infant and Young Child Feeding*. Fifty-Fifth World Health Assembly, Geneva: WHO.

Zargar, A.H., Laway, B.A., Masoodi, S.R., Bhat, M.H., Wani, A.I., Bashir, M.I., Salahuddin, M. and Rasool, R. (2005) Clinical and etiological profile of hyper-prolactinemia – data from a tertiary care centre. *Journal of the Association of Physicians of India* 53: 288–290.

9   Breastfeeding – a time for caution for Gujarati families

Alison Spiro

Breastfeeding is highly valued in Hindu and Jain Gujarati families, providing health, promoting perfect nutrition in a pure white, God-given fluid for the new infant. While feeding her child a mother is thought to transmit, through her milk, her own emotions, life force, *karma* and 'knowledge' of her ancestral heritage. After the birth, the woman and her infant's bodies are in states of transition between pregnancy and motherhood, intrauterine existence and life outside the womb, and as such are subjected to contradictions and dichotomies. At this time, the mother is both producing a pure, white food in the form of milk, and also excreting potentially polluting red blood. The infant's body is in a pure state after birth but may also have been affected by the impurity of the birth process. This ambivalent and transitional status of the bodies of both the newly delivered woman and her child makes them both vulnerable. They are cared for in the maternal home for forty days after birth, until this danger has subsided, and rituals are performed to protect them and other household members. At this time, women's bodies are sources of ultimate purity and extreme pollution. These contradictions and dichotomies became apparent during qualitative research I carried out in Harrow, north London and Ahmedabad, India for a doctoral thesis. The research was conducted with families that had young children, and the methodology used included participant observation and unstructured, taped interviews, which were transcribed, ensuring all names were fictitious to protect the identity of the informants. In this chapter I will examine the cultural imperatives to give pure, God-given milk, but also the potentially polluting effects of breastfeeding, through focusing on the bodies of Gujarati women and children and the dichotomies of purity and impurity, and positive and negative energies.

Purity/impurity

The body of a woman after delivery faces contradictions, through being seen as producing a source of purity in the form of milk and also of impurity in her blood loss. This ambivalent nature of her bodily status poses a dilemma for households, which on one hand have to care for her and her baby and provide her with optimum nutrition, but on the other hand have to protect themselves from her impurity.

After marriage, the young couple usually live with, or in close vicinity to, the husband's parents, that is, they are patrilocal. When the woman is seven months pregnant, many families perform a ritual during which rice is exchanged between her mother and mother-in-law, in the folds of their saris. This symbolises the joint responsibility they have for the unborn child and the last grains go to the woman's mother, who will assume the initial caring role after the birth. In the past, women may have returned to their natal home at this point, but most women in Britain go back to their husband's house until labour. The newly delivered woman and her child are taken from hospital to her parents' house where she will stay for the next forty days.

During this time, her mother provides her with special, nutritious foods designed to re-energise her body, which has become depleted during pregnancy and labour, and boiled water with added spices, called *sua*, to rid her body of impurities. In so doing, her mother will carefully control the entrances and exits to her daughter's body. She makes special foods, which are easily digested and high in energy and minerals. These foods are believed to improve the quality of the breast milk and help its flow into the baby. Some religious sects, notably Jains and Swaminaryans, will avoid garlic and onions, and vegetables that grow underground, because of beliefs about impurities and micro-organisms that exist there. Most households, Jains as well as Hindus, make *katlu* for new mothers, which is a food made from millet, nuts, honey, gum and ghee, and is thought to strengthen the woman's back after childbirth. Her mother will give her daughter's body a daily massage after she has massaged the baby.

The exits from the woman's body, in the form of blood and milk, will also be regulated by sanctions being put on the place where her physical body can reside. Her mother will suggest she remains in her bedroom for the first week until her blood flow reduces, so that she does not pose a danger to others in the household; although other members can enter her room, they should not touch her bed which is thought to be particularly polluting. After this time, she is allowed to move around the house, but cannot approach the household shrine, or enter the kitchen, or prepare food for the whole forty days. Older women in the household will direct the new mother to ensure her future health and that of her baby, at the same time protecting the household. A grandmother told me:

> 'Ladies in India work very hard. They support the family. They want to rest for twenty days after childbirth. They must not touch anyone and no one must touch anything belonging to them, especially their beds. Religion says she must not touch anyone and everyone prays for her. If you touch the woman, you cannot say prayers. She is unclean for forty days. For the first twenty days she cannot go in the kitchen and is given food in a separate plate. After forty days she can go to the temple.'

Food and its production have to be carefully regulated, because it is particularly vulnerable to both impurities and negative forces. Cooked food in particular, possibly because of its ambiguous status of being at a transitional state between fresh and digested food, could be easily spoilt by the mother's blood and then cause illness in the family. Mary Douglas has suggested that: 'The most dangerous pollution is for anything that has once emerged gaining re-entry' (Douglas 1991: 123). Pocock has also acknowledged the important role women play in controlling negative forces and impurities in the household.

> As cooks they are guardians of the religious purity of the family. At the same time they are subject to pollution by menstruation and occasionally by childbirth. Not only are they believed to be physically subject to pollution, but morally more subject to sexual temptation.
>
> (Pocock 1972: 12)

The infant's body, in contrast to his mother's, is in a state of purity after the birth and needs protection from both his mother's impurity and the evil eye or *najar*, which may come through the jealous look from an outsider. He will remain with his mother at his *nani* (maternal grandmother) and *nana*'s (maternal grandfather) house for the first forty days of his life, and will be washed, massaged and rocked by his *nani*. He drinks his mother's milk, which is a pure, life-giving substance, designed by the gods especially for him. In order to maintain the purity of his body, *nani* ties black threads around his ankles, wrists or waist, and may also put black spots on the soles of his feet, the palms of his hands, around the eyes, or behind his ears. These threads will protect his body extremities and prevent evil from entering. He is vulnerable to attacks from the evil eye, *najar*, through jealous looks from outsiders, or from over-indulgence by his mother *mithi-najar* (sweet evil eye). Protection of his body is also sought from the gods, who will be invoked in the six-day ritual, or *chhati*, which is led by the child's father's sister or *foi* and attended by close family and friends. Here the goddess Randalma is called upon to protect the child and the god of fate Vidhata is asked to write the child's future on a piece of white paper with a red pen; the white may symbolise the purity of the child and the red the auspiciousness of the god.

Here it is worth considering the colour symbolism used by Gujaratis and the accompanying cultural meanings. Red, the colour of blood, is the colour of the wedding sari and is auspicious at life-cycle rituals, symbolising fertility, success and happiness. It can, however, also be a colour that warns of danger and death. White, the colour of milk, symbolises purity and virginity, shown in the colour of the woman's sari before her wedding. The milk of the cow carries the meaning of ultimate purity, fit for the gods and offered to the gods in religious ritual. At the beginning of most ceremonies, the Ganesh Puja, the Elephant God, is washed in milk. Yoghurt or milk is included in most meals to aid digestion, but Dumont suggests it also sanctifies the meal and removes impurities that may have entered the food (Dumont 1980). White, like red, also has a contrasting meaning when used for the widow's sari as a representation of mourning and death. The meanings attached to the colours of the two fluid emissions from the woman's body after childbirth can be seen as ambiguous and contrasting, which reflects her status and demands vigilance and regulation.

The polluting effects of childbirth reduce over time and by the time the child is 40 days old they have subsided sufficiently for the mother to take a ritual bath and put on new clothes. The baby is also bathed and given new clothes, ridding him of any remaining impurities from his mother, and they are both taken to the temple for a blessing. The mother and her child can then return to her husband's family home, where her mother-in-law, the baby's *dadi*, will care for them. Vigilance is still required to protect them both from *najar*, the evil eye, especially when mixing socially with others outside the kin group.

Positive/negative energies

Breastfeeding itself carries with it contradictory messages through both transmitting the mother's positive *karma* in a pure, health-giving food for her child, as well as being a potential source of harm through her negative thoughts or *najar*.

Women of all ages have told me about their beliefs that emotions can pass through body fluids. At the beginning of my research, a group of elderly women insisted that breastfeeding was one of the most important things anyone can do for anyone else. They told me that breast milk is made especially for the mother's own child and is different from all other mothers' milk; it is part of her *karma*, or life force, and gives the child cultural messages about his or her cultural heritage. Through breastfeeding, a child learns about his or herself in the world. Women have also spoken about how the mother's thoughts and emotions pass through the milk. I met Hansa, a young mother born in India, when I was completing my preliminary research for my MSc (Spiro 1994), and she told me:

> 'Breastfeeding a child is thought to be one of the best things you can do. It is part of your *karma*, or life force. If you breastfeed someone, you do them a very big favour.'

Bina, a young mother from Uganda, and a friend of Hansa, continued by insisting that:

> 'You must feed your own milk; it is made especially for your child. If you breastfeed, the child knows his mother. If you bottle-feed he doesn't know his mother. If the bottle breaks, the child cries because the bottle is broken, but if the mother dies, the child does not care.'

A group of grandmothers I met at that time was in agreement that breast-feeding not only made babies physically strong, but also gave them a sense of their culture and knowledge of their ancestors. Here, they were indicating that breastfeeding is an embodied process where the milk contains elements of the mother's identity and heritage. Their views suggested a holistic body in which body fluids carry social messages and the breasts are connected to the emotions and the brain. Meera, a mother with two children, also thought that emotions could be transmitted through breastfeeding:

'Most people say that if you breastfeed and at the same time think good thoughts, the baby will grow up nicely, not like a hooligan who won't listen to his parents. If the mother is stubborn, then the kid tends to be stubborn too, I have seen it so many times in India.'

Millard and Graham (1984) have reported similar ideas about emotions passing through body fluids in pregnancy and breastfeeding, in their studies of women in rural Mexico. These embodied feelings have been lost to women in the west who tend to view their bodies as divided into somatic parts, through scientific discourse, where body organs are seen to be functioning independently of each other. They find it difficult to understand connections between the emotions and the physical body, let alone with the social body. For most Gujarati women these links exist, but are probably fading over time in Britain, with the influence of western education.

The other side of this dichotomy is that there is the possibility that negative, as well as positive, elements or energies pass to the child through his or her mother's milk. The transitional nature of the bodies of the mother and her child makes them both vulnerable to supernatural attack and so they require ritual protection. Van Gennep (1960) in his study of rites of passage and ritual argues that there are clearly defined stages in the process of rites of separation, threshold rites, and rites of re-aggregation. He emphasised that all rituals were associated with transition from one situation to another, and Victor Turner extended his argument and re-named the three stages as pre-liminal, liminal and post-liminal. The pre-liminal stage of the rite involves the novice being secluded or separated in some way, then passes to the liminal stage where the status of the participant is reversed and the weak become strong and the strong weak and there is social levelling. The attributes of liminality are always ambiguous; they are betwixt and between, neither here nor there. Rank and status disappear and passivity, humility and nakedness are apparent. Communitas arises out of liminality, when social structure appears to be no more and feelings of common humanity are expressed. For Turner, communitas has an 'existential quality; it involves the whole man in his relation to other whole men' (Turner 1969: 127). Mary Douglas also takes Van Gennep's theory of ritual and emphasises the danger of the transitional state, when the status of a person is changing from one to another. In my research, I found that the transitional states experienced in marriage, pregnancy, childbirth, breastfeeding and early childhood were dangerous times when supernatural attacks were more likely and ritual protection was needed.

> Danger lies in transitional states, simply because transition is neither one state nor the next, it is indefinable. The person who must pass from one to another is himself in danger and emanates danger to others. The danger is controlled by ritual which precisely separates him from his old status, segregates him for a time and then publicly declares his entry to his new status.
>
> (Douglas 1991: 96)

Breastfeeding occurs within a liminal time for mothers and their children, as it happens between intrauterine life and independent living for the child, and pregnancy and motherhood for the woman. Their uncertain statuses present dangers, requiring vigilance, caution and ritual. The child may be at risk through the mother transmitting negative energies through her milk. They both may be vulnerable to jealous looks from outsiders, which could attract *najar*, the evil eye. People suspected of casting the evil eye are usually outside the immediate kin group, but may be of similar status. They may look at the child in an envious way and inadvertently pass *najar* to him or her. As a result, the child may become ill or even die, refuse to eat, or his or her character may change. '*Najar* was usually unconsciously exercised and sprang from desire. If one was contented one did not feel desire and one's eyes could not hurt others' (Pocock 1973: 30).

Research carried out in India by Reynell (1985) reports that women in Rajasthan are also concerned about the evil eye, which is passed through a jealous look and can cause misfortune and death. Pocock was told by one of his informants of the strength of evil powers:

> A woman was once feeding her child and looked at it with great affection. Her mother-in-law, fearing for the child, suddenly directed her attention to the stone flourmill, which immediately broke in half. Here there was no question of envy, but of permanent evil eye unconsciously exercised.
>
> (Pocock 1973: 27)

Pocock described this different form of evil eye as a permanent one, but my research suggests that it arises when mothers show too much affection for their children in front of others. Gujarati women are discouraged from displaying affection for their children, for fear that they themselves may inflict *mithi najar*, the sweet evil eye, on their children. Kajol, a mother educated in Britain, told me that when someone boasts about their child or keeps looking at him or her lovingly then *najar* could be cast. It is different from the eye of jealousy, which comes from outside, but can still cause problems in the child, such as loss of appetite and illness. So rather than a 'permanent' evil eye, *mithi najar* is inflicted if the mother is too proud of her child, or demonstrates loving behaviour in front of others. Bhopal (1986) found that the views of Punjabi women in Glasgow were similar, and here *nazar* (evil eye in Hindi) was thought to cause fretfulness and loss of appetite in children. Here the gaze of a loving or malevolent person was thought to be responsible for transmitting the evil. Several tragic stories were told to me about the consequences of *najar*, during my research, often recounting disease and death in children. Sangita, a Jain mother, told me:

> 'I had a daughter who would have been twenty-six this year. When she was three years old, a neighbour and friend of my in-laws gave her the "look" and within an hour she had a temperature. We travelled to Leicester that evening and while we were still on the motorway, she stopped breathing and passed away. I still blame this woman for being jealous and passing the evil eye to her. Even today, I cannot speak to her. Many people today say they don't believe it, but when it happens to you, then you have to.'
>
> (Spiro 2005: 66)

Women in the kinship hierarchy will be consulted on the appropriate rituals needed to expel *najar*. These usually involve pungent substances similar to those used to prevent attacks, but in more severe cases special people with spiritual powers may be called upon. The risks of attack are highest soon after the birth but subside over time, although vigilance is still needed while the child is small.

Gujarati beliefs about the dangers posed by *najar* during breastfeeding were described to me by several women of different ages, and perhaps the most interesting came from Nikhita, who was educated in Britain and is a graduate. One evening, when her children were in bed, she told me about her family beliefs:

> 'Because we have this thing about the evil eye, Asian women will not breastfeed in front of other Asian women. They feel that the woman might cast an evil eye on their child, and then you will stop producing milk. They are cautious about who they feed in front of, and will probably restrict it to just direct family. If there is someone else there, they will not come out and feed their child. It is not the shame of showing a boob; it is out of fear of casting the evil eye. She may be jealous and think, oh, she's got a beautiful baby, or she's having milk and I couldn't do it; or it could be that she has a boy and I've got a girl, it could be a hundred and one things, and she could be from the most modern families.
>
> My mother-in-law told me not to feed in front of anyone, because we don't want anyone casting an evil eye on him. I would have breastfed

him if there were no other Asian mothers present. We don't think that
white people have the same jealousy.'

(Spiro 2005: 64)

Preventive measures have to be taken to protect the child and, as mentioned
above, the black marks that may be put on the child's body, which are made
of soot mixed with castor oil, are designed to make the child look less attrac-
tive to envious people. These may not be considered sufficient and other
rituals need to be performed to give added protection. Water or limes may
be passed around the child's head seven times each day, and pungent substances such as garlic and chilli may be burned and may also be passed over
the child's head. Once used, these fluids or solids must not be looked at by
anyone and are disposed of down a sink or thrown over the shoulder at a
crossroad. During my research, several mothers told me of the care they
took while breastfeeding their infants to avoid anyone watching them with a
jealous look, which could invoke the evil eye. There did appear to be a
generational change taking place, with the grandmothers believing in *najar*
more strongly than the mothers, but even so, most of the younger women
still practised the rituals. Seema expressed this change to me:

> 'There is a generation change. My mother-in-law believes in the evil eye
> more strongly than me. Older people believe that you have to pass a
> container of water, made of glass or steel, around the baby's head seven
> times in a clockwise direction. Then you take it outside the front door,
> not the back, to a crossroad and pour the water in the middle of the
> roads without looking at it.'

(Spiro 2005: 64)

Evil spirits and ghosts are thought to become trapped in gardens, so substances used to remove *najar* from the child are always taken out of the front
door. It is thought that once used in ritual to remove evil these liquids or
solids are highly dangerous and anyone looking at them could become
afflicted. Raheja reported similar findings in India: 'The negative qualities
that have been separated from the person are extremely dangerous until they
have been "moved away" and assimilated by the appropriate receptacle'
(Raheja 1988: 84).

Breast milk as a liminal substance, in between two bodies, carries with it
extreme danger. In addition, any substance which emerges from the body
and gains admission to another has the potential to carry with it serious
pollution (Douglas 1991). The status of breast milk as a body fluid that has
emerged from one body and is about to enter another requires cultural
action, ritual and convention, probably in all human societies. It can also
have implications as to where breastfeeding happens, who can watch, and
whether expressing milk is culturally acceptable. In Gujarati social groups,
it is the danger of *najar* being cast on the mother and her child that is the

concern when breastfeeding in front of those who are not close kin, and not the exposure of breasts.

Expressing milk may also pose problems because once the fluid has been separated from the body it is more vulnerable to evil attack through a jealous gaze, which will spoil the milk and make the baby ill. Indian women who feed formula milk to their babies through a bottle will often cover it with a cotton or knitted cloth, to protect it from direct view. Donated breast milk from a milk bank may be very problematical for Indian mothers, because of the personal qualities or negative energies contained in the milk. Meera, a Gujarati midwife, explained her views to me:

> 'There was a time when breast milk was so much in fashion; they were collecting it for milk banks. Then women started to think, do I really want to give my child milk from another woman, who might have a different kind of personality, different kinds of thoughts, do I want to use it? I feel the same way and I have no way of proving it, but I feel it so strongly. I would like to see some sort of research material that shows this is the case. The same with food, it doesn't matter what ingredients you have in cooking, if you don't have a portion of love in it, the food is never good.'

Here Meera is confirming the view that the breast milk itself contains the thoughts and feelings of the mother and is the medium through which they are transmitted to the child. Negative thoughts and energies from other women, who could be from different castes, ethnic groups, and cultures, could make donated milk unacceptable and could cause serious pollution.

Storing breast milk in a fridge or freezer may also not be acceptable to some Indian women, because once milk has been removed from the body it is vulnerable to jealous gaze from others and *najar,* which could make the baby ill. Formula milk on the other hand is seen as modern, scientific, containing pure elements of the cow, and as such may be more acceptable than expressed milk. Despite the cultural imperative to breastfeed, many Asian women are likely to give complementary formula milk rather than expressed milk (Hamlyn *et al.* 2002). Other women in the kin network, who have considerable influence, may doubt the adequacy of the mother's milk supply, and suggest she gives the baby formula as well. So although a new mother is supported initially in her desire to breastfeed, her female kin may doubt her body's ability to be the sole provider for her child. The strong network of inter-dependency in Gujarati kinship begins with the care of a newborn child, which is shared between the other women in the household who may also wish to feed him or her. Also, through daily massage, rocking and bathing, the baby may become attached to the grandmother or aunt more closely than to his or her own mother. As I suggested above, a close love relationship with the mother may be seen as a source of pollution through the *mithi najar* (sweet evil eye), and is discouraged.

Discussion

Scholars such as Mauss, Douglas and Dumont have focused on the body in an attempt to understand how the physical body is constrained and modified by social processes and categories. Marcel Mauss (1973) argued that every kind of bodily action or technique such as walking, feeding, washing and sex is a result of social learning. Mary Douglas identified two bodies, the physical body and the social body, and the continual exchange of meanings between the two; as a result the body itself becomes 'a highly restricted medium of expression': 'The physical experience of the body, always modified by the social categories through which it is known, sustains a particular view of society' (Douglas 1991: 93).

The way the woman's body is viewed by a society and the constraints placed on it will vary according to the meanings given to it. Douglas (1991) and Dumont (1980) have drawn on Van Gennep's rites of passage to suggest that cooked food may be seen as in a transitional state of being neither raw nor digested, and as such is vulnerable to pollution. Dumont explained why cooked food is more dangerous than raw food:

> This is perhaps because, by cooking, food is made to pass from the natural world to the human world, and one may wonder whether there is not here something analogous to the 'marginal state' in *rites de passage*, when a person is no longer in one condition nor yet in another, and consequently exposed, open in some way, to evil influences. In India itself most of these *rites de passage* correspond to an impurity, which expresses the irruption of the organic into the social life; now there is something of the organic in our case, as with excretion, and, with the necessary difference, there is not true impurity at least an exceptional permeability to impurity.
>
> (Dumont 1980: 140)

I have argued here that breast milk can also be seen as having uncertain status because of its transitional or liminal nature, as a fluid that is emerging from one body and entering another. It has not been cooked, but is in a state of readiness for easy digestion in another body and as such is probably more vulnerable to evil forces. Sanctions and controls are placed on the process of breastfeeding by societies, by restricting the place where it happens and who views it, and by making rules to control its frequency. It may be interesting here to consider why Gujarati women think that white people do not have the same powers to transmit the evil eye, which suggests that it is in some way culturally specific. In other cultural groups, other sanctions such as not breastfeeding in public, or strict time regimes, may be strategies that are applied, or they may be more subtle and hidden.

The liminal nature of the process of breastfeeding and the milk itself, as neither part of the mother's body nor that of the baby's, increases the danger associated with it. Gujarati women in Britain continue to view breastfeeding as a very special time for themselves and their children, but extra vigilance is required to protect the new mother and her child, so that the benefits of this pure food are realised.

References

Bhopal, R. (1986) 'The inter-relationship of folk, traditional and western medicine within an Asian community in Britain'. *Social Science and Medicine* 22(1): 96–105.

Douglas, M. (1991 [1966]) *Purity and Danger: An Analysis of the Concepts of Pollution and Taboo'*. London: Routledge.

Dumont, L. (1980) (1966 French original) *Homo Hierarchicus*. Chicago: Chicago University Press.

Hamlyn, B., Brooker, S., Oleinikova, K. and Wands, S. (2002) *Infant Feeding 2000*. London: Stationery Office.

Mauss, M. (1973 [1934]) 'Techniques of the body'. *Economy and Society* 2(1): 70–88.

Pocock, D. (1972) *Kanbi and Patidar*. Oxford: Clarendon Press.

Pocock, D. (1973) *Mind, Body and Wealth*. New Jersey: Rowman and Littlefield.

Raheja, G. (1988) *The Poison in the Gift*. Chicago: University of Chicago Press.

Reynell, J. (1985) 'Honour, nurture and festivity: aspects of female religiosity among Jain women in Jaipur'. Unpublished PhD thesis, University of Cambridge.

Spiro, A. (1994) 'Breastfeeding experiences of Gujarati women living in Harrow'. Unpublished MSc dissertation, Brunel University.

Spiro, A. (2003) 'Moral continuity. Gujarati kinship: women, children and rituals'. Unpublished PhD thesis, Brunel University.

Spiro, A. (2005) 'Najar or bhut – evil eye or ghost affliction: Gujarati views about illness causation'. *Anthropology and Medicine*: Routledge.

Turner, V. (1969) *The Ritual Process: Structure and Anti-structure*. London: Routledge & Kegan Paul.

Van Gennep, A. (1960) *The Rite of Passage*. London: Routledge & Kegan Paul.

Gujarati terms

The following are words used in the Gujarati vernacular:

chhati	six-day after-birth ceremony
dadi	paternal grandmother
foi	paternal aunt
karma	action which accumulates throughout life and attaches itself to the soul
katlu	special food made for mothers after giving birth
mithi-najar	sweet evil eye
najar	evil eye
nana	maternal grandfather
nani	maternal grandmother
sua	water mixed with spices, given after birth

10 The pollution of practice by tales from outside

Evidence for the denial of embodied understandings of feeding babies in the initial and ongoing learning of health professionals

Mary Smale

Globally and historically, breastfeeding has been initiated and sustained without medical intervention. Commercial and medical models of feeding, in collusion, came to dominate as twentieth-century hospital practices extended into the home. Apple shows how the scientification of breastfeeding and its substitute increasingly created cultural beliefs such as unreliable milk supply (Apple 1987). Marchant points to breastfeeding as an area in which it has been felt that midwives' advice may be influenced by their own experiences. So '[t]he legacy of misinformation that we all carry with us from our own earlier education' is acknowledged as 'still there in the health service psyche' (Renfrew 2004: 4). This suggests an urgent need for science to displace old tales now culturally embedded. However, Battersby suggests the impossibility of eradicating sources other than research-based understanding since midwives gain their knowledge of breastfeeding from a variety of sources (Battersby 2002). Some of the data collected during a training needs analysis undertaken from the Mother and Infant Research Unit in the University of Leeds between 1999 and 2001 contained material which suggests the need for an alternative to eradicating learning outside the clinical or academic setting.

Douglas writes of the need for rules about pollution 'whenever the organic erupts into the social' (Douglas 1975: 214). The data suggested implicit rules in relation to personal accounts of breastfeeding and their contamination of scientific knowledge by impure anecdote. Themes identified included the containing of stories to protect others from damaging ideas and 'dumping' feelings on others. This chapter offers evidence for concerns around conversations about breastfeeding among health professionals, considers the effect and meaning of the unspoken rules, and indicates the need for further research.

The main focus of the study was the perceived needs of respondents in relation to training and education for breastfeeding support. Initial interviews with expert educators and managers used open questions. These helped find routes to further subjects and set the agenda for a series of semi-structured questionnaires. Educators, managers and practitioners across a wide range of those involved, including midwives, health visitors, general practitioners, paediatricians, ancillary hospital workers and others, were interviewed. Respondents were sought, by as wide a set of invitations as practicable, in proportion to the extent to which they worked with breast-feeding women. Midwives were sought from different work settings. Interviews reflected the views of those with varying times since qualification. Mothers were also interviewed. Seventy-three individual and nine group interviews were conducted. A summary of each of the responses was written from notes, transcribed and returned to the respondent for correction and additions. Summaries therefore recorded the words from the perspective of the interviewer (e.g. 'You thought that . . .'). Key findings from this work have been published (Smale *et al.*, 2006).

Data revealed contrasting opinions about health professionals' learning via embodied experience. This was acknowledged as an important source of understanding, but there was considerable concern about passing on this knowledge to others in the health service. This was a similar finding to that of Battersby (2002). 'It is argued that the women's knowledge [in other peri-natal areas] is inferior to that gained from textbooks and other conventional sources used within health professional education' (Marchant 2004: 325). The possibility of sharing stories was asked about in relation to initial train-ing and when returning to work after motherhood.

Understanding this concern as a fear of the leaking out of personal under-standing into pure theory raises the possibility of seeing such stories as polluting. One respondent addressed the reconciliation of valued personal experience with some its dangers:

> You feel that people who have not breastfed should not help those who are . . . helpers who have breastfed must not be opinionated and force their views on others, but give information for an informed decision.
>
> (complementary practitioner)

'Real life learning'

Evidence from respondents

Almost all respondents with close experience of breastfeeding prioritised this as a source of learning. A few examples indicate opinions, mainly in response to the question: 'How do you feel you have learned most about feeding babies?'

> Completely through personal experience.
>
> (health promotion specialist)

> It is difficult to separate from your own experience. Personal experience is more important for you.
>
> (complementary practitioner)

Vicarious close experience was also seen as useful. One respondent explained her course gave:

> practical knowledge based on people's real life knowledge.
>
> (voluntary breastfeeding supporter)

Respondents sometimes felt that minimal initial educational input had been superseded by personal experience of breastfeeding.

> you feel you probably know more from being a father than from being a doctor.
>
> (university lecturer)

This learning included emotional and social aspects:

> it did help with mothers whose babies were separated from them, as yours was.
>
> (senior midwife)

> ... especially an appreciation of concerns such as 'Am I feeding enough?' How to know when a baby has had enough off one breast ...
>
> (midwife)

> your sister in law ... was pregnant young and fed her baby anywhere, being 'nicely arrogant' and normalising it 'gracefully' within the home and feeding in front of aunts and uncles whereas in your family it had been a total taboo.
>
> (health promotion specialist)

Respondents acknowledged missing experiences:

> Probably from books, as you had no problems yourself.
>
> (health visitor)

> Part of the problem is you have no personal experience.
>
> (nurse in cardiac ward)

A mother who had trained as a nurse identified aspects lacking in her training:

an idea of the emotional side of it from the mother's point of view. You . . . had no idea – for example you could not quite get your head round why women wanted to express.

(mother interviewed at home)

The legitimacy of personal experience was implicit in the response of a worker whose experience was of trying to breastfeed ill babies with little support:

You tell mothers that you breastfed.

(healthcare assistant)

There was incidental evidence from mothers too that authenticity was found in those with subjective experiences:

The first, and undisputed, suggestion was that all people offering help should have had to experience breastfeeding themselves . . . the group talked about the professionals who had breastfed themselves being the ones who understood how they felt and knew what they were talking about – personal experience like 'it hurts' . . .

A dietician/mother in the group said she would never again say 'it's a bit painful at first'.

(group of postnatal mothers)

This suggests that mothers were motivated, and able, to identify staff who had breastfed.

Competition for claiming the most authoritative information could be complex:

You feel health professionals often pay lip service to breastfeeding support . . . It is difficult to contradict their advice.

(lay breastfeeding supporter)

You relied on your lay knowledge and this was difficult from a point of view of standing your ground . . . Before . . . [voluntary] breastfeeding training . . . intimidated by midwives/health visitors with [an] approach to using bottle to give mums a rest – nothing in training to give confidence to stand ground.

(GP interviewed as volunteer supporter)

You feel you know more about breastfeeding than some health visitors and midwives and struggle not to interfere – for example when a mother had a fourth child after bottle feeding three babies you would like to have a conversation about her choice of feeding with her but felt it was not your role.

(social worker for drug-taking women)

For some, authoritative knowledge existed reliably inside the clinical setting only.

> In hospital most people should have enough professionalism to give help – it is worse in the public at large.

(team leader, paediatric surgical ward)

Mothers were only occasionally seen as providing useful information to others. Most practitioner respondents, asked for ideas about future training, focused on increasing research-based information, but one suggested:

> Sit with experienced breastfeeding women to get out of the first few weeks when new. See normal breastfeeding women, living their lives.

(midwife)

This knowledge was more generally kept back however. Despite professionals' feeling that informal and embodied learning outweighed academic training in usefulness for supporting women, there were considerable doubts about its articulation to women or to each other. With improved education there would be no need for anecdotal or embodied learning (or the involvement of voluntary support):

> Some [health professionals] identified that they had received no training either pre- or post-registration in the area of breastfeeding and that they were forced to rely on personal experience . . . or to use voluntary breastfeeding support services such as the National Childbirth Trust.

(facilitator of in-house training for health professionals)

The experience of mothers was only mentioned once as useful for mothers:

> You get mothers to come in and talk about feeding for pregnant mothers in parent craft.

(community midwife)

It was explicitly mentioned only once as a source of knowledge for a health professional:

> This comes from listening to women.

(health visitor)

The ignoring of women's experiences was sometimes regretted:

> One missed opportunity you felt was the use of experienced mothers to pass on knowledge.
>
> (manager)

However the improbability of women's input was generally assumed. No one mentioned learning from another health professional's own breastfeeding experience when asked about sources of learning, as suggested by Cantrill *et al.* (2003). One respondent regretted this:

> It is a shame that personal experience of breastfeeding e.g. of lecturers is not seen as valid knowledge.
>
> (midwifery lecturer)

A further question for those who had experienced breastfeeding was 'How was any opportunity given in training to spend time in considering this experience?' Recalling training over a long time span, between under one and over four decades since qualification, only two respondents spoke positively, both describing post-qualification training:

> On the [recent] two day course.
>
> (team support worker)

> In the M.Sc. there was a small amount in small group discussion, but only if safe, for example with other mothers.
>
> (health promotion specialist, trained as paediatric nurse)

Similar rules were identified in focus groups during the evaluation of a peer support project: 'if [health professional] participants did have personal experience of breastfeeding, this was entirely sidelined or silenced within their discussion' (Curtis *et al.* 2001: 28).

Educators' responses

A question about the inclusion of any opportunity for the consideration of personal experience was asked of educators: 'How is any opportunity given for each participant to spend time in coming to terms with their own experience of infant feeding?' The very few positive responses included:

> Not probably planned into sessions but may arise – as with bereavement such issues are covered as they arise.
>
> (midwifery lecturer)

> This comes up, for example a male student's wife 'failed' in breast-feeding. He felt women were not well supported in breastfeeding. He now says he will be able to support her better next time.
>
> (midwife involved in education of health staff)

Others indicated there was no time for such discussion, that this was not yet covered, or that it might happen in the future, with provision incidental rather than built in. It was notable that two respondents compared breast-feeding with loss, suggestive of a perceived similarity in level of emotional sensitivity.

'The intention of the professional education framework is to encourage research based evidence to supplant [these] more anecdotal influences' (Marchant 2004: 324). This it seemed was achieved largely by ignoring embodied or cultural experience.

The place of the personal in post-registration education

Post-registration provision (in a course reaching very few practitioners) provided useful opportunities for personal exploration but not without opposition.

> The course . . . includes time for debriefing centred on sessions about 'women, society and breasts'. This has proved challenging to some participants and has in the past met with criticism from a midwifery manager . . . also include[s] 'debriefing' sessions following experience of a number of women who were still very emotional about their breastfeeding experience . . . you are aware of midwives' needing to be aware of their own personal baggage where they did not receive good support and have feelings of guilt and failure.
>
> (midwifery lecturer)

Lifelong learning – opportunities for learning informally from those with experience

All those who had returned to work after having experienced, personally or vicariously, feeding a baby were asked: 'Were you given an opportunity to talk about your own experience?' A majority answered this question negatively:

> There was no opportunity given to consider this experience; it seems to be somewhat 'left in our family circle' and not discussed outside of that.
>
> (GP)

A further question was asked: 'Were you able to offer any insights to those who had not had such experience in a training context?' Responses were predominantly negative or appeared limited by barriers:

> No – you didn't push your experience on others.
>
> (community midwife)

> You were asked by the midwives to talk to mothers but no opportunity was offered to speak to fellow-workers.
>
> (GP)

Some reported sharing of experience after the birth of a baby, unofficially, or in particular, restricted forums.

> Informally . . . there was a delivery room for women with infectious diseases and midwives could talk about breastfeeding.
>
> (sister in paediatric ward)

> Only to those who would listen.
>
> (midwife)

> you felt it was inappropriate as you were in a new job when the baby was one and a half years old. You certainly don't talk about breastfeeding under those circumstances, because there is a stigma about feeding your baby at that age. You feel now that you would do so, but not mentioning being a mother is an issue in the workplace.
>
> (health promotion specialist)

These responses suggest a two-way cordon sanitaire around breastfeeding stories. One side protects those working with mothers and the mothers themselves while the other puts cultural embargoes on discussing breastfeeding, a bodily function. These barriers may have been part of the disintegration between different understandings of breastfeeding, as illustrated below.

Evidence for a split between theoretical and embodied or cultural understandings – the example of feasibility

An example of disintegration between official understanding and personal understandings is offered here. It was clear that almost all respondents in the study had a theoretical understanding of the almost universal feasibility of physiological breastfeeding, with the majority of practitioners answering the question below in a similar way: 'About what proportion of women do you feel can breastfeed?'

All women except with very retracted nipples, but you are informed that even these women can.

(GP)

Pretty well all women – the difficulty is our culture.

(special care midwife)

The majority offered percentages between 95 and 99 per cent. Only two respondents working with women gave lower answers ('75 per cent' and 'about 60 per cent').

In answer to another question – 'Are there any special things mothers have to do to be able to breastfeed?' – a minority offered a few conditions. Several placed emphasis on motivation and/or support:

No – just to have determined to do it and ask for support.

(health visitor)

A series of conditionalities emerged when considering breastfeeding as a real possibility. Some respondents explicitly recalled information given during training, some of which was perhaps now identified as incorrect:

Training suggested preparation, of the nipples, breasts, with breast shells. You were also told they must eat a lot with lots of protein and rest a great deal.

(health visitor)

Most answered for their own current understandings, revealing uncertainty about the effect of diet, tiredness or stress from older models of care and cultural beliefs.

Your understanding is that stress will hinder breastfeeding.

(complementary therapist)

if a mother is worn out her milk supply will not be as good.

(community paediatrician)

Another group of respondents explicitly juxtaposed these cultural condition-alities with a biomedical understanding of the demand and supply nature of milk production, engaging in a dialogue between different sets of beliefs:

Eat and drink regularly. Be healthy – they need calcium and lots of water. A balanced diet – and carbohydrate snacks – not too much caffeine. However this is to breastfeed effectively. Women in the third world breastfeed with no immediate problems.

(midwife)

You assume that the production of milk is based on mental well being. Being upset influences milk production.

> (health promotion specialist, trained as paediatric nurse)

The conditionalities put on breastfeeding here are reflective of cultural belief in the vulnerability of breast-milk supply, common in the UK. In practice they may lead women to feel powerless about subjective perceptions of low milk supply. No one mentioned specifically the idea of feeding when the baby asked for it and only one respondent mentioned attachment:

> Just to be helped to latch on.
>
> (recently trained midwife)

These inconsistencies between theory and personal/cultural understandings may perhaps illustrate not only education shortfalls but the result of leaving anecdotes unexplored.

Possible rationales for the denial of personal experience in learning and practice settings

Most explicit rationales for not sharing anecdotal or cultural experiences focused on the fear that incorrect advice could spread to mothers from those not purged, by good evidence, of unreliable secular learning. There was concern about the outside world contaminating the professional and thence infecting the cultural realm with the authenticity of professional endorsement.

> Midwives too are women, and may come from a bottle-feeding culture and their mothers did not breastfeed and they bring their own agenda and it shows in remarks like 'One bottle doesn't matter'.
>
> (midwife involved in the development of a post-registration course about breastfeeding)

Concerns about the authenticity of knowledge

Some initial open-ended interviews with managers and educators as well as practitioners showed the prioritisation of research-based knowledge. There was suspicion of embodied learning as potentially inaccurate. The response was to reduce the exposure of practitioners to its influence, stressing correct information needed for treatment.

'What do you feel are the really important issues which need to be looked at in the training of health professionals in relation to breastfeeding?'

> Current knowledge (not assumptions) . . .
>
> (midwifery lecturer)

There is a need to solve the possibility of people relying on their own experience or cultural myths.

(manager)

Your own aims are for people to have better theoretical knowledge based on research for example about fore and hind-milk and baby-led feeding and the prevention of sore nipples.

(midwife involved in development of post-registration course)

- origin of information – must be research-based, true and accurate, stopping the perpetuation of misinformation
- needs to be linked with research and to be updated
- trainers need to be both sure of content and also the psychosocial context for breastfeeding so that un-evidenced areas such as how women react to breastfeeding can be taught with understanding.

(university professor)

An implicit suggestion from the data was that personal and cultural knowledge might be erased or pre-empted by evidence-based understanding.

It is important to get to midwives early before they learn it wrong and hear anecdotal tales.

(special care midwife)

There is a responsibility not to project one's own experience or even pre-registration understanding.

(supervisor of midwives)

Fears may include the giving of un-evidenced practice advice because a treatment worked for the individual. There may also be concern that breastfeeding is seen as difficult because it was so for the helper.

Conversely there were worries about denying the difficulties of breastfeeding. The data revealed some fears of input into education or practice by those with 'an evangelical approach to breastfeeding'. One respondent's reply suggests that knowledgeable supporters were risky providers of knowledge for mothers:

You have had some exposure to the La Lèche League and find them 'a bit over the top' and feel they can be off-putting to normal women. They may know a lot but you feel they are too fanatical, for example about not giving a supplementary bottle when the alternative might be the end of breastfeeding.

(GP)

Fears of being seen, by reporting an uncomplicated (or even enjoyable) experience, to be insensitive may inhibit discussion among professionals. The result is that those who had managed their own breastfeeding successfully or who enjoyed the experience were likely to be silenced, reflecting a fear of passing on seemingly impossible expectations into the clinical setting.

Is the evidence for concern about informal learning justified?

Concerns about the feasibility of breastfeeding appear generally problematic for health professionals as mothers. Researchers found that a sample of Northern Irish midwives, initiating breastfeeding at a higher level than other women, ended feeding for similar reasons, including the perception of not having enough milk (McMulkin and Malone 1993). Battersby too found that being midwives did not prevent similar fears or problems to non-midwife mothers who breastfed, with few experiencing no problems at all (Battersby 1999).

Research has suggested that personal experience does affect practice and advice. Knowledge has been reported as best among health professionals who have breastfed themselves (Freed *et al.* 1996; Bleakney and McErlain 1996). Recent research with Australian midwives found that those who had breastfed for three months or longer were generally more knowledgeable than others (Cantrill *et al.* 2003). These findings suggest that, insofar as the findings from the studies are typical, ways to enable the sharing of experiences of those who have successful breastfeeding experience might be worth exploring among health professionals.

Little is known about the impact of negative personal breastfeeding experiences. Billingsley found from a small-scale study of midwives in training that some practice recommendations relating to personal experience remained after training (Billingsley 1991). Midwives who had bottle fed their own babies, for example, were more likely to suggest that mothers might change to bottle feeding if they encountered problems. It is known that attitudes are more difficult to change than knowledge (e.g. Bleakney and McErlain 1996). It is not known whether discouraging the sharing of personal experience during training and lifelong learning would be helpful or unhelpful where experiences were negative. Examples were not directly sought in the study. A paediatrician was reported by a mother to have responded to the giving of cups of formula by saying that it was 'ok to bottle feed if she wanted to do it . . . was good to breastfeed but that she did not and she was bottle fed herself and she was all right'.

Further explanations for boundaries

Maher sees breastfeeding rules as a way of 'inscribing' rules on women's bodies, in relation to wider issues, 'symbolic values and the structuring of social relationships' (Maher 1992: 165). The silencing of discussion about embodied breastfeeding experience could be read as a way of constructing rules about the behaviour of health professionals, for example at the liminal period of transition into professional status or at the return to it. Breastfeeding and working certainly did not sit easily together.

> A midwife just back at work has no right to breastfeed – she has to use their pump.
>
> (midwife)

> . . . there had been phone calls from distressed members of staff who had identified lack . . . 'in-house' support for midwives' breastfeeding, when returning to work, with poor facilities, attitudes and working practices and some colleagues making them feel uncomfortable expressing.
>
> (reunion of staff who had attended a post-registration lactation course)

It is possible that even talking about breastfeeding would breach a barrier between the professional and an emotional or embodied mother/not-mother. Those trained about breastfeeding may perhaps be seen as in need of socialisation into this understanding from the beginning, discouraging the leaking out of personal accounts into the training setting, with its possible vulnerabilities. This was not made explicit in the data, but the splitting of mother–midwife was occasionally mentioned, as here:

> [you] knew 'mother nature would take care of it' (for you the mother, not for you the midwife) and that, 'as a real person', nature would have it in hand.
>
> (midwife involved in development of post-registration course)

More speculatively it could be that helpers did not wish to be identified as gendered. Rodgers, in her study of a breastfeeding member of the House of Commons, suggests that a woman who is visibly pregnant or known to be breastfeeding is at her most explicitly female, engendering perhaps a fear of being revealed by association also as a woman out of place (Rodgers 1981).

Interpersonal and power issues

'Certainly caveats need to be made about the therapeutic use of self and the possibility is raised that distancing, although out of professional favour at least in nursing, may have its uses' (Meerabeau 1999). Keeping one's own story out of the picture can be respectful of the needs of the mother. It is also a way to maintain power differentials. Research into professional development for those involved in birth found that women wanted to hear of professionals' experience (McFarlane and Downe 1999). The right to ask questions or deny answers signifies dominance in any conversation. There may be a perceived need during training of those who will work with women to ensure there is distinction between a health professional, who speaks of policy and research, and a mother, who might deviate into the personal.

Marchant suggests that motivations for not exploring the subjective may be less therapeutically directed, questioning whether midwives are 'also collaborating with the general devaluation and marginalisation of women's health by society' when ignoring subjective explorations, becoming dominated by the 'male and medical view' (2004: 325).

Silence also disguises the fact that not all midwives have had personal experience of breastfeeding. Midwives' bodies may be in this way more identical and less idiosyncratic – uniform(ed) and in a shift system, replicable.

Alternative models of preparation

An awareness of a need to integrate personal experience was suggested occasionally, usually from outside health professions.

> Social work relies on women who have had children to use their own experience. But there is no debriefing so no recognition of how this influences other people. For instance if a woman had a negative experience of breastfeeding she won't be helpful to her clients.
>
> (social worker)

> You feel that so long as feelings are worked through in relation to any issue, including infant feeding, experience can be a strength and your staff do talk about their experiences.
>
> (women's health charity worker)

Some volunteer breastfeeding supporters are required to undertake 'rigorous reviews of (their) own feelings and assumptions' (Palmer 1993: 152). In a model of 'deep personal learning' prior learning needs to be integrated with physiology to make sense of the experience under consideration (Miller *et al.* 1994). Ongoing research in the area of breastfeeding support suggests it is important health professionals be given opportunities to review their own feeding experiences (Battersby 2002). Supervision, in a non-managerial model, additionally offers some supporters the chance to examine their own reactions, acknowledging that there may be 'leaking' from life events. Reviewing the differences between clinical and everyday situations is seen as useful, for example, for nurses in the area of sexual therapy (Meerabeau 1999).

The few people allowed this opportunity added spontaneous comments about the usefulness of this process:

> Lots of time given to debriefing own experience – 'imperative' – throughout.
>
> (voluntary supporter)

You were invited to share experiences and this was useful.

(recently trained health care assistant)

Possible advantages of sharing stories

- Identifying the results of supportive and non-supportive interventions in real life outcomes.
- Hearing others' attitudes, experiences and meanings in a safe group to broaden understanding.
- Practising communication skills, especially listening, with real situations.
- Being heard enough to avoid taking stories into the helping relationship – ready to focus on the mother rather than 'dumping' material on her.
- Understanding the origin of attitudes and choice of interventions so as to avoid replication of personal ways to 'fix' another person's concern.
- Increasing self-awareness necessary for working with others.

Hunter argues that midwives 'need fluency in the language of emotions, so that [they] can articulate feelings. Developing awareness of [their] own feelings should increase [their] insights into the feelings of others, thus enhancing the quality of [their] relationships with clients and colleagues' (Hunter 2004: 606). One of the results of earlier marginalisation of personal feelings, she argues, is to extend this to mothers and so render them invisible or peripheral.

A midwife who was also training as a voluntary supporter has examined the value of 'being allowed to consider who I am, how I breastfed my children, in an environment that was unsupportive to my choice'. She contrasted this process with the more objective expectations of her midwifery training, which was mainly clinically oriented. Professional training, by disregarding her previous experience, meant, 'I was expected to support breast-feeding mothers holistically whereas I had not had the opportunity professionally to reflect on my own breastfeeding experience.'

She explained that:

> 'I feel' was an alien phrase in my midwifery training. We were rather like observers in a cocoon who did not take part in what was happening around us – that's for the patient/client! I . . . presume that this approach was used to keep the patient/client relationship safe and not too personal.

She wished 'everyone supporting breastfeeding women professionally could go through a similar training' (Trewick and Smale 2003).

Conditions for considering experience

Lewis and Bradley have argued that health professionals could benefit from multi-disciplinary facilitated sessions about breastfeeding, as for infant death. They noted the complex feelings around how individuals were fed, concerns about diminishing women and suggest that a contented mother with her satisfied baby can provoke desires to be nurtured (1992).

The responses in the study suggested that any space for discussion needed to be safe. Repeated opportunities to integrate personal and cultural learning into other forms of education may be welcomed if offered by someone informed but outside health service or higher education hierarchies.

Research questions

The study looked at a wide sample of practitioners, with varying working histories. It was not easy to identify with any certainty how attitudes may be shifting from the need to contain contamination by personal accounts. If concern about breastfeeding talk remains as a way of socialising health professionals into learning to censor experiences, there is a need to know whether and how this works, why it might be seen as useful and whether it might do damage.

Other possible areas for enquiry include:

- The purposes served for the institution, the worker, and for mothers by discouraging anecdotal sharing.
- Lessons for women from containment of health professionals' experiences – about the acceptability of breastfeeding in wider society, including its status and links with sexuality.
- How silencing may create barriers behind which experience is unexamined, ready to be used inappropriately.
- Evidence about mothers' needs for and uses of knowledge of supporters' experiences.

Conclusion

The study indicated that pressure to ignore embodied feeding experiences had been common at key points. Increasingly peer supporters and midwifery assistants are involved in breastfeeding support. Identifying what kind of self-disclosure is useful and what is not could contribute to all training for support. It could be especially helpful to identify how the sharing of experience could be enabled safely as health professionals return to work after feeding experiences. One respondent was very clear:

> Because of . . . training it was possible to debrief and leave it at home.
> (voluntary breastfeeding supporter, during interview as a midwife)

Armstrong, training health professionals all over the world in UNICEF courses, found that at least three days were necessary to allow for resistance to practice changes due to a natural opposition to change to be overcome and for personal breastfeeding experience to be worked through before the new ideas and planning for change could begin (Armstrong 1990). One response to the fear of contamination of facts is to allow talk about research-based information only, ignoring embodied experience with its messy emotions. One problem is that by attempting to leave personal experiences in separate containment, however, they are in danger of leaking out, as reported here:

> I have to say it's best because it's Trust policy.
>
> (postnatal mothers' group)

Dr Elisabet Helsing (1975), a major contributor to the resurgence of breast-feeding in Norway, describes how midwives read books by volunteers, thus increasing their problem-based information about breastfeeding and success in feeding which they then passed on to mothers. The removal of barriers to a similar integration of embodied experience may have much to offer.

References

Apple, R. (1987) *Mothers and Medicine: A Social History of Infant Feeding*. Madison: University of Wisconsin Press.

Armstrong, H. (1990) 'Breastfeeding promotion: training of mid-level and outreach workers'. *International Journal of Gynecology and Obstetrics* 31(suppl 1): 91–103.

Battersby, S. (1999) 'Midwives' experiences of breastfeeding: can the attitudes developed affect how midwives support and promote breastfeeding?' *Book of Proceedings. 25th Triennial Congress of the International Confederation of Midwives*. Manila, Philippines, pp. 53–57.

Battersby, S. (2002) 'Midwives' embodied knowledge of breastfeeding'. *MIDIRS Midwifery Digest* 12(4): 523–526.

Billingsley, J. (1991) 'Midwives and breastfeeding – a health education challenge'. Dissertation submitted in part fulfilment of the requirements for the degree of Master of Arts in the University of Kent at Canterbury.

Bleakney, G.M. and McErlain, S. (1996) 'Infant feeding guidelines: an evaluation of the effect on health professionals' knowledge and attitudes'. *Journal of Human Nutrition and Dietetics* 9: 437–450.

Cantrill, R.M, Creedy, D.K. and Cooke, M. (2003) 'An Australian study of midwives' breast-feeding knowledge'. *Midwifery* 19: 310–317.

Curtis, P., Stapleton, H., Kirkham, M. and Smale, M. (2001) *Evaluation of the Doncaster Breastfriends 2000 Initiative*. Report to the Department of Health.

Douglas, M. (1975) *Implicit Meanings*. London: Routledge & Kegan Paul.

Freed, G.L., Clark, S.J., Harris, B.G. and Lowdermilk, D.L. (1996) 'Methods and outcomes of breastfeeding instruction for nursing students'. *Journal of Human Lactation* 12: 105–110.

Helsing, E. (1975) 'Women's liberation and breast-feeding'. *Journal of Tropical Paediatrics and Environmental Child Health* 21(5): 290–292.

Hunter, B. (2004) 'The importance of emotional intelligence'. *British Journal of Midwifery* 12(10): 604–605.

Lewis, E. and Bradley, E. (1992) 'Health service support of breastfeeding' (letter). *British Medical Journal* 305: 523.

McFarlane, S. and Downe, S. (1999) *The Southern Derbyshire Training and Education Project: Continuing Professional Development in the Maternity Services.* South Derbyshire Acute Hospitals NHS Trust.

McMulkin, S. and Malone, R. (1993) 'Midwives' personal experience of breast-feeding'. Paper presented at the International Congress of Midwives, Vancouver, Canada, May.

Maher, V. (ed.) (1992) *The Anthropology of Breastfeeding: Natural Law or Social Construct.* Oxford: Berg.

Marchant, S (2004) 'A woman's place – mothering and motherhood'. *MIDIRS Midwifery Digest* 14(3): 322–326.

Meerabeau, L. (1999) 'The management of embarrassment and sexuality in health care'. *Journal of Advanced Nursing* 29(6): 1507–1513.

Miller, C., Tomlinson, A. and Jones, M. (1994) *Researching Professional Education: Learning Styles and Facilitating Reflection.* London: English Nursing Board.

Palmer, G. (1993) 'Who helps health professionals with breastfeeding?' *Midwives Chronicle*, May.

Renfrew, M.J. (2004) 'Summary of the evidence'. *MIDIRS Supplement*, from joint NCT and Sure Start Conference, 30 March, 'Making breastfeeding a reality: sharing good practice and strategies that work'.

Rodgers, S. (1981) 'Women's space in a men's house'. In S. Ardener (ed.) *Women and Space: Ground Rules and Social Maps.* London: Croom Helm.

Smale, M., Renfrew, M.J., Marshall, J. and Spiby, H. (2006) 'Turning policy into practice: more difficult than it seems. The case of breastfeeding education'. *Maternal and Child Nutrition* 2(2): 103–113.

Trewick, A. and Smale, M. (2003) 'Making explicit previous cultural and personal learning about infant feeding during the training of those supporting breastfeeding mothers: "Like breaking down a jigsaw and putting it back together again"'. Paper given at University of Technology, Sydney, February.

Section 3

The dais

Section 3

The data

11 Understanding '*narak*': rethinking pollution

An interpretation of data from dais in north India

Janet Chawla

The MATRIKA research project

MATRIKA (Motherhood and Traditional Resources, Information, Knowledge, and Action) was a three-year participatory action research project in collaboration with four local NGOs during the years 1998–2001. MATRIKA is named after a group of female figures, usually either seven or eight, depicted in sculpture and myth as collective and semi-divine beings – and associated with mothering. The MATRIKA images include voluptuous beauties – one with an infant, theriomorphic (human body with animal head) figures and a wizened crone (for more detail see Panikkar 1997).

We drew up collaboration agreements with Action India (working in the slums of Delhi), Mahila Jagriti Kendra (South Bihar), Voluntary Health Association of Punjab (Fategarh District) and URMUL (Rajasthan) – in order to generate material that would be of use to the NGO as well as our own interests. The NGOs then called together dais who were considered by local women to be experienced and knowledgeable, for a series of three workshops. In these workshops we posed the question 'what does a woman need during pregnancy, birth and postpartum?'

Our initial methodology was derived from counselling – usually practised in a one-to-one setting – which we transposed to our workshops. 'Active listening', when practised by the interviewer or facilitator, allows the person (or group) to speak in a non-directed manner – with topics emerging from the informant/s rather than using a questionnaire with a specific agenda. Active listening also involves feeding back what has been understood by the researchers in order to allow the group/person to go deeper into the subject or refine or correct misunderstandings. Secondly, positive reinforcement involves recognising and appreciating behaviour which seems to the listener to have contributed to the speaker's own well being or the well being of those around her, particularly if gender or caste bias is involved. For example, if the family were biased towards the male children then protecting or taking care of a girl infant or child would be actively appreciated.

The attitudes of our team were crucial to the success of the research work. We consciously cultivated a team ethos in which we:

- were open to religio-cultural ways of thinking and doing 'health'
- assumed that poor, illiterate, low caste women could be skilled birth practitioners (for supporting data see Singh 2006)
- used our capacities for empathy and imagination to enter another world with different ways of knowing about the female body
- believed that birth is a normal and natural process
- understood that poverty compromises women's health apart from pregnancy and birth (for information and analysis see Murphy-Lawless 2003)

We realised that often dais have been made scapegoats for maternal mortality and morbidity and blamed for the effects of other macro-level processes. MATRIKA's workshop methodology reversed the common traditional birth assistant training model. We asked groups of dais to 'train us' by seeking to understand what they thought about and did to meet women's needs during parturition.

Our activities included role-plays, ritual drawings, body mapping, singing of birth songs, sharing of birth experiences (ours and theirs) as well as dais' life narratives. Group discussions, interpreting role-plays and other data, were at the heart of our activities. The lower-level NGO health workers were invaluable in helping us to understand the material we were receiving. Mostly drawn from local communities themselves, they, when given permission from those with 'authority', would explain and elaborate on the 'data'. We were able to access, and remain with, this alien (to us) information because we did not limit ourselves by separating data into mutually exclusive categories of 'medicine' and 'religion'. Rather we were receptive to diverse ways of facilitating birth, diagnosing and healing – to ritual enactments, notions of deities and demons, *bhut-pret* (ghosts and spirits) and the *nazar* or evil eye. We attempted to let the data speak the categories rather than the categories shape the data.

MATRIKA findings

At first, of course, dais seemed to want to impress us with their knowledge of the modern, biomedical approach. They spoke of the need for using a clean blade, taking the woman to the hospital if there were problems (when often there were no doctors or hospitals in the area). But as our sincere desire to learn and not 'teach' or criticise became apparent – and especially after our own enactments of the loneliness and confusion of a woman labouring alone in a hospital – they began to trust us and share what they really believed and practised. Ours was a collective effort: a group of researcher-activists interacting with a group of dais. We ate, slept, talked, sang and danced, produced drawings and plays together. Our workshop activities were a celebration of dais' cultural handling of childbirth. We were sometimes told that no one had ever called them together to share and enjoy like this.

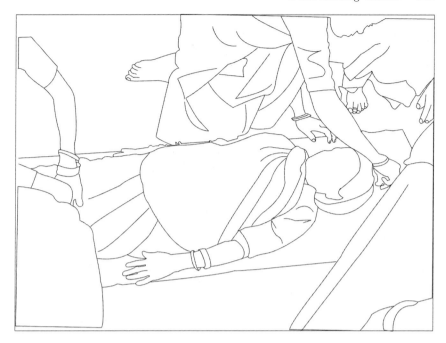

Figure 11.1

During body mapping sessions we would outline a woman's body (see Figure 11.1) and then generate terms, often terms of abuse, for parts of women's bodies. I repeatedly emphasised to our team that we were not generating the equivalent of a biomedical anatomy chart – but rather we were 'catching' women's stories, their words about and experiences with the body.

Motifs from rituals and ritual drawings emerged from Rajasthani dais when they were provided with felt pens and large swaths of paper (see Figure 11.2). Note the *swastika*, or *satiyas*, in the lower left-hand corner – a symbol connoting fertility and auspiciousness. Also the *sari* blouse hung on a tree in the seventh month – the spirit who lives there is evoked to protect the pregnant woman.

Our key research innovations included:

- No distinction made between the categories of 'religion' and 'medicine'.
- Returning to informants with our interpretive role-plays, drawings, posters – for clarification and correction.

A MATRIKA team member drew the poster of *Bemata* who dwells in *narak*, underground, a visual version of 'active listening' (see Figure 11.3). *Bemata* grows both babies in mothers' wombs and plants from the earth. Thus the postpartum 'bad' blood is shown here returning to the earth, completing the cycle. And in fact we have heard of families in Delhi slums who put sand

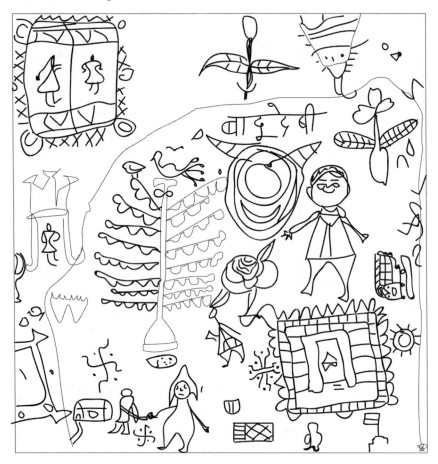

Figure 11.2

from the Jamuna River under the *charpoy* (woven rope cot) to absorb post-birth fluids. This drawing was shown to dais to make sure we had 'got it right'. Notice the 'three worlds' (*triloka*) of heaven (sky), mundane life (earthly plane) and *narak* (underground). In this way we were allowing categories like *narak* to emerge from the data, not producing data to fit into our own researchers' categories (for elaboration on *Bemata* and *narak* see Chawla 2003).

Narak quotes

The following quotes from our workshop transcripts present meanings of *narak*. The first series of quotes from Bihar speak explicitly, using the word '*narak*'. In other areas the meanings are more implicit in the practices and the 'dirtiness' associated with times of female fertility.

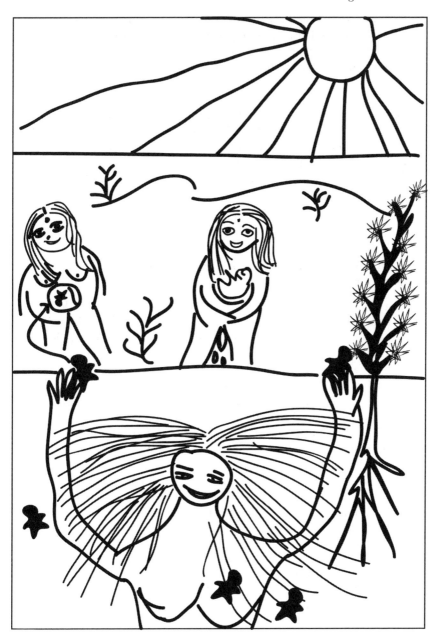

Figure 11.3

Girls are considered holy before puberty. The marriage of a young girl, who has not had her periods, is performed with her sitting on her father's lap. After puberty the woman is considered unclean, and is unholy, because she bleeds, and this is *narak*.

(Bihar)

On *Chhati* day the *narak* period ends. The *dai* checks if the umbilical cord has fallen off. Then she bathes the baby and beats a *thaali* (plate). After this the woman is bathed and wears new clothes. The *dai* cleans the room where the delivery took place and the woman was kept separately for six days. The dirty clothes of mother and child are washed. After this the *dai* is given soap and oil for bathing. All this is on the sixth day after delivery.

(Bihar)

The conflation of the female body and the earth – reclaiming *narak*

It is very tempting for us modern women to stand outside of ideas of the 'dirty' female body and critique them as archaic and misogynistic. Having listened carefully to dais' voices, and paid attention to Indian, indeed subcontinental, representation systems for almost thirty years I am now adamantly against doing so.

Although often translated as hellish or demonic place, *narak* can be understood as the site or energy of the unseen inner world – of the earth and of the body, particularly the fertile and bleeding female body. *Narak* has the connotation 'filth' but also signifies the fertility or fruitful potential of the earth and woman. So-called 'pollution taboos' are related to *narak* – where the idea of the sacred is radically separated from the reproductive potential of the female body. During menstruation and post-birth women are 'unclean'. However the dai speaks with a very different voice from the pundit about this uncleanness, this *narak*. To her the placenta, the ultimate polluting substance in the *shastra* literature, is spoken of reverently. It is no coincidence that dais are mainly from low and outcaste communities. Both caste and gender are involved in concepts of *narak*.

Despite the pejorative connotations of the word *narak*, the concept has allowed for abiding female spaces and birth cultures. In the 'male' or 'dominant' view these female times are 'filthy' or polluted, but they are also times when masculine, social and even familial demands on women are suspended. And traditionally older women guarded these spaces from any incursions – perhaps with the help of 'demons' and nether forces!? Within this imagistic representation, the nature of female bodily energy is understood as 'out of control' – women are presumed to be more emotional and have special physical needs at this time – so the usual social constraints are suspended. Of course we need to interrogate the priestly voice and de-sacralisation of menstruation and birth – but we should not throw out the baby with the bathwater. We should not ignore the traditional birth knowledge of India.

Conversely the fertility of land and woman is acknowledged and honoured. Both are 'fruitful' and this is not simply a symbolic device. Within indigenous medical traditions such as Ayurveda, and with the dais, a totally different ontological system is at work. Woman is not a 'symbol' of the earth. Nor is the earth a 'symbol' of woman. Rather they both partake of the same nature of fecundity. Just as the wind outside my window partakes of the same essence as the breath which flows in and out of my lungs.

During *narak* time, what is usually closed, the womb, is open, raw, vulnerable and bleeding. *Narak* allows for the imaging of the unseen – and the use of other senses, besides the visual, as well as the human capacities of empathy and imagination in diagnostics and therapeutics. And in fact *narak* is deeply implicated in the handling of postpartum care.

Postpartum care

> After delivery a woman is not given any grain or heavy food. This is called *narak* fasting. Grain is only given on the third day after all the dirty blood comes out. On first day, she eats biscuits with tea. She drinks warm water. Second day, heat-producing balls made out of ginger, pepper, turmeric, roasted rice, milk and jaggery (*saunth laddos*). On the third day, rice, dal and vegetables.
>
> (Bihar)

> It is called dirty blood because it has collected over nine months in the body. It is dark, smelly and clotted. It comes out first and then fresh clean blood comes out. With a little pressure and massage we take it out completely, and when the colour of the blood becomes clear like monthly cycle we believe that it is clean.
>
> (Punjab)

> *Gola* is baby's home. When the house becomes empty, only dirty blood is left. When this comes out there is pain. Hot drinks (of *ajwain*, *saunth*, *pipar* and *gur*) are given. This drink cleans the belly. After the baby is born, the *gola* roams around. This *gola* has taken care of the baby, now it must leave. If the pain is intense then warm fomentation is done and *gola* melts away (*pighal jata hai*). This is dirty blood and needs cleaning up.
>
> (Delhi)

Dais call the post-birth lochia 'bad blood' but they do not emphasise the pollution aspect of it. Rather the blood is 'bad' for the mother's health and needs to come out of the body. Both menstruation and postpartum bleeding are viewed as cleansing the body of 'toxins' and this view is congruent with naturopathic and other alternative and indigenous systems of medicine. My working hypothesis is that this blood is 'bad' because if it is retained it is bad for the woman's own health. Perhaps in the dominant world religions (Judeo-Christian-Islamic and Hinduism, or more correctly Brahminism) the concept of *narak* or 'hell' overlays previous meaning systems which had more to do with the health of women than the purity of priests.

Re-entering the social world and saying goodbye to *Bemata*

Women are ritually progressed from their status as 'unclean' differently and at different times within different religious traditions. Interestingly both the Leviticus text in the Old Testament of the Bible and the Dharamshastra writings – both of which concern themselves with ritual cleanliness in their respective traditions – specify a longer period of 'pollution' for a woman who has given birth to a female infant than a male infant. In the Indian context, birth is celebrated and the woman's 'confinement' gradually comes to an end.

> On the thirteenth day after birth, the new mother is allowed to enter the kitchen. (*Chauka Charhana*). Some do it on the seventh or eleventh day. Everybody celebrates. There is singing and dancing. On this day the new mother and the baby bathe and wear new clean clothes. She comes out to get everyone's blessing. Friends and relatives are invited and eat food together. The *dai* is given clothes, food and grain.
>
> (Punjab)

> On the day of the birth ritual celebration (*Chhatti* – sixth day) the woman wears everything that was taken off at the time of the birth. She puts on *bindi*, bangles, *henna* and nose ring. We make ritual drawings of swastika, worship *Bemata* and light a lamp. We make a foot impression of the mother on the floor and then the woman enters the main house. Till the fifth day *Bemata* roams around in the house. After the birth celebrations *Bemata* leaves, she goes to another house. The *dai* also goes to serve others.
>
> (Rajasthan)

To my knowledge there are no shrines, formal images, or textual references to *Bemata*. She is definitely a fleeting presence, invoked by women at the time of birth and sent off to another's home with postpartum ritual. According to the dais with whom we interacted, *Bemata* dwells in the realm of *narak*, deep within the earth. She is a Creatrix responsible for the conception, growth within the womb, and birth of human beings as well as the growth of all vegetation. In the image in Figure 11.4 *Bemata* was drawn on a charpoy leg along with the *swastika*, a common post-birth ritual drawing.

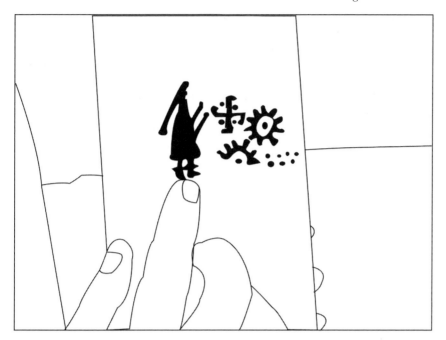

Figure 11.4

Contemporary relevance of *Bemata* and *narak*

Shakina, a Muslim dai working in a slum of Delhi, talked about birth time in a swirl of Hindu and Muslim references – a testimony to the syncretism of north Indian folk culture. And we found that Sikh, Christian and Muslim as well as 'Hindu' dais used the concepts and often the language of *narak* and *Bemata*.

> 'Look, sister, at the time of birth it's only the woman's *shakti*. She who gives birth, at that time, her one foot is in heaven and the other, in hell (*narak*).'

Shakina goes on to say:

> 'Before doing a delivery I get the woman to open all the trunks, doors and so on. I pray to the One above to open the knot quickly. I take of her *sari*, open her hair and take off any bangles or jewellery. I put the *atta* on a *thali* and ask the woman to divide it into two equal parts. Also I get Rs.1.25 in the name of *Sayyid* kept separately. But mostly I remember *Bemata*. Repeated I pray to *Bemata* "O mother! Please open the knot quickly."'

Invocations to Islamic and seemingly 'Hindu' figures (*Sayyid* and *Bemata*) accompany the 'sympathetic magic' of opening rituals. The untying of knots, opening of locks, doors and windows, loosening hair and removing bangles are common rites performed during labour throughout north India. This facilitation can be interpreted as an opening in the external word which is then mimicked or mirrored in the inner world of the maternal body. The manipulation of the external environment in this way serves as a permission and encouragement for the 'opening of the body'. The separation of the *atta* from one mound into two also imitates imaginatively the separation of the pregnant maternal body into two – mother and baby. When I first encountered these birth facilitations I noticed the parallel in guided imagery used in cancer treatments, when the patient was encouraged to imagine the T-cells and the immune system dealing with tumours. If internal imagery was effective, why should not externally manifest imagery also work?

Narak allows for a holistic and non-invasive diagnostics and therapeutics – health-promoting practices which do not violate the integrity of the body and facilitate the '*jee*' or life force. This concept then provides a mode of understanding and therapeutics which can negotiate and affect the inner body without violating the integrity of the skin/body/life force. And indeed the dais' health modalities are sophisticated in terms of emotional support and ritual practice. Their hands-on techniques include practical utilising touch (massage, pressure, manipulation, assisted squat, external version); natural resources (mud, baths and fomentation, herbs, *gobar* or cow dung); and application of 'hot and cold' (in food and drink, fomentation, heating lacenta to revive baby, birthing body as 'heated', etc.); isolation and protection (from household work and maternal, familial and sexual obligations).

This interpretation of *narak* is congruent with some dais' usage of the terms 'opening body' (labour), 'open body' (birth), and 'closing body' (post-partum) – for the entire process of birth time. These empirical terms stand in opposition to the factory model of birth (labour, delivery, failure to progress and false labour) implicit in many obstetrical terms. And interestingly the womb-bond between mother and newborn continues to be respected during this time – *Narak ka Samay*.

Implications for improving midwifery/dai training

MATRIKA findings about '*narak*' have great relevance to public health initiatives targeted at dais. As MATRIKA data have demonstrated above, dais say: 'Bad blood must come out.' Dai trainers say: 'Haemorrhage must stop.' Without reference to dais' indigenous medical ideas and cultural meanings, dai trainers assume that dais are ignorant and superstitious – and training effectiveness is compromised. In the context of postpartum care *narak* relates to the 'bad blood' that dais think must exit the body. That energy of the maternal body associated with growing the baby is signified by

the 'black blood' – this fluid emerges, signifying not only the uterus contracting, but also that the mother's body is transiting from holding the 'other' to
releasing the other. Sometimes we heard that the 'contractions' were the
womb 'searching' for the baby. Dais' imaging speaks a poetics of the body
that attributes consciousness, activity and sensation to the uterus – which is
totally absent in the biomedical framework. The understanding and use of
these concepts in dai training would significantly improve communications
on controlling haemorrhage postpartum, as well as preserve the respect for
indigenous meaning systems.

Furthermore, the *Bemata* figure encodes a process orientation towards
birth and postpartum while providing a framework for diagnostics and
therapeutics. In obstetrical practice the examination done immediately
after birth, 'the Apgar score', is used to assess the well being of the newborn.
It is a scale for measuring the infant's process of adapting to extra-uterine
life. But no such formal, process-oriented assessment is geared towards the
bodily functioning of the mother postpartum, the time the dais call 'the
closing of the body'. *Bemata* seems to function as a diagnostic system assisting
dais in their role as caretakers of mothers, especially crucial in the six-day
post-birth period.

Valorising the mother–infant connection – literally

The practice of not cutting the cord until the placenta is delivered is
common in all the areas where MATRIKA conducted research. Doctors
and health workers throughout the country also report it as the common
practice. Dais have the utmost respect for these parts of the female body
usually considered as waste products (by the biomedical system) or highly
polluting (by the Dharamshastras). It seems as though dais consider the
infant–cord–placenta as a package. They have been together for nine
months, cord and placenta functioning to nurture the foetus – why should
they be severed so quickly?

Dais say: 'Cut the cord after placenta is delivered.'

> If the baby is not active or does not cry then the *dai* rubs the cord,
> placing a coin or rice grain underneath it. By rubbing, heat passes to the
> baby. The baby often revives. Heating the placenta on a fire may also
> do this resuscitation.
>
> (Bihar)

> After birth, if the baby does not cry or is hardly breathing, or even seems
> stillborn, the placenta is used by placing it on a heated surface – pan or
> cow dung cakes. Life flows towards the baby most of the time. It is only
> after she knows that this is not needed that the cord is cut.
>
> (Delhi)

If the baby, once born, is not active, the placenta may be heated to stimulate the baby and bring it to life.

(Rajasthan)

But trainers and health education messages throughout the subcontinent are teaching dais to cut the cord right away.

We modern, 'educated' women have come to believe that 'pollution' taboos are atavistic relics of a misogynistic and patriarchal past – and that they should be superseded by 'scientific' understandings of the female body based on fact rather than superstitions. Our MATRIKA data, gathered by crossing boundaries and listening carefully, and respectfully, suggest that dais' knowledge and practice are encoded in a language, a poetics of the body – which differs radically from that of biomedical obstetrics, and is more congruent with other Asian medical/health/healing systems such as Yoga, Ayurveda, Tantra, as well as Chinese, Tibetan and even Greek/Islamic medicine.

In order to facilitate communications in training indigenous midwives, as well as reclaim aspects of indigenous Indian midwifery for use with more privileged women, MATRIKA recommends the development of criteria for evaluation of dais and their practices drawing on Ayurveda and other indigenous systems of health maintenance and healing. Rather than using the evaluation perspective of biomedicine, indigenous tools of assessment will allow the incorporation of a human resource base which can complement existing 'reproductive health' facilities and practitioners.

An entire legacy of midwifery knowledge will be erased unless we begin to learn to think and speak the language of '*narak*' (and develop dai-training materials dialoguing with that language). Or at the very least we should not cringe in disdain when we hear or observe women using these languages, or observing these practices. Finally, in the Asian subcontinent it is essential that we begin to include skilled dais in maternal child health programmes at all levels. Hopefully we will all be able to cross boundaries, listen carefully and help the world to be born more humanely.

References

Chawla, J. (2003) 'Negotiating narak and writing destiny: the theology of dais' handling of birth'. In N. Chitgopekar (ed.) *Invoking Goddesses: Gender Politics in Indian Religion*. New Delhi: Har-Anand.

Murphy-Lawless, J. (2003) 'How will the world be born: the critical importance of indigenous midwifery'. *Royal College of Midwives' Midwifery Journal* 6(10).

Panikkar, S.K. (1997) *Sapta Matrika Worship and Sculptures*. Delhi: DK Printworld.

Singh, A. (2006) ' "Her one foot is in this world and one in the other": Ayurveda, dais and maternity'. In J. Chawla (ed.) *Birth and Birthgivers – The Power Behind the Sharme*. New Delhi: Har-Anand.

12 Listening to dais speak about their work in Gujarat, India

Subadhra Rai

Women have always been healers. They were the unlicensed doctors and anatomists of western history. They were abortionists, nurses and counsellors. They were the pharmacists, cultivating healing herbs and exchanging the secrets of their uses. They were midwives, travelling from home to home and village to village. For centuries women were doctors without degrees, barred from books and lectures, learning from each other, and passing on experience from neighbour to neighbour and mother to daughter. They were called the 'wise women' by the people, witches or charlatans by the authorities. Medicine is part of our heritage as women, our history, our birthright (Ehrenreich and English 1973: 3).

Introduction

Polluting, *contaminating*, and *dirty* are common descriptors that identify dais' (indigenous midwives of India) work. Body fluids (amniotic fluid, blood, and vaginal discharges) are considered to be polluting and contaminating. Linked with *dirty* is the concept of *caste*. Dais are usually from the lower caste and considered to be polluting and therefore suitable for delivery work. Although the descriptors (often perceived to be imposed from outside) appear to lower the value of dais' work and degrade their image, my research shows that dais themselves promote these descriptors, but for entirely different reasons (Rai 2003). Dais use terms such as *charity*, *poonya ka kaam* (good work), and *dharm* (duty) to describe their work in the same breath that they use *dirty* and *polluting*, thus promoting the notion that despite the social and economic devaluations, they are willing to provide services to those who are in need. Within this context, their work becomes an act of selfless duty. The underlying message of selflessness is that money is not the prime motivator for delivery work. Dais have skilfully built their reputation to show that in spite of the social markers that relegate them to the bottom, they continue to do this work because of their concern for the poor. Another important factor is how 'dirty' work and pollution have enabled dais to apply some form of boundary around their authoritative knowledge. Describing their work as *dirty* allows dais to maintain a certain economic monopoly and power and create social reciprocity upon which they can call when needed.

Setting the context for women's work and health

In 'developing' nations, ensuring safe motherhood is the highest priority. Each year 600,000 women around the world die of complications related to pregnancy; less than 1 per cent of these deaths occur in the 'developed' countries (World Health Organization (WHO) 1998a, 2004). The direct causes of maternal mortality are infection, obstructed labour, hypertension, haemorrhage, and unsafe abortion (WHO 1998a, 2004). The indirect causes include poverty and inaccessible health facilities (WHO 1998b, 2000, 2004). In India alone about 125,000 women die each year from these pregnancy-related causes (United Nations Children's Fund (UNICEF) 1999). The majority of women who die are young, and often their deaths are preventable (UNICEF 1999). UNICEF noted that accurate data on India's maternal mortality are unavailable, and this in itself is a powerful commentary on the low priority placed on women's health. Statistics show that in India less than 25 per cent of deliveries occur in institutions, and in tribal areas about 10 to 15 per cent of women die on the way to hospital (UNICEF 1999).

In India dais conduct about 50 to 60 per cent of the deliveries (Swaminathan *et al.* 1986), whereas in Gujarat dais handle between 40 and 95 per cent (Chatterjee 1999; State Institute of Health and Family Welfare (SIHFW) 1999). The data illustrate dais' important contributions to the health care system, and, in particular, they show the extent of their workload. Furthermore, the data indicate that women have access to affordable and accessible labour and delivery services and other primary health care, an expressed goal of the joint WHO/UNICEF (WHO 1978) *Health for All* (HFA) Declaration. Interpreted another way, the statistics indicate that if dais were not present to meet the demand for delivery services, a vast majority of women would be without this maternity care. There is an increased realisation that despite the various health policies and implementations, the health care system has not met basic needs, especially for delivery services. Both the Government of India (GOI) and international agencies, however, continue to promote the framework of HFA because they perceive it as the most cost-effective (appropriate and accessible) agency to meet the health needs of the population.

Within this context, dais play a pivotal role in providing health care to women of urban and rural Gujarat. Previous studies conducted by WHO (Cabral *et al.* 1992a, 1992b, 1992c; Du Gas *et al.* 1979; Mangay-Maglacas and Pizurki 1981; Mangay-Maglacas and Simons 1979; United Nations Population Fund (UNFPA) 1996; Verderese and Turnbull 1975; Walt 1984; WHO 1982, 1995a, 1995b, 2004) and in India and Gujarat (SIHFW 1983, 1992, 1995, 1999; Swaminathan *et al.* 1986) have concentrated on the potential benefits to the healthy delivery of mother and child when indigenous midwives receive biomedical training. None focused on the effect of dais' work on their own health. In fact, discussions on indigenous midwives in India and elsewhere show that they themselves and those around them do not perceive midwives as formal workers, but rather as women assisting other women in the birthing process. Nevertheless, the low rate of institutional births in India indicates that dais play a key role in providing health care to women. Based on these observations, there are two reasons that this study on dais' work and health was critical and timely (Rai 2003).

The first is related to statistical proof that dais conduct a significant percentage of deliveries. Despite the evidence, dais are regarded as informal workers or helpers and not as part of the workforce. The second reason is to foster an understanding of the impact of doing work that is necessary but culturally unappealing: why do women work as dais, and what are the consequences of this type of work on their lives? If assistance during delivery is necessary to ensure that the birth process is uneventful, then it is important to understand why this work is undervalued both monetarily and socially. There appears to be a dissonance in perception between the actual contributions of dais and their status as workers, and the value of their work. In this chapter I explore the basis of this dissonance and attempt to provide some tentative answers to explain this dissonance with regard to the work of dais.

Women's work: a need for better valuation

Gaining an understanding of the parameters that define work (formal/informal, paid/unpaid) would profoundly affect the way that dais' work is evaluated economically. This is especially important in the current environment in which there is a move to institute UNFPA's 1994 *Reproductive and Child Health Programme* (RCH; GOI 1997) framework, which states that women's work plays a central role in their health. In view of this, both the Self-Employed Women's Association (SEWA),[1] a women's development organisation located in Gujarat, India, and the formulators of RCH have called for a broader definition of work. This call has important ramifications for the future development of dais' work. According to the *World Survey on the Role of Women in Development* (United Nations (UN) 1999), women are the ones who carry out the bulk of unpaid work, and in many countries female labour is still perceived as easily attainable and available when needed and dispensable when it is not. Thus how the Gujarat government evaluates and contextualises dais' work depends on (a) how it defines productive work, and (b) how it interprets the RCH framework in relation to work. The relevance of RCH to dais' work becomes apparent because the success of the framework is predicated on empowering women, providing them with choices through increased access to educational and health services, promoting skill development and employment, and removing barriers that impede women's access to stable income and work (GOI 1997).

The International Labour Organisation (ILO; 1996a) noted that women's contributions are underestimated because they do not have equal access to stable employment. This has led to the emergence of *ghost* work, also known as *invisible* work, in the domestic and informal sectors. The ILO predicted that if unpaid and invisible work by women were accurately accounted for, their levels of economic activity would increase by 10 to 20 per cent, and the GDP would increase by 25 to 30 per cent worldwide. Furthermore, the ILO found that in terms of work hours per week, the greatest gap between men and women is in Asia, where women work on average twelve to thirteen hours more than men. The ILO (1996b) noted that when the parameters of economic activity were broadened to cover the informal sector and non-market activities, the measured labour force activity of women in India rose from 13 per cent to 88 per cent. Informal work such as work in the home or subcontracted work is usually strenuous, is poorly paid, and offers few or no opportunities for training and reduced career advancements (Chandola 1995; ILO 1996b). Informal work usually parallels women's domestic roles and is devalued because of its feminised nature (Chandola 1995; ILO 1996a, 1996b; UN 1999). For all of these reasons, understanding dais' work beyond the statistical data, such as the percentage of deliveries conducted, is crucial. There needs to be a better understanding of the extent of their contributions and a more refined conceptualisation of informal work. Percentages hide the power relations that relegate dais to informal and marginal workers. A concerted effort is being made worldwide to monitor each country's human resource development because it has emerged as the most important variable in economic growth (UN 1999). The UN found that women significantly increased their participation in the labour force, entering informal employment under insecure and worsening economic conditions. Women worked longer and harder, both inside and outside their households; as a result, their welfare suffered because the increased burden of work exerted a heavy toll on their physical and mental health (UN 1999).

Why we work as dais: listening to dais speak

Myriad experiences, multiple perceptions – the profane intertwined with the sacred, and feelings of ambivalence linked with a sense of pride in doing good but dirty work. Dais' voices reveal all of these and much more. The multiple voices indicate that dais are a heterogeneous group who contribute varied work experiences and skills. Their heterogeneity gives them the freedom to interpret and reinterpret their work and identities within the strict social and health frameworks, and allows them to create multiple meanings and images that describe the body, delivery, and birth:

This is *God's work*.

(SAhd2)[2]

I am able to separate two lives, and therefore my soul is at peace.

(SAhd1)

Another dai expressed the following views about her work:

> How can I think this is good work? I do it out of necessity . . . for my stomach. I have no education, so there is no other work I can do. If I was educated like you *behn* [sister], then I too, would fly in a balloon and see America.

(SAhd6)

But the same dai also said:

> Because I am able to separate two lives from one and help the woman and her child, I am doing good work. My health is good because of this, and my family is blessed.

(SAhd6)

Others also expressed similar views:

> Dais' work is charity. I am saving somebody's soul, so my family is happy.

(NSAhd5)

> I like my Dai work compared to other work. I prefer Dai work because a Dai's work is a work of selfless duty. It is a reflection of my *dharm* [duty]. Whether you receive payment or not, it does not matter, so even when someone does not pay you, you do the delivery. So even if I don't get paid, at least I know her *atma* [soul] is satisfied, and she will praise and give me credit that I conducted the delivery well. Her *atma* blesses me when I do the delivery well, and the woman's family saves at least 500–1000 rupees. It does not matter if she [the woman] does not pay me. The government is bound to pay me 20 rupees for the delivery, and so I get the money from the government. At least the woman can use the money to buy *ghee* and her family can have enough for food to eat. And if she needs medicine, say for diarrhoea or for colic pain, then she does not have to go out. Otherwise, she has to pay 400–500 rupees for rickshaw fare and extra for medication or for transfusion or this and that. You can spend lakhs. But if you give her common medicines and she gets it at home, then she will be all right.

(SMeh7)

> For our stomachs. [Otherwise] who wants to put their hands in a dirty area? My husband cannot work because of weak knees, and he cannot

walk. My sons have left me, so my only source of income is from Dais' work.

(NSAhd6)

At the same time, their heterogeneity conveys a lack of unity among dais. For dais, their disunity remains a stumbling block because it hampers their ability to control outsiders' perceptions of their work. Multiple perceptions further indicate that there is no one unifying image that represents the dais or convey dais' interpretations of their work, which thus allows outsiders the freedom to attach labels that fit their own views about dais:

There are two groups of Dais: scavengers and birth attendants.

(SVAhd)[3]

Various images of dais have also led to outsiders' intervention in dais' work. This is exactly what has happened in India for the last fifty-two years (since 1957). Diverse dai training programmes initiated either by governments (state or central) or by nongovernmental organisations (NGOs) have been in place to train[4] dais so that they can provide women with safe delivery and birthing services. The overarching goal of all of these training sessions was to change dais' harmful practices:[5]

Dais' work is unscientific, and they must be taught to conduct deliveries in a systematic and scientific way.

(MO[Ad])

The intent was to replace their indigenous knowledge and practices. However, it is also important to ask whether dais could have taken advantage of this training to strengthen their position. In other words, was there a possibility that dais could subvert the effects of homogenisation of the biomedical training on their work, knowledge, and practice? More important, were the dais aware that they could carry out the subversion? It appears that they were unable to challenge the homogenisation, in part, because they did not perceive that they had the power to do so because they were (and continue to be) in the margins of the powerful biomedical system, which has the support of the government and international development organisations.[6]

Ideally, dais could have used the training process to organise and present a united front, because they were 'similar', and thus speak in one voice and situate themselves in a position of power to influence the wider decision-making mechanisms. But dais did not take advantage of this opportunity for a number of reasons, as noted above. It is interesting to note that the system that marginalises dais and relegates them as low-paid, informal workers could potentially provide them with an avenue to organise, strengthen, and be recognised as legitimate women health workers. But the authoritative knowledge of biomedicine continues to devalue dais' contributions and their indigenous learning and practice. The biomedical system seems to gain power through standardisation and mainstreaming knowledge within its own paradigm. Because dais do not fit biomedicine's perception of qualified health workers, dais (or traditional birth attendants (TBAs) as they are known in development and UN literature) are labelled 'non-skilled traditional birth attendants' (WHO 2004: 4)[7] or 'witches and charlatans' (Ehrenreich and English 1973: 3) or 'scavengers' (SVAhd). Proponents of skilled attendants want women to have 'effective, cross-culturally . . . holistic "women-centred care"' (WHO 2004: 3). Dais provide skilled, culturally appropriate, and women-centred care to women where there is none available, but they are not considered skilled attendants.

Despite the fact that their varied voices give the impression that they lack unity, in reality, dais' power is embedded within their multiple voices and perceptions. When they speak, their voices convey rich meanings and images that describe their work. Their multiple voices also create a framework that encompasses different individuals and defines their roles in relation to the birth mother and child, including the role of the woman within her family and in the community. Perhaps this is why dais did not take advantage of the opportunity to speak in one voice to strengthen their position. One voice could have restricted their use of different metaphors to describe their work and could have affected their authority to call upon reciprocal ties. The fluid indigenous system has enabled dais to learn and adapt from others and integrate that learning into their work. It is possible that dais understood this well and knew intuitively that rejecting the flexible indigenous system would mean rejecting their source of power. It is also conceivable that dais' lack of vigorous and sustained challenge against the continued efforts of the biomedical establishment, governments, and international aid agencies to replace their indigenous knowledge points towards a strategic action on their part to remain engaged with these entities. Thus, it appears that dais have subverted the power of homogenisation because they continue to speak of birth in multiple voices.

> Dais are able to do things that at times the health personnel are unable to do. There was a weak woman who needed a blood transfusion. The doctor said that she needed four pints of blood before the delivery could occur. During the night of Lord Krishna's birthday she began to experience labour pains at home, and at 6:00 a.m. she delivered a male child. I helped her, and then I applied an abdominal binder.
>
> (NSAhd13)

One SEWA dai related her experience:

> I am a member of SEWA, and apart from getting money from SEWA or blessings from people, there are no benefits from working as a dai. I have been subjected to untouchability. Some people say, 'Do not go

there, or here, or don't touch this or that, or don't touch the cloth' because I have handled the dirty things [placenta, cord, and amniotic fluid]. And for this I get Rs. 25, and so sometimes I feel sad, and so I say no to deliveries.

(SAhd8)

A SEWA dai noted that her community respects her because they need her:

I do not feel there are any benefits in Dais' work . . . When there is work [childbirth], people call me '*behn, behn*'; but after that no one calls me for many years.

(SAhd7)

But another dai observed:

We will receive blessings, because we have given peace to the woman.

(NSAhd13)

'But how can it be dirty when Vishnu lives in there?' The move to Sanskritise dirty work

A SEWA dai linked her polluting work with the Hindu deity, Vishnu:

As a Dai I am considered untouchable because I have to touch the dirt of nine months. But how can it be dirty when Vishnu lives in there? God [Vishnu] sits in there [the cord], so how can I say it is dirty? How can I be repulsed? I am not repulsed by it, and I am not dirty. The *Nag* [cobra, snake],[8] the nine-headed *Nag* when he fans his head [hood] is in there [the placenta]. I am narrating all these to you because you asked [me]. Otherwise, I would not discuss this.

(SMeh7)

In the previous section it was noted that dais' influence becomes apparent when we hear them speak. Where else can one find profane descriptions (*dirty, contaminating,* and *polluting*) combined with the sacred (Vishnu, *Nag, Atma, dharm,* and *poonya ka kaam*) in the same sentence and it still make complete sense? Linking both descriptions simultaneously convinces outsiders of the sacrifice that dais make for the greater good at the expense of their own well-being because they believe that they are doing their duty. The freedom and skill to create and recreate various images and metaphors that describe their work are apparent in dais' voices. So far, the negative images have prevailed because their work is often described from the viewpoint of biomedical workers and individuals of upper castes – groups who possess both formal and informal power. However, my research shows that dais, too, have promoted these negative images, but for entirely different reasons.

This has led to feelings of ambivalence: on the one hand, their work is necessary, and they are integral members of the health team; on the other hand, promoting negative images may be one strategy to create a boundary around their knowledge and work.

I also observed in the preceding section that dais' words hinder their ability to present a unified front to establish their authority. When this issue is examined closely, it is evident that dais' power lies within their cultural narratives and individualistic work approaches. SMeh7 may have used variations of metaphors (sacred and profane), but her narrative resonates with those of other dais because they are created within an established social, cultural, and religious framework. Seen in this way, it appears that dais are indeed speaking in one voice. The 'dirty' work perception provides dais with certain 'advantages'. They are able to establish boundaries that allow indigenous midwives such as SMeh7 to create parallelisms between polluted substances and sacred deities without fear or interference. It may also be that individuals (in the biomedical system or upper castes) do not perceive any threat to their social and economic standing from these comparisons.

Dais rely on the central tenet in South Asian socio-cultural and religious systems – that one must do one's duty – to explain the contradictions within their worldview about their work. Doing one's duty means fulfilling one's destiny, including performing particular work identified with one's caste no matter how unpleasant that task may be.[9] The *Bhagavad-Gita* is unambiguous on this:

> Know what your duty is and do it without hesitation.
>
> (Mitchell 2000: 51)

> The wise man lets go of all results, whether good or bad, and is focused on the action alone. Yoga is skill in action.
>
> (2000: 55)

> It is better to do your own duty badly, than to perfectly do another's; you are safe from harm when you do what you should be doing.
>
> (2000: 68)

The *Gita* is also clear on the ramifications of inaction. It states that 'not by avoiding actions does a man gain freedom from action' (Mitchell 2000: 62), which implies that performing one's duty (whether work or other responsibilities) is integral to one's well-being. Fulfilling one's duty is the beginning of the eventual release from the cycle of birth and rebirth and suffering. Carrying out the assigned tasks (no matter how unpleasant) contributes to the well-being of others and ensures a better birth for the individual in the next life. Thus in the South Asian context work is not merely a set of regulated actions but assumes spiritual connotations of *dharm* (duty, religion). There is a causal effect of work that goes beyond the present consciousness because the present is linked to the past and to the future. Understanding the spiritual context of action/work may provide some understanding of why dais do dirty work and at the same time have the desire to elevate their work and take pride in it.

Dais' attempt to spiritualise their work may have a more practical basis. Because most of their work and knowledge are oral-based, spirituality could provide a way for dais to reclaim their indigenous body of knowledge, one that is increasingly being eroded as a result of the government's sustained efforts to either phase dais out or 'convert' them into low-skilled biomedical health workers. Economics could be another reason to align with the sacred because it provides a layer of respectability and could lead to a better economic return. Whether dais acknowledge this or not, the amount of remuneration appears to be central to their grievances. The kind of payment and the amount reflect the level of power, control, and authority of their work and knowledge.

The overarching biomedical health framework obscures these denotations of dais' power because they do not fit within its definition of health and work. The exclusion of dais' narratives in the overall health paradigm has stripped dais of their authority as essential birth attendants, as promulgators of the tradition of birth and delivery, and as cultural teachers/healers/wise women. Indeed, biomedicine's dominance and suppression of dais are not new phenomena but form part of a larger movement worldwide to restrict and control women's knowledge. According to Ehrenreich and English:

> We learned this much: That the suppression of women health workers and the rise to dominance of male professionals was not a 'natural' process, resulting automatically from changes in medical science nor was it the result of women's failure to take on healing work. It was an active *takeover* by male professionals . . . The suppression of female healers by the medical establishment was a political struggle, first, in that it is part of the history of sex struggle in general. The status of women healers has risen and fallen with the status of women . . . It was a political struggle, second, in that it was part of a *class* struggle. Women healers were people's doctors, and their medicine was part of a people's subculture.
>
> (1973: 4)

The ascendancy of the medical profession and its dominance of women healers, the subsequent erosion of women's knowledge, and their struggles to maintain their legitimacy provide a good context for understanding dais' resistance through their metaphors and language. Dais' seemingly contradictory statements (as perceived by others) reinforce the importance of recording women's history and stories because they contain the underground or 'subversive' knowledge that has been ignored and suppressed. Furthermore, dais' narratives also tell of a unique way to adapt and challenge within a dominant system. Thus their statements on how they perceive their role in delivery work are critical elements in unifying disparate points of view, including the link between the sacred and pollution and dirt.

The emic explanation is also silent on why blood, which nourishes the foetus, amniotic fluid, which protects the foetus in the womb, and the placenta and cord, which ensure the development of the foetus, are considered polluting and dirty. If one follows the above perception through to its logical conclusion (at least for blood), then it can be assumed that blood oozing from a cut finger is also polluting. But this is not the case. Because not all blood is dirty and polluting, it can be presumed that only blood from the birth canal is dirty and causes contamination. The rationale for why this is so is not clear in the South Asian emic explanation. In the west, for example, the witch hunts to suppress women healers led to an aura of contamination associated with midwives. The church connected women with sex and condemned all pleasure in sex because it was thought to come from the devil. Thus women who were engaged in reproductive work and acts were considered evil and were perceived to possess magical powers that went against the teachings of the church (Ehrenreich and English 1973). This explanation may provide some clues to dais' marginal position in South Asia.

It appears that dais' untouchability[10] provides a powerful incentive for the upper castes to maintain the status quo and to ensure that work that is socially undesirable is carried out. And what better way to achieve this than to institutionalise work as religion and social obligation? It removes the possibility of a rebellion because it would require compelling reasons to question a system that is so ingrained and forms the basis for all social, cultural, economic, and political interactions.

Contamination, pollution, and *dirty* are words that describe bodily waste, and dais come into contact with them during their work. The pervasive association of these labels with dais' work means that their authoritative and intimate knowledge on birth are ignored. How could a body of knowledge be valuable when it is linked to unclean substances and work? The strict taboo appears to discredit dais' learning and healing roles and years of experience. Unlike biomedicine, which promotes the important role of bodily wastes in clinical and diagnostic work, the cultural interpretations appear to be diametrically opposite. The knowledge gained from urine, faeces, cord blood, and amniotic fluid is vital for the well-being of the mother and the foetus. Biomedicine has skilfully used the 'rational' science to co-opt the cultural connotations of pollution and dirty and has attached no stigma to biomedical health professionals working with body fluids. Indeed, the only time that biomedicine uses contamination is in the context of infection, another rational explanation, and it has devised methods to counter this.

Feminists have also noted that women's reproduction is a site for power struggles. Various images and metaphors are used to gain space and legitimacy for the woman and her multiple roles. Although the Hindu Trinity that represents creation, preservation, and dissolution is male-centred and represents power and authority, dais identify the essence of life with the female force – *Mataji* and *Shakti*. The common female deity that many dais evoke is *Mataji* (Mother Goddess). Dais believe that it is she who assists them in their work and that they receive blessings from her: '*I receive blessings from* Mataji *[Mother Goddess] and also get food. It is not I who does the deliveries, but it is through the* hands *of* Mataji' (SAhd6). This is not unexpected because dais perceive themselves as facilitators and mothers, as someone who guides both the woman and the child through their journey of giving birth and being born. *Mataji* and *Shakti*, the female essence and power and strength, seem to provide dais with the legitimacy to challenge the patriarchal principles that devalue their work, without any negative impact.

Ehrenreich and English (1973) observed that the exclusion of women healers has had more to do with political and economic monopolisation and less to do with superior medical knowledge replacing 'heresy'. In fact, the female anatomy, which is often blamed for all of women's 'backwardness', did not defeat women, but rather was used to support the rise of the male-controlled medical profession. In this regard, both the state and the church share responsibility.

Therefore dais' use of religious language, metaphors, and images is not surprising. They have done this through a process of emulation known as *Sanskritisation*,[11] which involves 'raising one's caste status within the framework of caste hierarchy by emulating the customs, traditions, norms and the lifestyle traditionally associated with the higher castes' (Bhatt 1975: 195). Although this term has been disputed as being unilateral and vague because it does not tell us what constitutes the imitation or why all Hindus are not completely Sanskritised ('raised' to a higher caste level) if the phenomenon has been occurring over millennia, its usefulness lies in the fact that it connotes the strength of the tendency to imitate and the direction of the imitation (Dumont 1970). Bhatt reiterated that, today, Sanskritisation has become unimportant compared to politicisation: 'The changing aspirations and demands of caste associations clearly show the shift from Sanskritisation to politicisation and modernisation for raising the position of the caste group' (1975: 196). Many 'backward' or low castes are taking advantage of the central government's special assistance to educate or organise themselves as collectives for business ventures or in other fields. However, this does not mean that lower castes do not emulate or change their lifestyles, because emulation occurs continuously in all societies and at all levels (Bhatt 1975).

Bhatt noted that the important change is that Brahmans or any other high castes no longer provide the model of emulation; instead economic and political models provide the framework for upward mobility and emulation. However, dais' narratives indicate that there are exceptions and that Sanskritisation continues to encourage emulation. The Brahmans' spiritual knowledge, interpretations, and rituals provide key characteristics for dais to emulate. Aligning their 'dirty' and 'polluting' work with the highest form of work (serving God) provides evidence that their work, too, is godly. Dais seem to imply that, like the Brahmans, they are the *authoritative figures* in the birthing process. Sanskritisation appears to allow dais to reclaim their authority and further establish the fact that they are able to conduct births, work that was deemed impossible in the biomedical world. Put another way, dais' alignment with the sacred and as authoritative figures challenges the notion that they are unskilled and illiterate. They seem to reject the cultural notion that their work is 'polluting,' 'dirty', and 'contaminating'. Indeed, they could even say that they are in touch with the divine much more closely than anyone else is, including the Brahman, because they handle the placenta and the cord.

As the facilitators of life (and lives), dais' use of male godly images such as *Krishna* (the Vishnu incarnate) and Vishnu, the preserver of life, who lives in the cord and the placenta, is understandable and offers multiple layers of meanings. First, identifying women's work with male figures is significant in the patriarchal system. Males occupy a higher socio-cultural position than women do. Linking delivery work with the work of the Hindu priests (male-dominated) means attempting to co-opt the male authority. In doing so, the dais are trying to counter the ideas of contamination and pollution of the woman's body and replace them with notions of the divine, temple, and *Shakti*.

Dais appear to position themselves as preservers of life and not destroyers. This is the second layer of meaning. Through Vishnu, they attempt to refute biomedicine's claims that dais contribute to high infant and maternal mortality rates. Because Vishnu resides in the placenta and the cord, it is unthinkable that dais would destroy life. The cord is not cut until the essence of life flows into the child and the child begins to breathe. To facilitate this flow, the dai massages the placenta, the implication being that, like the male priests, dais also have sacred rituals to ensure that life is respected and continues.

The third layer of meaning is related to payment. Because people generously offer money and other in-kind gifts to the Brahman priests to intercede between humans and the gods, dais, too, intercede between birth and death. The separation of one life into two may be difficult without their intervention. In the context of Sanskritisation, dais' work is sacred and requires years of learning and apprenticeship, just as that of the Brahman priests does. Dais contend that they deserve the same social respect and generosity because they are fulfilling their duty and religion.

Why is our work not valued? Doing good work in a dirty space: continuing to listen to dais speaking about their dirty work

Over time, the process of Sanskritisation may enhance the image of dais and increase the value of their work. In the meantime, it is important to address why they are not compensated adequately for their good work. Dais assert that because they are doing work that people avoid, they should be recognised for their contributions and sacrifice. Implicit in their statements is that if they did not perform this work, women would be deprived of delivery care, which would affect their health and that of their unborn child, an observation borne out by UNICEF's (1999) statistics on India. On the other hand, community members have used the same socio-cultural framework to counter dais' claims that their work is unique. They view dais' involvement in delivery work as women fulfilling their duty – women helping other women – and not as something extraordinary. Therefore society is not obliged to reward dais beyond what is ordinarily expected. The implication is that dais' work is ordinary and part of life.

The dilemma that dais face is that the emic explanation that gives them the authority to describe their work as a sacrifice, *poonya ka kaam*, and *dharm* also devalues their work. Dais have been unable either to translate the social merit of their work into a higher financial value or to convince society that their work deserves more respect. Listening to dais speak shows that they are aware of this disconnection. At the same time, they continue to promote the notion of charitable work and believe that low or no payment is acceptable. However, this noble idea works against them. It allows those who are unwilling to pay for the service to justify their refusals:

> In one case a doctor told the family that the woman needed an intravenous infusion, and the cost of the whole treatment [childbirth] would be Rs. 8000, but I did her delivery at home. The family only gave me Rs. 400. I asked for Rs. 500, and they refused me. They were willing to give the doctor Rs. 8000 but not the Rs. 500 that I asked.
>
> (NSAhd13)

> I have to be [satisfied]. What can I do? Especially if it is a poor household, then I get a lot of blessings. I do not ask for money. If they give of their own free will, I take it. How can I ask for money from a poor household if they have only one meal a day?
>
> (SAhd8)

> What can we do if they do not give? There are no benefits. Who will give us any benefits? If people pay, then we have some benefits. If they do not, then we do not have any. They give Rs. 1000 to hospitals, and yet they give us Rs. 10. I did not even get Rs. 5 for an entire night's work.
>
> (SAhd8)

A non-SEWA dai noted that delivery work affects her health and that the monetary remuneration that she receives does not compensate for the long-term effects on her health:

I handle nine months of dirt and heat, faeces, urine, and it affects me, so I wish they would increase the money.[12] At the private hospital they have to pay Rs. 4000, so they should at least pay me Rs. 500 per delivery. I have to clean all the dirty stuff and clean the place and wash their clothes.

(NSAhd14)

Apart from the economic issue, the question also highlights the contradictions found in the ideal of doing good work. For example, if good work ensures societal well-being, should the venue of the work impact the intrinsic value of the work? More important, what is the impact on the individual who does good but dirty work? In the case of dais, the location of their work is considered to be unclean. Should their delivery work, which benefits society, be perceived as menial work and of low value because it is performed in an unclean space? It is because of dais that poor women have access to maternity care. Exploring the concept of good and how it relates to work would be a useful beginning to understanding why dais' good work has negative connotations.

On the other hand, dais' untouchable work has hidden advantages. Because of the nature of the work, dais appear to maintain some form of economic monopoly and knowledge boundary. Their charity work allows them to create reciprocal ties with families who are unable to pay them for their delivery work. At least in the arena of delivery work, low-caste women form the majority, and as a group they have the potential to wield some form of power to define who they are and what their work involves. And despite the negative connotations of being a birth attendant, delivery work provides many women with an avenue to earn income when there may be no other. The in-between space that dais occupy gives them the freedom to move between their indigenous and biomedical knowledge/space to re-create a collective body of knowledge. The freedom to interpret and reinterpret using unique metaphors and images means that dais are creating their own authoritative knowledge. In light of this, it would be interesting to explore whether the taboos of delivery and birth are created by the women themselves to keep the men away, rather than outcomes of patriarchy.[13] This is a plausible assumption because dais have created another layer of meaning that connects pregnancy and birth with the divine, an idea that may not be accepted in the mainstream socio-cultural framework. When the dai states that Vishnu lives in the cord and the placenta, one wonders whether she means that the woman is in a divine state. How does Vishnu's abode in the woman for nine months (which is considered sacred) align with the concept of dirt and stale air/wind in the woman? One wonders whether these statements are variations of subversive knowledge or an underground movement by dais to gain control. These questions need to be explored further, but what is obvious is that dais' dirty and polluting work is a product of cultural interpretations that are fluid and changing.

Dais' journey to legitimise their work through Sanskritisation is an attempt to move away from the negative connotations that continue to devalue their work. It would be interesting to listen to their voices in the future to observe whether they have been successful in this regard. The notion that there is a divine being in something dirty is an important one and could lead to a shift in dais' power and status. Future work could explore whether there have been any changes in dais' cultural interpretations, whether the insertion of the divine had provided dais with the authority to counter society's and bio-medicine's negative perceptions of their work, and whether the new cultural interpretations could withstand the powerful movement by the biomedical establishment (which has the support of the state) to phase dais out of the health care system.

Dais appear to be selective about those to whom they reveal their new interpretations. In itself, this is a strategic move because it allows them to gauge people's reactions to their 'new' knowledge. Thus it is interesting that SMeh7, who associated her work with Vishnu, would tell only me about this link and not others. One wonders whether her sense of trust was linked to the fact that, because I am an outsider, I would accept her interpretation of her work. Or could it be that, as a researcher, I am in a strategic position to spread her interpretation of her work to a wider audience and thus elevate the image of dais' 'dirty' work.

Their voices indicate that they know that it is critical to speak a common language to convince people of the value of their work. *Poonya ka kaam* and *dharm* are two such words/phrases that they have used constantly to portray themselves as women who have their community's welfare at heart, and, because of this, they continue to engage in delivery work despite the negative impact on them. Their work therefore assumes the attributes of a selfless duty and godliness. These confer prestige on their dirty work. I would like to end this chapter with dais' voices. Their voices convey the conflict, pride, and happiness that they feel in who they are and what they are doing:

> No, I do not get any benefits from this. I want my daughter to study and be educated. It depends on her abilities and brains. If she wants to be a Dai, so be it. Otherwise she has to do housework. We get what we put out in terms of our effort. I consider it [Dais' work] beneficial only if I receive over and above what I put out in terms of money, vessels, cloths, grains, and so forth. I work as a Dai because of my children and for our stomachs. I am uneducated, so I have to do this. Otherwise, if I were [educated], I would do something else.
>
> (NSAhd8)

> A private doctor in my area does not want women to have deliveries at home, so she tells them that the child's presentation is not normal. She advises women to have their deliveries at her clinic. In this way she earns about Rs. 2000. But those who are poor, how can they afford this?

I conduct their deliveries at home, and she [the doctor] becomes angry. She asks me why I conducted the delivery at home. I take whatever the family gives me, whether it is Rs. 10 or Rs. 100, depending on the family's income. I am not greedy, but I do need the money for my family expenses. But it is not my duty to exploit people.

(SAhd8)

I have a stomach, and I need money to meet my household expenses.

(SAhd6)

I have to go [to work as a dai] because my family is poor . . . Only if you work will you get food; otherwise there is no advantage.

(NSAhd11)

I am able to comfort the woman, and she feels happy. So I feel happy and satisfied.

(NSAhd8)

It is good to help.

(SAhd5)

I feel that I have an obligation because I have learned it [delivery work].

(SAhd9)

Notes

1 SEWA is the organisation to which I was attached while I conducted my doctoral fieldwork from 1999 to 2000.
2 I use codes to protect the identity of the dais and to maintain their confidentiality. All quotations are from the doctoral research that I conducted in Gujarat, India, from 1999 to 2000 (Rai 2003).
3 The Head of the Department of Paediatrics, Civil Hospital, Ahmedabad, made this distinction during the discussion at a state-level conference on RCH in Gujarat in 1999. She made the point that even within dais' work there is a hier-archy. The state-level health officials included Gujarat's health minister and members of various NGOs, and I also attended this meeting, which provided me with the background for my research.
4 Dais' training through apprenticeships and learning through doing and obser-ving is not recognised as formal training and learning. The training here refers to learning and attaining competency in managing birth and delivery by mastering biomedical procedures. According to the joint statement by WHO/ICM/FIGO:

> A **skilled attendant** is an accredited health professional – such as a midwife, doctor, or nurse – who has been educated and trained to proficiency in the skills needed to manage normal (uncomplicated) pregnancies, childbirth and

the immediate postnatal period, and in the identification, management and referral of complications in women and newborns.

(WHO 2004: 1)

This definition has also been endorsed by UNFPA and the World Bank (WHO 2004).

5 In her groundbreaking book *Birth in Four Cultures: A Cross-Cultural Investigation of Childbirth in Yucatan, Holland, Sweden, and the United States*, Brigitte Jordan (1978/ 1993) pointed out that not all biomedical procedures are beneficial to women (e.g. putting women in a lithotomy position during delivery); rather, they are a means of facilitating and helping the work of the biomedical practitioner. Despite this, the biomedical system supports this practice and others because it has convinced everyone of the *benefits* of the lithotomy position to women. Brigitte Jordan called this 'authoritative knowledge'.

6 According to WHO/ICM/FIGO:

Investing in strategies based *solely* on TBAs has historically caused governments to delay the development and implementation of strategies for ensuring that skilled attendants are available to all women and newborns. To avoid falling into this trap, the decision to incorporate TBAs into the strategy for the provision of skilled care should be an interim step of a longer-term plan for training and providing sufficient skilled attendants.

(WHO 2004: 8)

WHO noted that young and able TBAs should enrol in midwifery programmes or become auxiliary midwives to support skilled birth attendants.

7 A TBA is one who is a 'traditional, independent (of the health system), non-formally trained and community-based provider of care during pregnancy, childbirth and the postnatal period' (WHO 2004: 8).

8 In Hindu cosmology the cobra, just like the cow and the monkey, is revered. The cobra is often associated with Lord Shiva. In other cases, one can also see in various icons Vishnu reclining on the coiled body of the nine-headed cobra. Vishnu and Shiva, together with Brahma, make the Hindu Trinity.

9 Here I am referring to the Hindu tradition because most dais were Hindu; however, the concept of doing one's duty and work is practised by most South Asians.

10 The caste system is a complex structure based on the *Jajmani* system, in which trades and work have been prescribed and passed down from generation to generation. So ingrained is this system that the surnames of individuals in each of the castes and subcastes further indicate their work and trades. The caste system is independent of the economic level. In most discussions the four main caste groups identified are the Brahmans, Kshatriyas, Vaishyas, and Sudras. It is believed that these caste groups emerged from the different body parts of the Brahma, the god of creation. Thus the Brahman emerged from the mouth and the head, the Kshatriyas from the arms, the Vaishyas from the thighs, and the Sudras from the feet (Mulder 1995). Below these castes are the Untouchables, whom Gandhi named *Harijans* or 'Children of God'.

11 *Sanskritisation* was first conceptualised by the Indian sociologist M.N. Srinivas in his study of the Coorgs of south India in 1952.

12 It is believed that conception and pregnancy enclose the 'stale air/wind'. When birth occurs, the stale air or wind of nine months affects the eyes. Dais believe that their weak eyesight is a result of being constantly exposed to this dirty wind/ air.

13 I would like to thank Dr Susan James for sharing her many wonderful ideas and our rich discussions during my PhD studies.

References

Bhatt, A. (1975). *Caste, class, and politics: an empirical profile of social stratification in modern India*. Delhi: Manohar Book Service.

Cabral, M., Kamal, I., Kumar, V., and Mehra, L. (1992a). *Training of traditional birth attendants (TBAs): a guide for master trainers*. Geneva: WHO.

Cabral, M., Kamal, I., Kumar, V., and Mehra, L. (1992b). *Training of traditional birth attendants (TBAs): a guide for TBA trainers*. Geneva: WHO.

Cabral, M., Kamal, I., Kumar, V., and Mehra, L. (1992c). *Training of traditional birth attendants (TBAs): an illustrated guide for TBAs*. Geneva: WHO.

Chandola, L.M. (1995). *Women in the unorganised sector*. New Delhi: Radiant.

Chatterjee, M. (1999). Concept paper of Dais' training at SEWA. Unpublished paper, Ahmedabad, India.

Du Gas, B., Mangay-Maglacas, A., Pizurki, H., and Simons, J. (1979). *Traditional birth attendants: a field guide to their training, evaluation, and articulation with health services*. Geneva: WHO.

Dumont, L. (1970). *Homo hierarchicus: the caste system and its implications* (M. Sainsbury, trans.). London: Weidenfeld and Nicolson.

Ehrenreich, B. and English, D. (1973). *Witches, midwives, and nurses: a history of women healers*. Old Westbury, NY: Feminist Press.

Government of India (1997). *Reproductive and Child Health Programme: schemes for implementation*. New Delhi: Ministry of Health and Family Welfare, Department of Family Welfare

International Labour Organisation (1996a). *ILO Convention on Home Work: Eighty-third session, June 4, 1996: Ratification of treaty on homebased workers, Article (1)*. Retrieved February 2002, from http://www.homenetww.org.uk/conv.html

International Labour Organisation (1996b). *Remuneration for women's work: a curious paradox*. Retrieved February 2002, from http://www.ilo.org/public/english/bureau/inf/pkits/women2

Mangay-Maglacas, A. and Pizurki, H. (eds) (1981). *The traditional birth attendants in seven countries: case studies and utilisation and training*. Geneva: WHO.

Mangay-Maglacas, A. and Simons, J. (eds) (1979). *The potential of the traditional birth attendant*. WHO Offset Publication No. 95. Geneva: WHO.

Mitchell, S. (2000). *Bhagavad Gita* (S. Mitchell, trans.). New York: Three Rivers Press.

Rai, S. (2003). The work and health of dais: the effect of authoritative perception on indigenous midwives of Gujarat, India. Unpublished PhD dissertation, University of Alberta, Edmonton.

State Institute of Health and Family Welfare (1983). *Modular refresher training programme for Dais in maternal and child health: 6 working days*. Ahmedabad, India: Author.

State Institute of Health and Family Welfare (1992). *Report on Dai training*. Ahmedabad, India: Author.

State Institute of Health and Family Welfare (1995). *Intensive modular training programme for trainers of active trained Dais in maternal and child health: 3 working days.* Ahmedabad, India: Author.

State Institute of Health and Family Welfare (1999). *Report on Dai training under [the] celebration of Ma-Raksha Mahotsav.* Sola, India: Author.

Swaminathan, M.C., Naidu, A.N., and Krishna, T.P. (1986). An evaluation of dai training in Andhra Pradesh. In A. Mangay-Maglacas and J. Simons (eds) *The potential of the traditional birth attendant* (pp. 22–34). WHO Offset Publication No. 95. Geneva: WHO.

United Nations (1999). *Executive summary of the world survey on the role of women in development.* Geneva: UN. Retrieved March 2001, from http://www.un.org/documents/ecosoc/docs/1999

United Nations Children's Fund (UNICEF) (1999). *A programme for children and women in India: plan of operations 1999–2002.* New Delhi: Government of India/UNICEF.

United Nations Population Fund (1994). *International Conference on Health and Population Development.* Retrieved March 2001, from http://www.undp.org/popin/icpd

United Nations Population Fund (1996). Support to traditional birth attendants. *Evaluation findings* 7: 1–9. Retrieved November 1, 2005, from http://www.unfpa.org/monitoring/pdf

Verderese, M.D.L. and Turnbull, L.M. (1975). *The traditional birth attendant in maternal and child health and family planning: a guide to her training and utilisation.* Geneva: WHO.

Walt, G. (1984). *The supervision of traditional birth attendants.* Geneva: WHO.

World Health Organisation. (1978). *Report of the International Conference on Primary Health Care, Alma-Ata.* Geneva: WHO/UNICEF.

World Health Organization (1982). *Training and use of auxiliaries in the provision of nursing/midwifery care.* Copenhagen: WHO Regional Office for Europe.

World Health Organization (1995a). *Guidelines for training traditional practitioners as primary health care workers.* Geneva: WHO, Division of Strengthening of Health Services and the Traditional Medicine Programme.

World Health Organization (1995b). *Traditional practitioners as primary health care workers.* Geneva: WHO, Division of Strengthening of Health Services and the Traditional Medicine Programme.

World Health Organization (1998a). *Safe motherhood fact sheet: maternal mortality.* Retrieved February 2002, from http://www.safemotherhood.org/facts

World Health Organization (1998b). *Safe motherhood fact sheet: measuring progress.* Retrieved from http://www.safemotherhood.org/facts

World Health Organization (2000). *Gender, health, and poverty.* WHO Fact Sheet No. 251. Retrieved February 2002, from http://www.who.int/inf-fs/en/fact251

World Health Organization (2004). *Making pregnancy safer: the critical role of the skilled attendant: a joint statement by WHO, ICM, and FIGO.* Retrieved September 30, 2005, from http://www.who.int/reproductive-health/publications

Additional resources on indigenous midwives:

Bailey, P.E., Szaszdi, J.A. and Glover, L. (2002). Obstetric complications: does training traditional birth attendants make a difference? *Pan American Journal of Public Health* 11(1): 15–23.

Department for International Development (2004). *Reducing maternal deaths: evidence and action: a strategy for DFID*. Retrieved September 30, 2005, from http://www.dfid.gov.uk/pubs/files/reducmaternaldeath.pdf

Lule, E., Ramana, G.N.V., Oomman, N., Epp, J., Huntington, D. and Rosen, J.E. (2005). *Achieving the millennium development goals of improving maternal health: determinants, interventions and challenges*. Retrieved November 1, 2005, from http://www.sitesources.worldbank.org/healthnutritionand population/resources/

Subramanian, T., Charles, N., Balasubramanian, R., Sundaram, V., Ganapathy, S., Dharmaraj, D. *et al.* (1996). Role and acceptability of traditional birth attendants (*dais*) in a rural community in south India. *Indian Journal of Preventive and Social Medicine* 27(3 and 4): 109–116. Retrieved September 30, 2005, from http://www.medind.nic.in/imvw/imvw11196.html

Training of traditional birth attendants (n.d.). Retrieved September 30, 2005, from http://www.cedpa.org/publications/pdf/savingmotherslives6.pdf

United Nations Population Fund (2004). *A skilled birth attendant at every birth: consensus and concerns*. Regional workshop on skilled birth attendants in South and West Asia, Islamabad, Pakistan, April. Retrieved September 30, 2005, from http://www.unfpa.org.np/pub/sba.report.pdf

United Nations Population Fund (n.d.). *Ensuring skilled attendance at births*. Retrieved September 30, 2005, from http://www.unfpa.org/mothers/skilled.att.htm#top

World Health Organization (n.d.). *Global action for skilled attendants for pregnant women*. Retrieved September 30, 2005, from http://www.who.int/reproductivehealth/publications/global.action.for.skilled.attendants/mpr.global.action.pdf

13 Shame, honour and pollution for Pakistani women

Margaret Chesney

By making women the objects of fear and something to be avoided as unclean, it is possible to reduce the cultural status of women. As such any biological advantage is demoted to the state of cultural disadvantage, once this has been achieved they are then converted to biological disadvantage.

(Montague 1999: 82)

Background

This chapter draws on findings from an empirical study which aimed to explore the life and birth experiences of women who have given birth in Pakistan (Chesney 2004). Seventeen women told their birth stories within in-depth life-story framed interviews: seven were recruited through acquaintances in the Punjab district of Pakistan and ten from an over-fifties club in a town in the north of England. Further contextual data were gleaned from participant observations undertaken during nine field trips to Pakistan and two focus groups at the over-fifties club. The methodology was interpretive ethnography (Denzin 1997) with an anthropological underpinning. Reflection was an important part of the research methodology; a contemporaneous research diary was kept. Analysis was undertaken using adapted frameworks from Alasuutari (1995), Polkinghorne (1995) and Childress (1998).

The key theme to emerge from the data surrounded the dai (untrained traditional birth attendant), her influence on the birth experiences of women, her work and her life. The sub-themes from the research that sourced this chapter are boy preference, shame and honour, and menstrual and childbirth bleeding. The stories told by the women about the dai relate to her position in the family and her defiling role at childbirth.

Boy preference

Preference for boy children emerged as a theme from the women's life and birth stories. Within this, a generation difference was also evident; the younger generation felt that:

'elders wanted sons so they could be looked after in their old age'

(B)

The older generation recognised that there were fewer babies these days, so:

'As long as there is one of each, the girl is valued.'

(N)

The findings were framed around the use of family planning by sex composition of living children. The acceptance of contraception was found to be higher amongst women who had one or more living sons. Contraception was the source of F's concern when her second daughter was born:

'My mother never said she was pleased my daughter was healthy . . . my mother-in-law say you must have another [baby]. When I came here [UK], we had another girl and my husband said, "these are our boys, so we don't want to have any more". He said have an operation . . . I did not know what to say, I told my friend and she said "why can't he do that [be sterilised], if he had operation so . . . in case he needed more children he can't blame you". I wasn't clever enough to tell this until she gave this idea. He kept saying to me have an operation . . . He asked me to go to the doctor to arrange . . . the doctor would not do his [husband] operation [sterilisation] just in case my death then he needed more [male] children . . .'

(F)

N's first four children were girls and

'With each girl my mother-in-law treated me worse'

(N)

Having four girls was linked to the divorce of I's daughter:

'I have two girls, she [daughter] has four and is now divorced, when she got two girls the family were anxious to have the boy . . .'

(I)

Being born a girl into a Muslim family in Pakistan brings with it a responsibility to the family, both natal and 'real'.

'I didn't go to secondary school you know, when I was twelve. I was going to primary school . . . then my mother very ill . . . she nearly dies and there is nobody to look after my brothers and sisters. My mother said "sorry you cannot go to school I need you to help me", *then* I help others and look after my brothers and sisters . . . hard working, cooking and cleaning . . . *I like it . . .*'

(F)

F was not aggrieved that she had to give up school; instead she took pride in caring for her siblings. Much as N, a second wife, was content to hand over her son to her husband's first wife as a sign of gratitude that he had rescued her from the life of a non-person, as a widow who had to return to live and be dependent upon her parents, brothers and their wives.

The views of the women interviewed spoke of the constraints of life as a woman and the 'specialness 'of being able to give birth:

'Nothing else to do really, we have the special mechanism . . .'

(C)

This statement was made in the context of a restricted social life compared to her boy cousins.

'Even in our family [enlightened] . . . now the boys . . . of . . . you see Afiz . . . he is the same age as me . . . all the girls, even Sabrina at sixteen . . . she is so much mature than the eldest . . . it is so obvious in the family . . . he will be running up and down in his car and everything . . . the girls are just sort of . . . "sit there".'

(N)

It would appear that from birth the value of being a girl hangs on the birth order and gender of the siblings, assigning status to both the mother and the child. Once there is a son then the girl is valued and takes on a special status and role in childcare and the upkeep of the home. It is the man's responsibility to 'provide' and to communicate with the world outside the family.

Menstruation, fertility and vulnerability

The picture around menstruation worldwide emerges as complex and contradictory. Douglas (1966) raised the question of why it is that menstrual rather than other bleeding is regarded with disgust or feared, out of proportion to its actual ability to harm or infect. Kristeva (1982) distinguishes between bodily fluids that are polluting and those that are not, linking menstrual and post-delivery blood to excrement. The blood of menstruation and childbirth is called 'Haram' in Punjabi or 'Narak' in Hindu. Both terms loosely translate as dirty. Menstruating and postnatal women are widely seen as unclean and a source of contamination.

'Menstrual and postnatal blood is "Khunda hoon" like you would think of eating dog.'

(N)

Following menarche, women remain alienated from their sexuality, silenced by the shame of it, segregated from the family.

'I could no longer sit on my father's lap.'

(Petcheski and Judd 1998: 286)

'I don't know . . . my mum . . . she said . . . right . . . just put this [sanitary towel] here and sit down and behave like a lady . . .'

(N's granddaughter)

'I just thought I had dirtied my undies . . . it can be so embarrassing.'

(N)

The following parable epitomises the 'ownership' and responsibility of the father and husband for their daughter and wife:

She is like an unripe fig, or a ripening fig, or a fully ripe fig, While she is yet a child, and a 'ripening fig', these are the days of her girlhood, and during these times her father is entitled to aught that she finds, and to the work of her hands and he can annul her vows. As a fully ripe fig she is past her girlhood, when her father has no more rights over her (Mishnah, Niddah). Her husband then takes on these rights.

(Norris 1998: 70)

Further to this Ben Shira recounted:

The only value a daughter can offer is negative, she is the treasure of sleeplessness' worrying over her prospects and his (father's) reputation. In her youth, lest she pass the flower of age, and when she is married lest she be hated, in her virginity lest she be seduced, in the house of her husband lest she prove unfaithful, in her father's house lest she becomes pregnant and in her husband's house lest she becomes barren. So much that marriage does not bring relief.

(Norris 1998: 71)

Shira's quotation depicts the vulnerability of the family when there is a post-menarche daughter living at home unmarried. In Pakistan a daughter's first menarche directs the parents' thoughts towards marriage. Until married, the girl is potentially able to bring shame on the family; this would be considered unforgivable and would affect the marriageability of other members of the extended family. This window of vulnerability has the potential to be extended when the family live in the UK, as marriage is not allowed until the age of 16 and a girl may have reached puberty some years earlier.

Gaining sins, shame and honour

After puberty,

> 'As a girl going out . . . you were gaining sins . . .'
>
> (F)

After a long pause, I asked, 'going out, do you mean *meeting a boy?*' to which F nodded. When asked what she did from the age 15 (her menarche) until she got married aged 19, F's reply demonstrated the responsibility her mother took to prepare her for her future role as a wife.

> 'sort of . . . went to a centre . . . we used to learn Arabic and the meaning of the Qur'an . . . my mother bought lots of embroidery and sewing and cooking . . .'
>
> (F)

Once menarche occurred, F was restricted from 'going out' and the final preparation for her new role as wife, housekeeper and mother took place. The segregation of women from men in the household was never more apparent than when visiting a home in Pakistan. 'Mixed company', that is, women and men unrelated to one another socialising, was frowned upon and it was common practice to be shown into the women's quarters (usually at the back of the house) whilst the men would be entertained in another room. If women were to go out of the house, a chaperone was seen to be essential.

Pakistani girls' behaviour is governed by honour (izzat) and its potential loss and the multiple negative connotations of shame. However, sharm is a term that is used in both the negative (shame) and positive (honour) sense. This constituted an important sub-theme that emerged from the women's words. The post-pubertal daughter of a GP friend in Pakistan was chaperoned at all times because her parents believed that her honour (and marriageability) would be lost or affected if she was seen in the 'wrong company'. Honouring one's parents is a strong norm in a traditional Muslim family and would be considered positive sharm. The depth of social control of behaviour, not just women's, is epitomised in a quotation from one of the many interpreters of Qur'anic principles:

> 'Women's status and dignity is not a matter for negotiation in the Islamic context. Not only are all forms of exploitation of the women's image directly prohibited, but are indirectly discouraged by imposition

of rules of modesty in dress, behaviour and demeanour, which applies to men as well.'

(Abedin 1996: 73)

It would appear that family honour, negative sharm and loss of izzat are the responsibility of the community as a whole, both men and women, It is the women that are held to account, with men being responsible for monitoring, protection and punishment.

Sending a daughter to Pakistan to arrange a marriage may be perceived as protecting her from western norms and the promiscuous behaviour of western teenagers. It is also true that although young men appear to have freedom to socialise in their teen years, they stay at home after marriage, taking on the responsibility of caring in monetary terms for their elders and the marriages of their sisters. They do not have any more say in the selection of a marriage partner than young women do (Jeffery *et al.* 1988). Thompson (1981) found it possible that negative sharm and the consequential loss of honour (izzat) gains some of its emotive force from its association with physical modesty. Almost from the time a child can talk, great stress is laid on girls concealing their genitals; this is the first way they are taught to express sharm.

> 'Even though my daughter is . . . [unable to verbalise the rite of passage (menstruation) her daughter has reached] . . . like her body is changing, but mentally she is a child . . . so we tell her to sit properly or, when she run . . . you know . . . cover her body . . . [her breasts do not show] that is a part of growing up . . .preparing her . . . she does mentally become prepared . . .'
>
> (N)

> 'My daughter will sit there something like that [with her legs splayed] and I will say, close your legs, it does not look nice, or, don't keep touching your knickers . . . it would not look nice in public to be doing that . . .'
>
> (N)

Accepting the restrictive gendered role highlights the complexities that exist for a third-generation Pakistani girl in the UK. Her life spans at least two cultures and three generations. She will be living in a home where values, roles and rules are such that she cannot go out on her own and must not socialise in mixed company for fear of losing the family izzat in the community. She must not question elders and must accept the family choice of a husband; thereafter she will live with her in-laws, obeying their rules. She will not have to work outside the home or be responsible for the family's income. The parents of children educated in a society which has values that are considered immoral must suffer agonies of worry that their children may be drawn into the culture of western youth. It is not surprising that some parents choose to send their children back to live with the families in Pakistan. The irony is that most of the women who came to the UK came to give their children a better education and chance in life, that is, after they were married.

Marriage and sharm

An agreement must be made between the couple before they come forward for marriage – no one can force them to get married (Salahi 1993). The marriage itself requires a commitment by the bride or her guardian. However, it is inevitable that there will be times when opinions differ. The bride-to-be is required to have retained her chastity and her future husband must retain her honour. It is not permissible for a man and a woman to be alone in a closed room if they are not related (Salahi 1993: 90). Choice does not always involve other options, as the retired midwife identified.

> 'Nobody gave me a choice, they do ask if it is OK, this is not a choice . . . you have to say yes because if you say no they have to find someone else . . .'
>
> (I)

Positive sharm is predominant; respect for her parents' choice takes precedence over a girl's own. Often from the very birth of a girl, the family begins to look for an appropriate marriage partner. Some families look first within their own extended family. A colleague midwife, who was brought to the UK by her parents when she was aged 5, said:

> 'We knew there was no one in our extended family of an appropriate age [for marriage] . . . so my parents had to look outside the family to friends of relatives. My parents gave me a choice of three [men to marry], I said I wanted someone who had lived in the UK. Subsequently however, my father's eldest sister in Pakistan, wanted a distant relative, so I had to take her choice, I would not upset my mother and father. We have already arranged that my husband's younger brother is to marry my sister (they are both aged eleven now).'
>
> (S)

An arranged marriage does not come with a guarantee of success. Breakdown can create reverberations through a whole extended family network, especially if the couple are related. The shame of divorce is linked to the loss of family honour (izzat) (Khan 1999).

D told a graphic story about how her eventual marriage was affected by her sister's divorce.

'My sister got divorced, my eldest brother-in-law threw her [his wife] out because she could not conceive, yet he was found to have a child in another village . . . I said I do not want to get married . . . my wedding was a secret . . . my Nakah [part of marriage ceremony] was held in a car, my father did not want anyone to know.'

(D)

Also convoluted family relationships evolve in proportion to the number of wives the husband takes. R, answering for her mother, said:

'She laughs when you ask . . . she has not had a good marriage . . . it is a joke . . . it has gone past . . . he is her first cousin . . . her mother and his mother are sisters . . . it is all so complicated . . . he has always been coming and going.. . . . he went to Pakistan and got divorced there and sent mum the divorce papers . . . he came back and wanted to live with her and she said no way . . . he has done before, married two other wives and she has taken him back . . . he now lives with me . . . he has divorced his third wife . . . he is a sad man, he used to be popular at one time he had lots of money and his own business . . . the women only married him for his money, when he had no money he came back to mum and she always accepted him . . . now if she cooks she will send some round [to our house] for him.'

(R)

B admitted that having one troubled marriage in the family affects the marriages of the other women. However, she also very clearly said that it was not her responsibility to be concerned. The men, father and brothers, take on that responsibility.

S, speaking for her mother, said:

'It was very late [when her mother Bas got married] aged twenty-eight years, this is because her father died when she was thirteen or fourteen, her mother was scared what might happen . . . they were still worried with what happened to my aunt . . . [divorced].'

(S)

The social and economic significance of marriage and the marital relation-ship was confirmed in the words of the women, and marriage was indeed a very important part of their narrative. For the second- and third-generation Pakistani girls and women in the UK, living and retaining a religion and culture that is radically different from the country of residence creates many challenges. Some of the first-generation immigrants to the UK, who followed their husbands, had no need to learn the language because they stayed within their own community, shopping and socialising within the commu-nity. However, the second and third generations were educated in the host culture and would often be living and socialising across a dual cultural system with confounding norms and values. This created a problem for the first-generation elders who found it difficult to understand the norms and values of the school and social environment of their children.

Carroll, a lawyer who has done considerable work on Islamic divorce, particularly with women who are seeking divorce in the UK, concentrated upon the effects on women and found that: 'Muslim women were forced by ignorance and social pressure to subject themselves to an interpretation of Islamic law that is harsher than it is for women in Pakistan' (1997: 97). Not only were women disadvantaged socially through divorce, but also financially. If they applied for a divorce the husband often would demand the return of the marriage jewellery or a substantial financial settlement. Muslim women are not entitled to a divorce without the husband's consent and no Muslim marriage can be dissolved without the husband pronouncing a talaq, which begins the divorce proceedings and is the utterance of the phrase 'I divorce you' once. (This is spoken due to the marriage being a verbal contract and thus its dissolution is normally verbal.)

When a man intends to divorce his wife he has to make sure that she is not in her menstruation period and that the two of them had not had sexual intercourse during the period of cleanliness after the bleeding. It is forbidden to effect a divorce if sexual intercourse has taken place. From the moment of the talaq there starts a waiting period that lasts three menstrual cycles. If the woman is pregnant, then the waiting period is until the birth. During this time the wife stays at home but is no longer obliged to do housework. If there is a change of mind within the waiting period then the couple need not have a fresh marriage or pay another dower. If they do not reunite, then at the end of the waiting period, the woman returns to her parents' house. She is not entitled to maintenance but if she has custody of the children, the husband should support them.

To summarise, the woman's position in Pakistani society moves from the non-person position of a prepubescent, unmarried daughter without 'true' family through the spiral of defining and defiling of menstruation to become fertile, and prior to marriage attracts a huge potential for bringing shame to the family. Following the all-important arranged marriage, she moves on to be defined at childbirth. When defined as being the mother of a son, then she has her own true family. The person seen to be most important in the life and birth experiences of the women in the research was the dai.

The dai and the family

A direct translation of the term 'dai' in the Urdu dictionary is 'midwife'; however, the dai is a traditional birth attendant (TBA), not formally trained. There are midwives (relatively few) who have undertaken a minimum of twelve months' recognised training (Pakistan Nurses Association 1992). Women in the research used the terms dai and midwife interchangeably. Global confusion around terms and definitions of TBAs led to a study by WHO (1992), which did little to clarify the issue. Literature from Pakistan (UNICEF 1989) further confuses, as it classifies 'trained' dais and midwives collectively, with no mention of the TBA.

If the definition of midwife is taken literally, from the old English '*wif* (with) *woman*' (Collins 1994), then the dai is indeed a '*midwife*' in that she is the person '*with woman*'. The statistics to uphold this are recorded by Fikree *et al.* (1998), Chawla (2000), Kamal (2000) and Kasi (2002), each confirming that between 75 and 90 per cent of women who give birth in Pakistan are attended by the dai. This situation is complex, as senior female family members also attend women in labour, they thereby gains skills, and they exercise a role commensurate with their position in the family. The mother-in-law or other female member of the family having already made the diagnosis of labour, a decision to call the dai is made. She will then undertake duties that no one else is prepared to undertake in assisting the woman to give birth. The word 'dai' can be used to describe both roles. According to one study, 'the best dais appear to be the woman's mother or mother-in law' due to their 'knowing' the birthing woman well. This role would be that of adviser and supporter, rather than that of delivering the baby and dealing with blood and the placenta. If there is a dai who happens to be a relative she will also attend the birth; however, another dai may be called (if the family can afford it) to undertake the defiling work of touching the genitals (undertaking vaginal examinations), cutting the cord, dealing with the placenta and cleaning up the blood. Roles appear to be clearly delineated in terms of pollution.

Jeffery *et al.* studied birth in Binjor, in northern India and found that the roles of the relative and dai are directly opposite to the family and midwife roles in the west.

> It is inappropriate to regard the dai as the expert midwife in the contemporary western sense as it is the senior relative, usually the sas (mother-in-law), who manages and directs the actions of the dai.
>
> (Jeffery *et al.* 1988: 108)

The mother as the dai, providing care only for family members, is one of the many complexities within the social fabric of the Pakistani community. Comments made by the women in the study about the dai and the family relationship all had a common theme:

> 'My mother was a dai, but only for the family.'

> 'She know everything, you know, my mother, even though she was uneducated.'

> (D)

'The dai was my dad's auntie . . . she live in our street, only a few homes away, she is looking at me.'

(F)

'The dai was very kind, she delivered all my brothers [I got six and one sister].'

(Fi)

'Yeh . . . they [dai] looked after her [grandmother] . . . the family system . . . most of the family used to look after her when she was in labour . . . The women in the family . . . because it was quite a big family they looked after her . . .'

(S, granddaughter of T)

It was evident from the women's narratives that dais are trusted, special and influential members of the female community. The term bhajee (sister) was used by the women about the dai to denote the same respect that is accorded to the eldest sister. The dai is not usually directly related to the woman, however; she is called the 'family dai'; she is the one that all the family call. She is usually from the same community or village as the labouring woman and her family.

'She, the dai is in the same village, her mother was also . . .'

(Bs)

Although not usually connected by blood, marriage or kinship, the connection is through the trust established through reputation. It is usual for the dai to be from the poorest and lowest group in the community, on the same level as the dung woman, who makes and sells fuel cakes from animal dung. The dai's position in society is that of a woman who needs to work; who does not have the support of a man. The role is often undertaken following widowhood.

'My sister became a dai; it was the only way to "get some money".'

(N)

It could be argued that the 'dirty' part of childbirth and the dai's role therein makes her essential to the birth, as no one else is prepared to take on what she does. In Bangladesh, where the family is too poor to call a dai outside the family the woman herself is asked to undertake the most defiling task of cutting the cord.

Abedin offers a perspective on the dai that encompasses the dialectic of essential yet dangerous.

The dai is the most exploited yet the most resourceful; the most ignored yet the most indispensable, the most vulnerable yet the most valuable.

(Abedin 1996: 86)

These descriptors were used by Abedin to illustrate the situation for Islamic women. As such they exemplify life for most Pakistani woman.

The dai as dangerous and blamed, yet powerless

The view of the dai as dangerous, upheld by Jeffery *et al.* (1988), is linked to her profoundly polluting role, that of cutting the cord, touching the genitals and inserting a hand into the vagina. From my experience of birth in hospitals in Pakistan, I would suggest that there was evidence of 'dangerous practice' performed by 'trained' staff in the hospitals in Pakistan. These same staff attributed these practices to dais in women's homes and labelled them as dangerous. Examples were: administering oxytocin without monitoring the foetal heart, instructing the woman to push when her cervix was not fully dilated, applying fundal pressure in the second stage of labour and stretching the woman's vulva manually. Whilst obstetric opinion in the UK would see these practices as dangerous wherever they occurred, in Pakistan they were seen as dangerous when practised out of place. In the hospital, the status of the place and the practitioners meant that these practices were accepted there.

Women were admitted to the hospital, supposedly 'dai handled'. One woman had a badly bruised vulva when the baby's head was not even in the pelvis. Another woman was *in extremis* from obstructed labour because the baby lay in the transverse and she had been in labour for many days. Many women were admitted with their babies dead inside them with histories of multiple injections and having suffered long labours in the home. There was however no proof that dais were responsible; the woman did not say the dai had stretched her or delayed her transfer to hospital. It is probable that the dai did the stretching, as a relative would never touch the genitals. The dais, however, may have been under instruction from the mother-in-law. In addition, any delay in transfer is likely to have been due to decisions made by the mother-in-law or senior relative not the dai, the lack of funds for travel and treatment, or the poor reputation of the hospital.

Emergency management of birth in the home has been the basis of most TBA training programmes. However, it is my observation that such programmes have mainly been designed, planned and delivered by hospital-trained staff who may themselves have never worked in the rural areas. This may account for the programmes being largely unsuccessful in changing practice or improving mortality rates (Brasseur 1992). A very recent randomised controlled trial undertaken in the Sind Province of Pakistan by Jokhari (2005) involved a three-day training programme for TBAs (dais). There was a 3 per cent reduction in the mortality rate for the intervention

group. An initial review of the methodology raised questions about the
record keeping and training of the personnel collecting the data. The validity of research of this nature is compromised because of a relative lack of
knowledge of the rural poor, a lack of consistency in the training message
and a lack of understanding of the dai's indigenous practice (Chawla 2000).
Training programmes can assume an infrastructure that does not exist.

There is however a strong belief that the risk of death in childbirth could
be reduced if fully trained and supervised midwives were placed in villages.

> Professionally competent midwives can bring down the maternal death
> rate. The evidence exists to show that the countries that have utilised
> competent midwives to provide maternal health services brought down
> their maternal death rates much quicker than those who did not.
>
> (Kamal 2000)

There are as yet insufficient trained midwives to meet the workforce needs in
hospitals in Pakistan, let alone supply the rural areas. Even if the cultural
safety issues could be resolved to enable students to have a placement in the
villages and the curriculum included community midwifery, there is no one
to teach or mentor the students. There is also the additional problem of
working after marriage being socially and culturally unacceptable.

Chawla (1999: 167) questions whether trained traditional birth attendants can be expected to reduce overall mortality and morbidity rates 'in
the presence of poverty, illiteracy and discrimination'. When exploring the
expectations placed upon the untrained dai, it is evident that she is not in
control of the decision to transfer to hospital; it may be to her credit that she
does not abandon the woman.

In the context of the belief system that considers the dai as essential for
birth, it would appear that her presence ensures that someone undertakes
the dirty work. However, the dai is judged by external standards such as
mortality and morbidity rates and is subsequently blamed for the appall-
ingly high morbidity rates. It would appear that the wider public health
issues, such as poverty, are not factored into the causes of the high morbidity
and mortality rates.

Chawla, in her text on maternity in colonial and post-colonial countries,
reports that dais would continue 'to practice in dangerous cases when there
is no other alternative, if the family did not blame them' (1999: 164). In the
absence of anyone else to take on their role, this seems a reasonable conclusion. Yet dais are rapidly becoming scarce, due to the social repugnance of
their work and possibly the potential for blame. The daughter of a dai in the
research study would rather do any other work than become a dai:

'I am too frightened to take a case.'

(S)

Conclusion

Pollution has been shown to be one thread in the lives of women in Pakistan, particularly the dai. Being born a girl, to be 'on loan' to her birth family until marriage, she will be both blessed and polluted by the blood of menstruation to hold the responsibility of two families' honour. Following which she will experience birth, which is both defining and defiling, attended by a woman considered to have the lowest position in Pakistan society.

The stories collected included examples of dais acting to save lives and of them lacking the authority to influence the actions of others. Sometimes they feared blame from families, though they were rarely blamed by those they cared for. When complications arose, it was the family, not the dai, who took the decision and bore the cost of transferring the woman to hospital. Nevertheless, the dai was often blamed by the hospital for the woman's condition on admission. With the growth in obstetric authority, in the absence of widespread obstetric services, the role of the dai seems to extend to containing blame as well as pollution.

Status, education and gender influence how far blood defiles those who handle it. Doctors, surgeons and female obstetricians also 'deal with' blood. All doctors are highly educated and respected; they are not considered fouled by the handling of blood. Cultural norms associated with blood and pollution have served to keep men out of childbirth; the bleeding woman and the dai are outside the domain of men. Most, if not all, of the obstetricians in Pakistan are women. Muslim women and their husbands prefer that women be attended by female doctors. Although a strongly patriarchal society, the door to a woman's life and birth is kept firmly closed to men. This fact alone may be responsible for the lack of national interest in maternal health and well-being.

References

Abedin, S.M. (1996) Women in Search of Equality, Development and Peace. A Critical Analysis of the Platform for Action. Fourth World Conference on Women, Islamabad, Pakistan. *Journal of Muslim Minority Affairs* 16(1): 73–98.

Alasuutari, P. (1995) *Researching Culture.* London: Sage.

Brasseur, O. (1992) *United Nations Population Fund.* National Committee for Maternal Health, August: 2.

Carroll, L. (1997) Muslim Women and Islamic Divorce in England. *Journal of Muslim Minority Affairs* 17(1): 97–115.

Chawla, J. (1999) Hawa Gola and Mother-in-law's Big Toe. *Midwifery Today,* Winter: 54–59.

Chawla, J. (2000) Crossing Boundaries and Listening Carefully. *MATRIKA – Motherhood and Traditional Resources, Information, Knowledge and Action. Final Report, January 1997–March 2000.* Pakistan.

Chesney, M. (2004) Birth for some women in Pakistan, defining and defiling. Unpublished PhD thesis, University of Sheffield.

Childress, H. (1998) Kinder Ethnographic Writing. *Qualitative Inquiry* 4(2): 249–264.

Collins (1994) *English Dictionary*, 3rd edn. Glasgow: HarperCollins.

Denzin, N.K. (1997) *Interpretive Ethnography: Ethnographic Practices for the 21st Century*. Thousand Oaks, Calif.: Sage.

Douglas, M. (1966) *Purity and Danger*. London: Routledge.

Fikree, F., Jafarey, S.N. and Kureshy, N. (1998) A Community and Hospital Based Study to Examine the Magnitude of Induced Abortion and Associated Gynaecological Morbidity in Karachi Pakistan. *MotherCare*. Karachi: Aga Khan University.

Jeffery, P. Jeffery, R. and Lyon, A. (1988) *Labour Pains and Labour Power*. London: Zed.

Jokhari, A. (2005) An Intervention Involving Traditional Birth Attendants, Perinatal and Maternal Mortality in Pakistan. *New England Journal of Medicine* 352/ May: 2091–2098.

Kamal, I. (2000) *Situation Analysis of Midwifery Training in Sindh*. UNICEF.

Kasi, A.M. (2002) Pakistan's Federal Health Minister's Address to the International Day of the Midwife. *National Committee for Maternal Health Newsletter*, August 2.

Khan, A. (1999) Mobility of Women and Access to Health and Family Planning Services in Pakistan. *Reproductive Health Matters* 7(14): 39–47.

Kristeva, J. (1982) *Powers of Horror: An Essay on Abjection*. New York: Columbia University Press.

Montague, A. (1999) *The Natural Superiority of Women*, 5th edn. London: Altmira.

Norris, P. (1998) *The Story of Eve*. London: Picador.

Pakistan Nurses Association (1992) *History of Nursing in Pakistan*. Pakistan Nursing Council.

Petcheski, R. and Judd, K. (1998) *Negotiating Reproductive Rights. International Reproductive Rights Research Action Group*. London: Sage.

Polkinghorne, D.E. (1995) Narrative Configurations in Qualitative Analysis. In J.A. Hatch and R. Wisniewski (eds) *Life History and Narrative*. Washington DC: Falmer.

Salahi, A. (ed.) (1993) 'Our Dialogue'. The Religious Editor, Arab News, Jeddah. Apkar, Pakistan.

Thompson, C. (1981) A Sense of Sharm: Its Implications for the Position of Women in a Village in Central Asia. *South Asia Research* 39–53.

UNICEF (1989) *Statistical Profile of Women in the Punjab*. Prepared by the Punjab Economic Institute, Shaheen Attiqurehman, Lahore.

WHO (1992) *Traditional Birth Attendants*. A Joint WHO/UNFPA/UNICEF Statement. WHO, Geneva, 11.

Section 4

Leakage and labelling

14 Gynaecology nursing: dirty work, women's work

Sharon C. Bolton

Introduction

Gynaecology is an area of health care that is essentially a woman's world: women nursing women who are experiencing uniquely women's 'problems'. This world defines the gendered experience of nursing, that is, women in a women's job carrying out women's work (Porter 1992). It is also a world that receives scant public recognition due to its association with the private domain of women's reproductive health or, more specifically, 'the catastrophic disintegration' of women's sexual body (Martin 1990: 75). Many issues dealt with on a daily basis by gynaecology nurses are socially 'difficult': cancer, infertility, miscarriage and foetal abnormalities; or socially 'distasteful': termination of pregnancy, urinary incontinence, menstruation and sexually transmitted disease. The 'tainted' (Hughes 1958) nature of gynaecology gives it the social distinction of 'dirty work'. Like many occupations, nursing work, women's work and dirty work are inextricably linked due to an association with the private realm (Lawler 1991). This is never more clearly explicit than in gynaecology, due to its connection with the 'failure and dissolution' of women's bodies (Martin 1990: 75), especially the stigma associated with failed pregnancy (McQueen 1997). And, despite being acknowledged as a distinctive area of health care, gynaecology nursing remains a specialism without specialist status (Webb 1985). The ambiguous position of gynaecology in the 'status hierarchy' of health care, however, does not deter gynaecology nurses from declaring their work as 'special', requiring distinctive knowledge and skills (McQueen 1997; Webb 1985).

There can be little doubt that recourse to women's 'special skills' is a potentially precarious strategy, especially in a feminine profession such as nursing. It pre-supposes essentialist notions of what it is to be a woman: that not only are women more caring, sensitive and emotional than men but that they are also weaker, timid and irrational (Segal 1987). The concept of 'woman' has some legitimacy as a source of shared understanding amongst women (Assiter 1996), but unfortunately many of its defining characteristics are frequently associated with the powerless and subordinate. In setting feminine knowledge, against masculine knowledge, women are actually positioning themselves as the 'second sex' (de Beauvoir 1983; Gherardi 1994) – an inferior status supported by their subordinate position to male health care professionals in a medical division of labour which continues to celebrate and sustain a masculine vision of professional expertise (Davies 1996). Little wonder that it is declared that 'the problem for nursing has been and continues to be the problem of gender' (Witz 1994: 23), and that nurses are repeatedly blamed for perpetuating their inferior status (Mackay 1990).

To completely dismiss the usefulness of claims to uniquely female knowledge would, however, be to assume that the cultural resource of woman is a static category that exists in a different space from the male. It is to imagine that women are discursively defined by the ideology of the feminine, trapped in a symbolic universe, a 'mode of impossibility' (Jardine 1997: 80), from which there can be no escape. And it is to believe, though rarely openly acknowledged, that gender becomes a fixed attribute, a 'universal and historical construct' (Butler 1990; Gherardi 1994: 595; Weedon 1997). These are familiar themes in contemporary feminist thought which, whilst in vehement denial, actually have the same essentialising and universalising qualities as an argument based on biological difference (de Beauvoir 1983; Daly 1979; Firestone 1979).

It is suggested here that this 'negative paradigm' (McNay 1999) is not supported in the scenario portrayed by data collected, over a period of several years, from a group of gynaecology nurses in a North West NHS hospital. In confirmation of previous studies (McQueen 1997; Webb 1985), the gynaecology nurses in this study display how they actively celebrate their status as women carrying out 'dirty work'. Shared meanings are achieved by 'doing' gender and the nurses claim that only they, as women, are able to nurse the gynaecology patient and do it well. Through the use of ceremonial work that continually re-affirms their 'womanly' qualities the gynaecology nurses establish themselves as 'different', as 'special', as the 'Other'.

The gynaecology nurses actively pursue the ideology of 'the good woman/ the good nurse' (Mackay 1990; Abbott and Wallace 1990), but they are not passive, not entirely powerless and do not exist in a separate symbolic universe. The nurses actively 'do' gender by being kind and cruel, gentle and aggressive, emotional and rational, and so the list goes on. They know only too well their position in the stark medical division of labour and the very real consequences of it. Yet their persistence in ensuring the provision of quality health care to women has had a major impact on formal procedure and the attitudes of senior doctors and management. In the day-to-day lived reality of the women's world of gynaecology the multiple meanings of many symbolic universes and past experiences are simultaneously used as cultural resources. That is, gender is a dynamic and continuing process, a distinct social accomplishment that is achieved through the lived experiences of women *and* men (Davies 1996; New 1998; West and Zimmerman 1987). The category of woman and women's identification with it, therefore, is a movable feast (McNay 2000; Pollert 1996; Segal 1987). Thinking about gender in this way displays the 'contradiction, opposition and dynamic' (Pollert 1996: 655) involved in carrying out women's work and dirty work and highlights how spaces are created where the status quo can be challenged and, however gradually, ultimately changed.

Methodology and background

Qualitative data presented in this chapter forms part of a longitudinal study looking at the effects upon the nursing labour process of changes in the management of British public sector services. The focus of the study is a group of gynaecology nurses working in a large North West trust hospital. Fieldwork has been a continuous, though often sporadic, project conducted over a period of several years using semi-structured interviews and observation in two surgical wards and the associated out-patient clinics. Informal contact with clerical staff, cleaners, doctors and managers has also been a valuable source of data. Indeed, it is often the casual conversations which provide the greatest insight into the complexities involved in nursing work, as do the observed reactions of nurses to particular incidents and their interactions with doctors, managers and patients.

The specific group of forty-five gynaecology nurses included in this study exemplifies a particularly close occupational community which may not represent all nursing communities. All staff on the gynaecology unit, with the exception of doctors, are from the local, racially and economically diverse, area. They can be safely described as coming from predominantly white, working-class backgrounds, and many accounts, especially from the older members of staff, reflect a celebration of their origins. Over half of the nurses have worked together for an average of fifteen years, with the length of service for senior staff being between twenty and twenty-five years.

Within the social network of the hospital many of the gynaecology nurses are renowned for their 'in the face' attitude, their 'bolshiness', their 'manic' sense of humour and their close-knit community. They have created their own coping mechanisms, their own methods of letting off steam and their own ways of asserting their collective identity – an identity based not only upon shared experiences of the gendered nature of nursing work and a mutual confidence in their status as health care professionals but also a belief in their distinctive position as gynaecology nurses.

Women's work

Nursing is commonly associated with the ideological feminine qualities of being loving and kind, and the vocational drive to care for people. Whilst wanting recognition for their technical skills and unique knowledge, nurses continue to identify with and willingly regenerate the stereotypical image of the 'angel of mercy'.

Nursing is something I felt I wanted to do for a long time. I always felt I wanted to care for things: people, animals whatever.

(Senior Staff Nurse, July 1994)

I'd always wanted to be a nurse from being tiny. I know it sounds twee, but I wanted to help people. I suppose everybody says that. But I also did it for self-gratification as well, because it gives me a feeling of belonging and being important in the community. I suppose my reasons are quite selfish really.

(Ward Sister, July 1994)

Their comments confirm the underlying social expectation that nursing is a vocation, involving altruism and an overwhelming drive to 'care' for people, rather than offering a career involving choice and skill. This sense of vocation and commitment to the value of caring for people is seen as belonging to an essentially 'women's world'. The nursing workforce is 90 per cent female[1] and nurses frequently defend the status of nursing as 'women's work' by citing examples of how they feel 'men just couldn't do the job':

I do think nursing is gender specific, especially on gynaecology. It would be extremely difficult for a male nurse to give the same kind of support. I'm not saying it's impossible, because I feel that would be too big a generalisation. There are some male nurses that would be able to give good practical care, but I feel the emotional care would not be of the same quality.

(Ward Sister, July 1994)

Some nurses add to this and express concern about men having a role to play in gynaecology services and the delivery of health care in general:

I have very mixed feelings about male gynaecologists, not just male gynaecology nurses. I really feel that men should be horse doctors and not let loose on people at all! They would be all right treating animals because they only have to worry about the technical skills involved and not about the patient's emotional well being.

(Ward Sister, July 1997)

I think women would be much better at delivering all forms of health care at all levels. Most of the consultants are male, I'm surprised at that. They do try and understand patients' problems, but often it comes across in a patronising manner. They just don't have what it takes. I do think they're in the wrong job. Why don't they stick to being engineers or something? I think it's a strange world that gives men these jobs and women have difficulty getting there, especially in the top ranks.

(Senior Staff Nurse, July 1994)

From the above statements it can be seen that those interviewed appear to have been attracted into nursing because of the possibility of using skills they feel they already possess as women. They draw on gender as a symbolic resource in order to assert their claim concerning their possession of uniquely feminine qualities such as being loving and kind and having the drive to care for people. However, this 'special' knowledge is also gained through their practical experiences as women, daughters, partners and mothers. The physical intimacy and the domestic duties that are commonly regarded as the work of a nurse rely on women's lived experiences of a gendered division of tasks, first in play and, ultimately, in paid and unpaid labour.

The assumed proclivity of women towards this type of work, however, belongs very much in the symbolic realm. For instance, the caring instinct, seen as an essential prerequisite for nursing, is often equated with the maternal instinct (Lawler 1991; Porter 1992; Whitbeck 1993). The ideology of the 'natural mother' is fundamental to the image of the nurse: 'the world turns to women for mothering, and this fact silently attaches itself to many a job description' (Hochschild 1983: 170). Many nurses on the gynaecology unit feel their status as mothers does give them deeper insights and, therefore, make them more skilled at managing certain emotionally charged situations. This is clearly linked to the way nurses continually refer to miscarriage and termination of pregnancy as the most demanding but also the most rewarding aspect of their work. Whilst believing that their drive to care is instinctual, the nurses are also very aware that these 'insights' are drawn from their everyday experiences as mothers:

> I think being a mother gives me an added edge when coping with certain situations on the ward, and not just because some patients behave like naughty children! I think I understand better some of the difficulties many of our women patients are experiencing. I'm not just talking about the emotional difficulties, but the social difficulties; like are the children being cared for? How could a male nurse have insights like these? Of course it is not necessary to have gone through an experience to identify and empathise with a patient's experiences, but it must help. As a working mother I feel I could nurse on a male ward and understand how patients feel, if they have concerns about their jobs and their families for instance, but I don't think it can work the other way. I don't think a male nurse can come on here and understand the concerns of the women patients.
>
> (Ward Sister, July 1994)

The nurses, in line with other studies concerning caring labour, view their work as highly skilled, not only technically but also in the way they are able to care for patients (James 1989; Latimer 2000). However, the notion of caring as a skill has proved to be problematic. Since the elements of efficient caring are seen as being rooted in the natural sphere of a woman's abilities, they are 'invisible' skills that are not rendered visible when used in the productive sector (Bolton 2004; Tancred 1995). Caring labour is not categorised as skilled work because the world of 'work' is still defined in terms of men's experiences of productive labour. This is clearly highlighted in the way nurses are described as 'semi-professional' (Etzioni 1969) or 'feminine professional' (Lorentzon 1990). Gender ideology expects nurses to 'care' without questioning what it actually entails. Hence, no monetary or status value is placed upon the 'women's work' of nursing (Abbott and Wallace 1990; Bolton 2004; Lawler 1991).

Unwittingly, the nurses appear to strengthen the ideology that women and caring go hand in hand. In celebrating their ability to offer care to patients they rely on the essentialist notions of women's 'difference' – their identities as women carrying out women's work and their status as 'caring' professionals are inextricably linked. The nurses actively do gender as they draw on the category of 'woman' and their own experiences in the domestic sphere in order to constantly create and re-create the image of the altruistically motivated caring professional. Caring labour is integrated into every dimension of their daily practice, but it is not the only element of what it takes to be a nurse (Latimer 2000).

Dirty work

In a 'non-touching culture' the requirement for nurses to endure close physical proximity to patients and carry out body care activities has meant that elements of nursing have an association with 'dirty work' (Lawler 1991). For the gynaecology nurse this association is much stronger. The women's world of the gynaecology unit is an area of health care that deals with infertility, reproductive cancers, terminations of pregnancy and miscarriages, most of which are uniquely 'women's problems' that normally remain firmly in the private domain (Martin 1990; McQueen 1997). As de Beauvoir describes, except as objects of male desire, women's bodies do not 'have reference to the rest of the world' and are not afforded positive value: 'The feminine sex organ is mysterious even to the woman herself, concealed, mucous and humid, as it is; it bleeds each month, it is often sullied with body fluids, it has a secret and perilous life of its own' (de Beauvoir 1983: 406).

The gynaecology nurses in this study feel their attention to the bodily realities of women's reproductive health renders their work unique, unrecognised and often socially taboo. They are fully aware that one of the potentially most 'mysterious' and 'perilous' products of a woman's body is a dead or dying and/or malformed foetus. A nurse describes how her feelings when handling a dying foetus moved from repugnance, to acceptance and then to a real involvement in the process:

When I first started this job I would do anything not to have to deliver the dead foetus and dispose of it or have to dress it etc. My stomach would heave and I'd feel a sense of despair for each and every one. I thought this is one of the worst jobs I've ever done in nursing – the touch, the smell, ugh, just everything about it. I then managed to block it off for a while but now that I'm used to the physical aspects of the handling I really want to care for the foetus and ensure that it's recognised and remembered as a lost life. The very fact that parts of our job aren't very nice is what makes it so important.

(Staff Nurse, July 2000)

In its connection with 'dirty work', the work of the gynaecology nurse can be classified as 'physically, socially and morally tainted' (Hughes 1958: 122): physically tainted due to its association with the body, death and abnormality; socially tainted through the regular contact with unmentionable topics such as termination of pregnancy, incontinence, infertility and sexually transmitted disease; and morally tainted because what should remain private and invisible is made public and rendered visible. As Ashforth and Kreiner usefully point out: 'the common denominator among tainted jobs is not so much their specific attributes but the visceral repugnance of people to them' (1999: 415). The nurses on this particular gynaecology unit are very aware of public perceptions of their work:

People don't seem to know what we do in gynae. I suspect they don't really want to know. They ask what you do and you say 'I'm a nurse'. They say 'Oh, that's interesting. Where do you work?' I say 'gynaecology' and they just say 'Oh'. End of conversation.

(Staff Nurse, June 1999)

For the gynaecology nurse it is the 'dirty' nature of their work that makes it special. They view their work as 'significant and honourable' (Ackroyd and Crowdy 1992; Ashforth and Kreiner 1999) and defend its status as a specialist area requiring special skills:

That could be my baby in there and I like to think that if it was, someone like me would be seeing to it. That is a woman and a mother. Some think that because it isn't a full term pregnancy then it's not human. But it is and we have to remember that. I hear tales about how it used to be, taking babies away like you would someone's gallstones and I'm appalled. That's going back to a time when we had less say in how patients were to be treated. With male doctors in charge it's little wonder things like that happened. I think the clinical nurse manager and the senior sister have done a wonderful job of making people aware of the basic humanity of the situation. It's not always easy for us, but if you want an easy job don't come on here in the first place.

(Staff Nurse, May 1997)

This nurse draws on her lived experiences and identity as a mother and also the caring image that this implies. Her symbolic resource, however, does not equate with the patriarchal feminine. She recognises the need for caring, nurturing and self-sacrifice but also displays a determination, decisiveness and sometimes apparent ruthlessness that are not normally associated with the 'ideal' woman. Ambivalence when dealing with patients undergoing late terminations due to social reasons often leaks out and nurses pass cruel comments between them or are observed to be more abrupt in their dealings with some patients. Yet most frequently, nurses are relaxed and open in their interactions with each other and with patients. They are very tactile, openly embracing each other or stroking patients' arms or holding their hands. These are the complexities and contradictions involved in the 'conduct of care' (Latimer 2000) and represent a clear example of the combination of the caring and instrumental, so aptly described by Strauss *et al.* (1982) as 'sentimental work'.

In doing 'dirty work' the nurses also 'do' gender but there is little sense of being tied into a particular symbolic universe. The nurses seek to enhance their status by referring to the feminine qualities that make their work special but, as the following statement shows, they actively dissociate from any notion of women being passive, irrational or weak:

Sometimes I get really mad. No one has any idea what we do for these women. It's a closed world and who wants to know about ugly dead babies – the common attitude is 'well, she can always have another one'. That's not the point is it? And then, of course, what we do for these women is not recognised as anything special – it's just something that we do. Midwives deliver live healthy babies in a routine way and get the title of 'practitioner' and are seen as being superior to us and yet they won't do what we do. Yes, they do have stillbirths sometimes and they follow much the same procedure as we do, but they don't deal with abnormalities like we do and social late terminations and all the connotations this holds for the patient. It's because midwives are supposed to have a higher range of technical tasks than we do, so they get more money and status and what we do for these women is seen as something that a nurse will do naturally. But could you do what we do? There are not a lot of people who could. I know I said a man couldn't do this job, but a lot of women couldn't do it either. You have to really, truly care and yet at the same time be able to cope with caring too much and remain professional. If that's not a skill I don't know what is.

(Staff Nurse, May 1997)

For the gynaecology nurse women's work and dirty work represent skilled work that requires uniquely women's knowledge. It allows them to celebrate their identity as 'woman'. They grasp every opportunity to have it recognised as such, with some success. Their determination that women who miscarry should have the same care and attention as women who give birth to full-term, healthy babies has now received national recognition.[2] Their now formalised procedure for dealing with an aborted foetus does not fit with a task-centred, masculine model of health care – the babies are bathed, dressed, photographed and presented to the grieving parents. The language of the procedure recommends 'care', 'warmth', 'gentleness' and 'sensitivity'. Yes, they are confirming this type of work as 'women's work', but there is a growing appreciation, supported with material resources, of it as contributing significantly to the quality of women's reproductive health care and it has had a major impact on various health professionals' approach, including senior doctors and management.

The lived experiences of the gynaecology nurses serve to alter what it means to be a woman (Pollert 1996; McNay 2000). They are small steps in a small world but they are not insignificant. For instance, the changes they have instituted in the care of women who have miscarried have given parents (fathers and mothers) the confidence to unwrap their grief away from the safe haven of the gynaecology ward. They are no longer made to feel ashamed of giving birth to a malformed or unviable foetus; the father is no longer excluded as a bystander. They are both able to see their baby as a beautiful lost child. In turn this helps to dissolve the socially 'tainted' aura and feminine mystery surrounding such an event.

Conclusion

This particular nursing community is distinctive – special. This, of course, can prove to be a methodological weakness. Not all nursing communities can be thought of in this way. However, it is the distinctiveness of this group of nurses that highlights, so very well, what it is to 'do' gender. They are women in a women's world and, in many ways, exemplify the symbolic woman. This is especially paradoxical for the gynaecology nurse. More importantly, perhaps, these nurses represent far more than a cultural construction; they also show how the category of woman is historically and socially embedded. These nurses cannot be reduced to discursively defined characters playing on a symbolically constructed stage. Their lives are not just made up of abstract signs but based on lived experiences. Some draw upon their understanding as mothers, some as carers of their own mothers, some on bitter memories of an impoverished childhood. They also identify their work and their own status as health care professionals in relation to others in the structured divisions of health care. Whilst continually proclaiming their work to be special they are aware that they are defined as of lesser 'value' in relation to junior doctors who carry the mantle of the male medical model of health care and in their relation to the sanctified status of the midwife as the legitimate guardian of healthy and productive female bodies. For many this would merely mean that the nurses, whilst they may identify themselves as autonomous subjects, are actually caught up in a gender system that involves an endless re-production of the same (Butler 1990). What is the use of opposition or alternatives when there is little likelihood, and definitely no 'final guarantee', that anything will change (Weedon 1997)? The way the gynaecology nurses celebrate their status as 'feminine professionals' would appear to endorse this 'negative paradigm' (McNay 2000).

Nevertheless, though failing to resist the ideological image of the patriarchal feminine, they do resist its subordinate position in a differentiated social order. The nurses featured in this study highlight how the shifting category of 'woman' does not stand alone, female experience (as diverse as it is) shares the same space and cultural resources as the male and will have an impact upon it, thus showing how even the smallest acts may 'transcend their immediate sphere in order to transform collective behaviour and norms' (McNay 2000: 4). This is confirmed in the way the nurses have introduced new ways of dealing with the 'dirty work' involved in failed pregnancy. They have brought into the public realm an oft misunderstood human tragedy and created new understandings that have now been translated into formal policy and procedure and widely accepted as 'best practice'.

The voices of the gynaecology nurses highlight how their lives are made up of both symbolic and material dimensions. In 'doing' gender the nurses seek to utilise their 'special' knowledge and experience to change the women's world of reproductive health. In their celebration of women's work and 'dirty work' they actively define a distinctive kind of 'other' with which they can challenge the status quo.

Acknowledgement

This is a revised and shortened version of an article originally published in *Gender, Work and Organisation*, 2005, vol. 12, no. 2, pp. 169–186, with generous permission of the publisher.

Notes

1 Though it is well documented how men hold a disproportionate amount of senior posts (Davies 1996; Porter 1992).
2 This particular gynaecology unit was one of the first in Britain to informally introduce different ways of dealing with miscarriage in the early 1980s – that is, different from the male model of health care where distance was maintained and dead babies taken from mothers straight after birth and their bodies disposed of by the hospital. The gynaecology nurses' innovative ideas have been endorsed by

SANDS (Stillbirth and Neo-natal Death Society) and now fully adopted as procedure by NHS hospitals.

References

Abbott, P. and Wallace, C. (1990) *The Sociology of the Caring Professions*. Basingstoke: Falmer Press.

Ackroyd, S. and Crowdy, P. (1992) 'Can Culture be Managed? Working with "Raw" Material: The Case of the English Slaughtermen'. *Personnel Review* 19(5): 3–13.

Ashforth, B. and Kreiner, G. (1999) '"How Can You Do It?" Dirty Work and the Challenge of Constructing a Positive Identity'. *Academy of Management Review* 24(2): 413–434.

Assiter, A. (1996) *Enlightened Women*. London: Routledge.

Bolton, S. (2004) 'Conceptual Confusions: Emotion Work as Skilled Work'. In C. Warhurst, E. Keep and I. Grugulis (eds) *The Skills that Matter*. London: Palgrave, pp. 19–37.

Butler, J. (1990) *Gender Trouble: Feminism and the Subversion of Identiy*. London: Routledge.

Daly, M. (1979) *Gyn/Ecology*. London: Women's Press.

Davies, C. (1996) 'The Sociology of the Professions and the Profession of Gender'. *Sociology* 30(4): 661–678.

de Beauvoir, S. (1983) *The Second Sex*. Harmondsworth: Penguin.

Etzioni, A. (1969) *The Semi-Professions and Their Organization*. New York: Free Press.

Firestone, S. (1979) *The Dialectic of Sex: The Case for Feminist Revolution*. London: Women's Press.

Gherardi, S. (1994) 'The Gender We Think, the Gender We Do in Our Everyday Organizational Lives'. *Human Relations* 47(6): 591–610.

Hochschild, A. (1983) *The Managed Heart: Commercialization of Human Feeling*. Berkeley: University of California Press.

Hughes, E.C. (1958) *Men and their Work*. Glencoe, Ill: Free Press.

James, N. (1989) 'Emotional Labour: Skill and Work in the Social Regulation of Feeling'. *Sociological Review* 37(1): 15–42.

Jardine, A. (1997) 'Notes for an Analysis'. In S. Kemp and J. Squires (eds) *Feminisms*. Oxford: Oxford University Press.

Latimer, J. (2000) *The Conduct of Care: Understanding Nursing Practice*. Oxford: Blackwell Science.

Lawler, J. (1991) *Behind the Screens: Nursing, Somology, and the Problem of the Body*. Melbourne: Churchill Livingstone.

Lorentzon, M. (1990) 'Professional Status and Managerial Tasks: Feminine Service Ideology in British Nursing and Social Work'. In P. Abbott and C. Wallace (eds) *The Sociology of the Caring Professions*. Basingstoke: Falmer Press.

Mackay, L. (1990) 'Nursing: Just Another Job?' In P. Abbott and C. Wallace (eds) *The Sociology of the Caring Professions*. Basingstoke: Falmer Press.

McNay, L. (2000) *Gender and Agency*. Cambridge: Polity Press.

McQueen, A. (1997) 'Gynaecology Nursing'. *Journal of Advanced Nursing* 25: 767–774.

Martin, E. (1990) 'Science and Women's Bodies'. In M. Jacobus, E. Fox Keller and S. Shuttleworth (eds) *Body Politics*. London: Routledge.

New, C. (1998) 'Realism, Deconstruction and the Feminist Standpoint'. *Journal for the Theory of Social Behaviour* 28(3): 349–372.

Pollert, A. (1996) 'Gender and Class Revisited; or, the Poverty of Patriarchy'. *Sociology* 30(4): 639–659.

Porter, S. (1992) 'Women in a Women's Job: The Gendered Experience of Nurses'. *Sociology of Health and Illness* 14(4): 510–527.

Segal, L. (1987) *Is the Future Female? Troubled Thoughts on Contemporary Feminism.* New York: Peter Bedrick Books.

Strauss, A., Fagerhaugh, S., Suczek, B. and Wiener, C. (1982) 'Sentimental Work in the Technologized Hospital'. *Sociology of Health and Illness* 4(3): 255–278.

Tancred, P. (1995) 'Women's Work: A Challenge to the Sociology of Work'. *Gender, Work and Organisation* 2(1): 11–20.

Webb, C. (1985) 'Gynaecology Nursing: A Compromising Situation'. *Journal of Advanced Nursing* 10: 47–54.

Weedon, C. (1997) *Feminist Practice and Poststructuralist Theory.* Oxford: Blackwell.

West, C. and Zimmerman, D. (1987) 'Doing Gender'. *Gender and Society* 1: 125–151.

Whitbeck, C. (1993) 'The Maternal Instinct'. In J. Trebilcot (ed.) *Mothering Essays in Feminist Theory.* Lanham: Rowman and Littlefield.

Witz, A. (1994) 'The Challenge of Nursing'. In J. Gabe, D. Kellener and G. Williams (eds) *Challenging Medicine.* London: Routledge.

15 Containing the 'leaky' body: female urinary incontinence and formal health care

Joanne Jordan

Introduction

In this chapter I use two sources of data to examine conflicting definitions of female urinary incontinence (FUI) and the consequences of this conflict for the provision of continence health care: first, the contents of a range of written material given to patients attending specialist nurse-led continence clinics, including general health promotion literature as well as more specific (in)continence literature; and second, data derived from interviews with ten specialist continence nurses/advisers (SCNs) working in a range of community and community/acute Trusts. Combining the evidence from both sets of data, I demonstrate the presence of conflicting understandings of FUI, how these understandings are embedded in underlying cultural expectations of the female body and, finally, how these meanings come together to inform the provision of continence services. I show how the interplay of conflicting understandings of FUI contributes to a situation in which different health care professionals communicate 'mixed messages' to women about incontinence, thereby serving to militate against coherent service provision.

Background

Although there is no universally accepted definition of urinary incontinence (Continence Foundation 2000), the International Continence Society (ICS) defines urinary incontinence as 'the complaint of any involuntary leakage of urine' (Abrams *et al.* 2003: 38), while the Department of Health's (DoH) definition outlines incontinence as 'the involuntary or inappropriate passing of urine and/or faeces that has an impact on social functioning or hygiene' (DoH 2000: 7). The lack of uniformity, as well as the content of the definitions offered above, highlights an essential problematic: while the ICS definition makes leakage of urine categorically a 'complaint', the DoH definition is more ambiguous, endorsing the notion that incontinence can only be defined by individuals (unspecified) on the basis of their personal assessment of the degree to which loss is '*inappropriate*', as well as its level of '*impact on social functioning or hygiene*'.

The reported prevalence for urinary incontinence in women varies widely (Dolan *et al.* 1999; Dolman 2001; van der Vaart *et al.* 2002), with van der Vaart *et al.* quoting studies which report anything between 14 and 71.5 per cent. This variation in part reflects the disparities in definition alluded to above, as well as heterogeneity in age, subjects, methodology and the effects of under-reporting, a phenomenon typically related to the embarrassment or stigma associated with the condition (Dolan *et al.* 1999; Continence Foundation 2000). Currently, incontinence of the urine and faeces costs the National Health Service (NHS) approximately £424 million pounds per annum in terms of care; in the region of £80 million worth of absorbent products alone are purchased by the NHS annually (Thomas 2003). The figure of £424 million, which is widely acknowledged as a conservative estimate of expenditure, represents approximately 0.85 per cent of the total cost of the NHS (Thakar *et al.* 2003).

It is only in the past two decades that urinary incontinence has become the focus of systematic non-clinical research attention. However, this research has tended to focus on psychosocial impact, to the detriment of other aspects of the social and cultural context in which urinary incontinence is experienced (Peake *et al.* 1999). In terms of psychosocial impact, research has highlighted the overall detrimental effect on quality of life, including in terms of, for example, psychological well-being, social interactions and activities, and impact on family, including carers (Coyne *et al.* 2003; Fultz *et al.* 2003, 2005; Lee 2004; Shaw 2001). According to Mitteness and Barker (1995), increased attention to urinary incontinence since the beginning of the 1980s has been fuelled largely by a rising elderly population, resulting in a disproportionate number of psychosocial studies being targeted at this group. Significantly, there has been even less attention paid to the social and cultural context of the treatment/management of urinary incontinence, including in the context of service delivery. Given its emphasis on services and the 'gendered meanings' (Peake *et al.* 1999: 269) of urinary incontinence which inform these services, this chapter thus contributes new insights into how FUI is understood and responded to within formal health care and the implications of this understanding for the care women receive.

Female urinary incontinence, biomedicine and the pursuit of 'normality'

The dominance of the biomedical model as the central paradigm of medical care is, by now, well documented. In outlining the model's fundamental principles, Blaxter (2004) highlights how, typically, care proceeds on a set of assumptions about the body and the processes through which disease/ illness occurs. Of particular relevance is the notion that disease and illness represent deviation from a *normal* state of affairs, with the medical profession determining the standards of normality against which the presence (or absence) of disease and illness is judged (Lupton 2003). The setting of such standards of 'normality' is evident in the written literature given out to patients using continence services. This written material is of two main types: generic leaflets designed, for the most part, by pharmaceutical companies and interested organisations such as charities, and specific leaflets designed at the local level by incontinence staff themselves, primarily specialist nurses. Space restrictions permit only a few examples taken from a range of such material.

> In a normal bladder, the bladder muscle only contracts when you decide to urinate, usually when the bladder is full. In detrusor instability the bladder muscle contracts without warning.

> Adults usually go to the toilet between four and seven times a day, and no more than once during the night. When we feel the need to go to the toilet, we can usually hold on until it is convenient for us to go.

> Most women have some leakage of urine during pregnancy but most bladder problems get better after delivery. Pelvic floor exercises can help with these problems and can be done before, during and after pregnancy . . . Some women develop stress incontinence after the menopause. Even before the menopause, some woman (*sic*) may notice that stress incontinence becomes worse before a period. Occasionally, stress incontinence occurs after having a hysterectomy and some operations on the bladder.

> The normal bladder fills and empties 4–6 times each day depending on how much you drink.

> Most people empty their bladder 6 times a day. It is considered normal to get up once at night to pass urine.

> Stress incontinence means leakage when you cough, sneeze or exercise . . . It is most usual in women and is caused by a weak bladder outlet and pelvic floor muscles.

> Many common problems are caused by an overactive bladder . . .
>
> * some people may not get there in time so they have an accident (called **urge incontinence**)
> * needing to go very often – more than 7 times a day (called **frequency**)

The above statements set the standards by which bodily working and, by extension, personal behaviour, are to be assessed as 'normal', and thus, as 'problematic'. They represent a cogent means by which the health care profession establishes the basis of the 'problem' of incontinence through a linking of standards of (female) normality with bodily dysfunction. What are ostensibly a range of neutral medical categories become conflated with social norms, in that correlations are established between 'proper' biological functioning and 'proper' social conduct; for example, the medical category 'frequency' serves as a social norm guiding the frequency with which women are expected to, that is *should*, visit the toilet, in this case, no more than seven times in a day.

The normative equation of 'normal' biological functioning with appropriate or acceptable social behaviour is further evidenced by the systematic referencing of the notion of bodily *control*. Thus, the value and validity of such control are underscored, in large part by drawing attention to the negative impact of 'losing' control, in this case by not being able to prevent the leakage of urine from the body. Not only are unambiguous statements made concerning the need to regain, and means of regaining, control over bladder and bowel function, but the use of such words as 'weak', weaknesses', 'improve', 'learn', 'choice' and 'embarrassment' further endorses the idea that incontinence represents a departure from what is 'morally acceptable' behaviour. In this regard, Kirmayer's insistence on the importance of metaphor in expressing underlying 'affectively charged emotional schemata' (1992: 337) is instructive because it enables insight into how the language used in the written literature expresses basic cultural imperatives, in this case, that of the 'moral' (autonomous and contained) self.

Through the provision of detailed instructions about what can be done to cure or alleviate incontinence, which accompany the information given about its causes, the onus is placed firmly on the individual (woman) to adopt the means (primarily by following the written and verbal advice offered by specialist continence practitioners) by which she can achieve continence and, thus, behave in accordance with relevant norms of personal bodily control and hygiene. The following extracts give some flavour of the ways in which the importance and means of achieving bodily control are communicated in the written literature.

> Emptying your bladder is under your control and you can choose the time and place.

> A bladder retraining programme will help you learn how to control your bladder by gradually encouraging your bladder to hold more urine and to empty only when it is convenient for you.

> Pelvic floor exercises strengthen these muscles and enable you to improve the control of your bladder and bowels.

> Does your bladder leak when you cough, sneeze, laugh or jump? Losing control of the bladder, even just a little, can be upsetting and can cause embarrassment and discomfort.

Usually the pelvic floor muscles are able to stop leakage of urine or bowel motion, but sometimes weaknesses occur and the muscle sags. This may be due to childbirth, lack of exercise, the change of life or just getting older. Weak muscles give less control, and you may leak when you cough, laugh, sneeze, or exercise.

Bladder retraining is all about you taking control of your bladder, not the other way round.

The preceding analysis has used written evidence to establish the bifurcate conceptual status of urinary incontinence. On the one hand, it is located firmly in the medical domain, as the written leaflets spell out its physiological status as a manifestation of bodily deterioration. On the other hand, it is positioned just as firmly in the social domain, as a personal problem of lack of bodily control and the transgression of conventions governing social behaviour. Throughout, the notion of the *particular* vulnerability of the female body to physical decline as a result of menstruation, bearing and nurturing children and the menopause is evident. However, what is also evident is a discourse emphasising that this vulnerability need not, necessarily, compel a trajectory of female bodily degeneration. In a nutshell, urinary incontinence can be cured. Using data from interviews conducted with SCNs, the remainder of this chapter examines the current tension between these two views of FUI as they inform the provision of health care: on the one hand, as a biological 'inevitability', and, on the other, as 'predictable' but not necessarily prescriptive of how women need experience their biological and social selves.

The data from interviews is, in the context of the analysis presented here, treated as a valid means of inferring knowledge and behaviour occurring outside of the immediate context of the interview (see Silverman 2001 for a discussion of the different ways of using interview data). Adopting this approach, and using thematic content analysis (Green and Thorogood 2004), a number of related contributory factors, all linked to the ways in which FUI is conceptualised and treated/managed within the formal health care system, are evident.

Treating urinary incontinence: a focus on the individual and conservative care

As indicated in the preceding analysis, for the purposes of diagnosis the SCNs approach FUI using an essentially biomedical understanding. Accordingly, FUI is seen as a symptom (or set of symptoms) of some underlying physiological dysfunction, whether this be, for example, a weakening of the pelvic floor muscles, post-menopausal oestrogen deficiency or an overactive bladder. Again, in line with a biomedical approach, a range of examinations and investigations, varying in their degree of technological complexity and invasiveness, are used for the purposes of clinical assessment, diagnosis and decision-making regarding appropriate care-giving. However, it is at this point that the SCNs' employment of, and dependency on, a biomedical model of care starts to wane. Thus, in contradistinction to the wholesale 'technological imperative' typically associated with biomedicine (Nettleton and Gustafsson 2002), SCNs are painstakingly selective in their use (including in terms of referral) of technologically driven treatments, instead being firmly committed to a range of conservative measures pursued over the long term, with referral onwards for other, typically more invasive forms of treatment only being undertaken as a last resort. Simply put, there is no rush to surgery in the care offered to women by SCNs. Instead, in line with the messages conveyed in the written literature, it is the women themselves who, at least in the first instance, are expected to make a commitment to curing *themselves* of their incontinence with the support and encouragement of the SCNs. It is in this context that, depending on the identified underlying cause(s) of incontinence, the SCNs use two initial forms of treatment: pelvic floor exercises and bladder retraining (behaviour therapy).

> 'They don't go onto urodynamics until everything else has failed, like they do behaviour therapy . . . And put them onto pelvic floors, give them healthy lifestyle . . . Wouldn't start into it [the medication] immediately, for stress incontinence I'd make sure they start their pelvic muscles because that would be the baseline of all management . . . and I would start them, I would look into their lifestyle, reduce their tea and coffee, bladder retraining.'

> 'It really takes 10–12 weeks to see a benefit, some more than others that have been motivated and done it correctly, you will see a better improvement. If we see good improvement and . . . we will keep them on . . . I would certainly keep them a minimum of six months, so I would and maybe if they feel things to them are cured, I'll bring them back and review them maybe six months later.'

> 'And, probably do a combination of treatments where we'll try to modify the fluid intake, try to do a toileting programme, a bladder retraining programme, plus pelvic floor muscle exercises because . . . none of those things will cause her any harm and all three are necessary regardless of what her problem . . . Most definitely we would try conservative treatments first.'

> 'I personally think that the simpler it is the better. So if you can make it simple, so if you can treat a patient using nothing more than bladder retraining and pelvic floor exercise and get success then that's what you should be doing. I am not one of these people who sticks every urge incontinent patient on medication, I don't think it's appropriate. I will

introduce medication if we're having a problem, you know, and the patient isn't moving forward . . . It's as long as they need basically . . . I would only refer them on if they're not progressing but if they're progressing, no matter how slowly, I'll stick with them.'

Of course, the practice of placing the responsibility for the achievement of health on the individual (patient) has been comprehensively critiqued from a number of different positions (Bunton *et al.* 1995; Foucault 1988, 1991; Lupton 1995; Rees Jones 2001). From the SCNs' perspective, however, while they acknowledge that their treatment focuses attention on individual women, requires considerable ongoing effort on their part, and is subject to scrutiny over an extended period of time by the nurses themselves, they see this as intrinsically appropriate, in that it both enables women to become continent and, more fundamentally, 'liberates' them from a health care system which both trivialises FUI and makes it subject to an overly medical approach through, for example, a 'rush to surgery'. Two specific mani-festations of the trivialisation of FUI were the focus of considerable SCN criticism: first, in terms of the marginalisation of incontinence in the context of health care education, training and provision; and, second, in terms of the attitudes of health service personnel, most notably GPs.

'Because continence is not one of the major health problems that the DoH . . . that's where the monies are poured into. We're like a subsidi-ary of the elderly. We're not!! It's [continence] very very important . . . And I don't think it [continence] will ever get a high profile, not unless we have a female PM who has had lots of children!'

'There was a lot of patients in the community that DNs were only going into purely for continence issues and they were only being reviewed every six months and with their case loads being so big it was the bottom of the pile and a lot of the time they either weren't reviewed or it just wasn't a priority . . . And they were just, there was no active treat-ment sought.'

'It [the service] is more of a high priority now and it's more recognised. They [women patients] were going to GPs and GPs were saying "Agh, its just your age, its just part of life" . . . They [GPs] now have realised they have a continence service and they're now very willing to refer them to us.'

'And we've tried, we have been fighting a losing battle with the GPs, but the GPs still tell them they're sending them for pads, right. So . . . but they have now got the message that they will not get pads so they just don't come.'

'generally the referrals that we get are based on patients looking for products because nobody knows that you can be treated or the GPs are saying things like "ach, what do you expect, you're 45" or "you've had five children" and therein lies our problem because we, in this Trust, have moved away from just throwing packets of pads at patients and offering them treatment but we can't get the GPs to move with us. They're still saying to patients "ach, I'll refer you for a wee packet of pads".'

'My biggest problem are the GPs, I still get referral letters saying "Mrs such and such needs pads". When women go to their GP they should be telling them what can be done for them . . . giving them the proper information . . . not saying "Right you are, you need pads, I'll refer you to the incontinence team".'

'When I walk into a surgery, I can hear them [the GPs] saying "Oh, here comes the wet nurse!" . . . That's still the attitude many GPs have, that we're a pad service for people who are incontinent.'

The above statements make explicit the SCNs' awareness of varying degrees of apathy, even muted opposition, on the part of some health professionals to the proactive promotion of continence. They highlight a set of cultural assumptions that normalise the gendered nature of FUI, thereby relegating it to the world of 'women's troubles' and, consequently, rendering it relatively trivial and worthy only of reactive management (typically, the use of pads) rather than proactive treatment. Of course, not all colleagues were so characterised, and even in relation to those they considered indifferent to their work, some of the SCNs could identify a trend towards increased acknowledgement of the validity of continence promotion. Although not made explicit by any of the SCNs, the link between what they identified as individual examples of the trivialisation of FUI and its systematic marginalisation within the formal health care system is clear; both are founded on the same cultural assumptions that promote what Peake *et al.* (1999: 274) call the 'gendered inevitability of incontinence', leading to its downgrading in terms of both individual practitioner and institutional prioritisation. Indeed, it is only in the last ten years or so that specialist continence services have emerged; the SCNs could account for this emergence, not on the grounds of any considered clinical and/or policy prioritisation, but, much more prosaically, because of the need to reduce Trust spend on absorbent products. Some of the SCNs were personally responsible for monitoring this spend; while none of them objected to this component of their work, at no point was it ever proposed as a justification for their efforts to promote continence, the latter always being portrayed as an entirely valid end in itself.

SCNs saw their work as doubly frustrated on the grounds that significant numbers of women, both patients and others whom they perceived as unlikely to avail themselves of continence services, shared the same set of cultural expectations of FUI as identified for some health service colleagues. Care needs to be taken not to overstate this phenomenon; alongside the dissenters, SCNs identified significant numbers of women who acknowledged the validity of conservative treatment and followed, sometimes enthusiastically, personal care programmes. However, one issue in particular brought into sharp relief the chasm of understanding separating SCNs and those women who refused to concur with recommended treatment, namely, the prescription of absorbent products. While SCNs saw the issuing of 'pads' as something to be done only in specific circumstances, and *not* issuing them as an effective means of encouraging women to work towards continence, they described how many women validated their incontinence as something to be expected and accommodated, and viewed pads as an entirely appropriate means of such accommodation. Professional colleagues, in particular GPs, were implicated in the perpetuation of this mindset.

'But there's a lot come where they only come . . . "I'm here just because I want my pads, I don't want any active treatment."'

'Depends how motivated the patient is . . . just depends on the motivation. And you know how motivated the patient is when she comes to you with that chart all filled in . . . Like I have them coming and they come to me and they think I'm a quick fix for pads and I don't give out pads on the first visit . . . I don't give out pads, I'm not a pad supplier . . . I tell them that and those . . . the ones who are not motivated, you don't have coming back. They DNA [do not attend].'

'Because I'm not treating . . . I'm only mopping incontinence, I'm only a mopper-up. My gut feeling, my training would go against what I'm doing. Like, you know, I was never trained, with my specialist course, I was never trained to give out pads to mop up. I was there to treat and manage and to contain those 30 per cent that can never resolve to dryness.'

'I have them [patients] coming and coming and coming and eventually I do, hopefully, I get them round to my . . . not to my way but the benefits of continence promotion. You know, the ones that keep going on, the ones that don't want, don't come back . . . I don't know what they're doing honestly, borrowing their mothers', their aunts' or buying sanitary towels or what . . . There's a certain core, and you know the minute they come through the door that they're looking for a quick fix . . . surgery or tablets, they want a magic wand.'

'It's just a cultural thing, the older, older population, it's just part of ageing. They accept what their mothers have told them in the past or the GP, they have literally accepted their word as gospel.'

While the SCNs voiced frustration at those women who asked for pads and who, on being refused, subsequently failed to attend clinic appointments, their rationalisation of such behaviour tended not, at least ostensibly, to be based on individualised 'blame-making'. Rather, as the above quotes exemplify, their accounts of the 'clash' of perspectives portrayed women more as 'victims' of a set of cultural expectations and of a health care system which continued to promulgate these expectations. Thus, they perceive a diminution of the female body as well as the social experience of womanhood, accompanied by an over-reliance on medical capability, so that women are cheated on two counts: first, in terms of being given equivocal messages concerning whether FUI is a medical problem or a 'normal' consequence of childbearing and/or ageing; and, second, in that, based on a misguided belief in the supremacy of medicine to cure, women are lulled into believing that their urinary incontinence can be eradicated through the application of technology.

Cognisant of the need to transform the knowledge and attitudes of a significant number of women *and* professional colleagues, the SCNs highlighted the importance of extending their work beyond the strictly clinical to encompass education and training, as well as their frustration that the demands of clinical work, in the context of endemic under-resourcing of continence services, prevented them from so doing. Indeed, at times the descriptions by SCNs of the type of knowledge transfer activity they would ideally like to pursue cast them in the proselytising, even evangelical, role of 'ridding' both women and fellow health care practitioners of a mindset that accepts incontinence as 'part and parcel' of being a woman.

'My wish list? Reducing my clinical role, doing my administration, keeping up to date, instead of reacting to be more proactive and to go round the schools and have a pelvic muscle exercise programme incorporated into 15 year old girls' education.'

'There's at least 50 per cent of women out there who we could help but we're not seeing. My aim is to get into schools . . . teach 15 year old girls before I retire from incontinence . . . to go round the schools and teach that because that's where the groundwork in pelvic floor should be taught.'

Summary

The preceding analysis has highlighted that there is no such thing as a gender neutral understanding of FUI and how it should be treated/managed within the health care system. Descriptions of their work given by SCNs bear testimony to the influence of a medical discourse that constructs (engenders) the female body as reducible to physical decline and which, in turn, uses the normalisation of physical decline as the justification for discrimination in health care. However, these descriptions also highlight the SCNs' involvement in a growing scrutinisation of and resistance to this particular discourse and the set of health care practices it sponsors. While the work of the SCNs certainly is informed by biomedical understandings of the female body, FUI and the extent/ways in which this incontinence may be cured or alleviated, they do not see themselves as advocates of a biomedical enterprise but as using their specialist knowledge to actually *reduce* the dependency of women on medical intervention. An important part of this project centres on informing and *reforming* the ways in which FUI and, by extension, the female body and the social experience of womanhood are understood within the health care system. The SCNs acknowledge that some women will require ongoing management in the form of, for example, the provision of absorbent products, and, equally, that some women for whom conservative management does not work will require some degree of technological intervention. However, they are clear that the majority of women can maintain and/or regain continence in the right circumstances, these circumstances involving a mixture of being appropriately informed, taking responsibility for their own health through, for example, undertaking relevant pelvic floor exercises, and having access to health care which values and upholds a notion of womanhood as not based on the inevitability of physical (and social?) decline.

Regulation or emancipation? The work of specialist nurses in the promotion of continence

Taken as a whole, the efforts of SCNs in the promotion of continence allude to an essential sociological dilemma. On the one hand, it could be argued that these efforts are empowering women to take authority over their personal biological and social life trajectory and, in the process, creating a distance between themselves and medical scrutiny. On the other hand, the very same work could be seen as enhancing the dominance of the medical profession in that the SCNs are targeting a condition capable of being managed (through, for example, the use of pads) without any clinical input at all. Such questioning raises the issue of how far and in what ways the work of the SCNs is contributing to a medicalisation of FUI? Further, even if it is the case that their work does promote such medicalisation, is it then simply a case of 'reining' in the authority of the SCNs so that, for example, women are enabled to manage their incontinence entirely within the social domain?

The orthodox medicalisation critique proposes that medicine has become increasingly powerful despite an apparent lack of effectiveness in crucial areas (such as the eradication of chronic illness) as well as a range of iatrogenic side effects (Illich 1976). As a result of the accumulation of power, an ever growing array of what could otherwise be seen as 'everyday' aspects of life (eating, drinking, sexual intercourse, 'naughty' behaviour in young children) has come under the authority of medicine. The increasing medicalisation of social life has made medicine central to the setting of standards by which what is to be considered 'normal' and 'deviant' may be judged. In so doing, medicine has become an institution of social regulation by determining appropriate and/or responsible behaviour and sanctioning that which it deems otherwise (Zola 1972).

Latterly, a more nuanced understanding of medicalisation has gained precedence (Heitman 1999; Lupton 1997; Williams and Calnan 1996). Accordingly, rather than seeing medicine as a quintessentially repressive institution (and promoting a view of patient interests 'pitted' against those of the medical profession), analyses have highlighted some of the more positive aspects of biomedicine (Lupton 1997) and have demonstrated mutuality in the medicalisation of social phenomena encompassing the activities of both the lay and health professional populations (Giddens 1992).

Lupton (1997: 96) suggests that,

> In concert with liberal humanist ideals, critics argue that becoming 'medicalised' denies rational, independent human action by allowing members of an authoritative group (in this case the medical profession) to dictate to others how they should behave . . . 'medicalisation' is positioned as something which should resisted (*sic*), in favour of some degree of 'de-medicalisation'.

From this perspective it is hard to see how the education, training and health care work of SCNs could be anything other than a contribution to the medicalisation of FUI, often in the face of considerable resistance on the part of women patients (through, for example, their insistence on the provision of pads and/or their withdrawal from service use). The SCNs seek to cast an ever widening authority over the ways in which women manage themselves (for example, in terms of educating young girls about the need for lifelong pelvic floor muscle exercising) as well as when they engage with the health care system (for example, in terms of being denied pads).

However, looking at the feminist uptake of medicalisation (for example, Ehrenreich and English 1974; Martin 1987), a different view of SCNs' promotion of continence across the entire gamut of their activities is possible. In varying ways, feminists have critiqued the medical profession as a largely patriarchal institution which has advanced particular definitions of illness and disease to maintain the relative inequality of women by highlighting their physical and emotional weaknesses as well as their susceptibility to ill-health (Lupton 1997). Such institutional demeaning of women's biological and social functioning has been apparent throughout the preceding analysis – for example, in the ways in which both GPs and women treat FUI as 'womanly inheritance' (Peake *et al.* 1999: 283) – and has been shown to be the target of significant challenge on the part of SCNs.

More specifically, Emily Martin (1987) has argued that representations of the female body and its routine functions as inherently abnormal or deviant are intrinsic to medical discourse. Based on the testimonies of SCNs, the same process of 'deviancy by definition' appears to be at play in the context of health care offered to women experiencing urinary incontinence. Consequently, and despite the dangers of individualisation inherent in the adoption of regimes of health care premised on education and the (self) promotion of health, specialist continence nurses may be seen to be involved in an essentially positive realignment of 'what counts as a legitimate body' (Shilling 1993: 145). Thus, their work can be seen to de-legitimise the notion that a biologically dysfunctioning female body is acceptable, that it is okay for women to 'leak', and in so doing to challenge the view of the female body as inherently deviant, and, thus, to promote a set of cultural expectations around the essential validity and social worth of 'femaleness'.

In their analysis of women's experiences of urinary incontinence, Peake *et al.* draw attention to a multiplicity of social meanings regarding the 'engendered body' (1999: 258). However, their analysis tends, in the end, towards a more uni-dimensional view of meaning-making in that they highlight the predominance of an understanding which 'normalises' female biological dysfunctioning and associated disease and illness. Whilst not disagreeing with their observations, I want to argue that the picture is necessarily more complicated by suggesting that the 'engendered body' has become a site of conflict within formal health care. There are (at least) two contrasting sets of understandings of the biological and social female in operation: one which emphasises vulnerability, the inevitably of bodily decline and the need for acceptance of such; and another which acknowledges vulnerability, but only the potential for decline and not at all the need for acceptance of such.

Ultimately, then, the work of SCNs might be seen as contributing to the de-medicalisation of FUI on a number of different fronts, not least because they advocate the empowerment of women patients through 'taking (back) control' over their health by engaging in preventive health activities. Paradoxically, the extent to which women themselves crave such empowerment is debatable; the significant numbers of women who, according to the SCNs, seek a surgical 'quick-fix' or prefer to use pads than to work towards continence suggest a situation which calls for a more finely grained analysis than the orthodox medicalisation thesis enables. Thus, the (de)medicalisation of FUI cannot be seen to be the outcome of the activities of one group in relation to another but rather the outcome of the interplay between a relatively loose set of ways of thinking and doing that criss-cross lay and health professional populaces. On the basis of this reading, the work of SCNs in the promotion of continence is unlikely to be either straightforward or easily accomplished.

References

Abrams, P., Cardozo, L., Fall, M. *et al.* (2003) The standardisation of terminology of lower urinary tract function: report from the Standardisation Sub-committee of the International Continence Society (update). *Urology* 61: 37–49.

Blaxter, M. (2004) *Health*. Cambridge: Polity Press.

Bunton, R., Nettleton, S. and Burrows, R. (1995) *The Sociology of Health Promotion: Critical Analyses of Consumption, Lifestyle and Risk*. London: Routledge.

Continence Foundation (2000) *Integrated Continence Service: A Source Book for Continence Services*. London: The Continence Foundation.

Coyne, K.S., Zhou, Z., Thompson. C. *et al.* (2003) The impact on health-related quality of life of stress, urge and mixed urinary incontinence. *British Journal of Urology International* 92: 731–735.

Department of Health (2000) *Good Practice in Continence Services*. London: Department of Health.

Dolan, L.M., Casson, K., McDonald, P. and Ashe, R.G. (1999) Urinary incontinence in Northern Ireland: a prevalence study. *British Journal of Urology International* 83: 760–766.

Dolman, M. (2001) Continence issues. In G. Andrews (ed.) *Women's Sexual Health* (2nd edn). Edinburgh: Baillière Tindall, pp. 456–480.

Ehrenreich, B. and English, D. (1974) *Complaints and Disorders: The Sexual Politics of Sickness*. London: Compendium.

Foucault, M. (1988) 'Technologies of the self'. In L.H. Martin, H. Gutman and P. Hutton (eds) *Technologies of the Self: A Seminar with Michel Foucault*. London: Tavistock.

Foucault, M. (1991) Governmentality. In G. Burchell, C. Gordon and P. Miller (eds) *The Foucault Effect: Studies in Governmentality*. London: Harvester Wheatsheaf.

Fultz, N.H., Burgio, K., Diokno, A.C. *et al.* (2003) Burden of stress urinary incontinence for community-dwelling women. *American Journal of Obstetrics and Gynaecology* 189: 1275–1282.

Fultz, N H., Jenkins, KR., Østbye, T. *et al.* (2005) The impact of own and spouse's urinary incontinence on depressive symptoms. *Social Science and Medicine* 60(11): 2537–2584.

Giddens, A. (1992) *The Transformation of Intimacy: Sexuality, Love and Eroticism in Modern Societies*. Cambridge: Polity Press.

Green, J. and Thorogood, N. (2004) *Qualitative Methods for Health Research*. London: Sage.

Heitman, E. (1999) Social and ethical aspects of in vitro fertilisation. *International Journal of Assessment in Health Care* 15(1): 22–32.

Illich, I. (1976) *Limits to Medicine. Medical Nemesis: The Expropriation of Health*. Harmondsworth: Pelican.

Kirmayer, L.J. (1992) The body's insistance on meaning: metaphor as presentation and representation in illness experience. *Medical Anthropology Quarterly* 6: 323–347.

Lee, J.J. (2004) The relationship between gender and the psychological impact of urinary incontinence on older people in Hong Kong: an exploratory analysis. *Ageing and Society* 24: 553–566.

Lupton, D. (1995) *The Imperative of Health: Public Health and the Regulated Body*. London: Sage.

Lupton, D. (1997) Foucault and the medicalisation critique. In A. Petersen and R. Bunton (eds) *Foucault, Health and Medicine*. London: Routledge, pp. 94–110.

Lupton, D. (2003) *Medicine as Culture: Illness, Disease and the Body in Western Societies* (2nd edn). London: Sage.

Martin, E. (1987) *The Woman in the Body*. Boston: Beacon Press.

Mitteness, L.S. and Barker, J.C. (1995) Stigmatising a 'normal' condition: urinary incontinence in late life. *Medical Anthropology Quarterly* 9: 188–210.

Nettleton, S. and Gustafsson, U. (2002) Introduction. In S. Nettleton and U. Gustafsson, *The Sociology of Health and Illness Reader*. Cambridge: Polity Press, pp. 1–10.

Peake, S., Manderson, L. and Potts, H. (1999) 'Part and parcel of being a woman': female urinary incontinence and constructions of control. *Medical Anthropology Quarterly* 13(3): 267–285.

Rees Jones, I. (2001) Habermas or Foucault or Habermas and Foucault? The implications of a shifting debate for medical sociology. In G. Scambler (ed.) *Habermas, Critical Theory and Health*. London: Routledge, pp. 163–181.

Shaw, C. (2001) A review of the psychosocial predictors of help-seeking behaviour and impact on quality of life in people with urinary incontinence. *Journal of Clinical Nursing* 10: 15–24.

Shilling, C. (1993) *The Body and Social Theory*. London: Sage.

Silverman, D. (2001) *Interpreting Qualitative Data: Methods for Analysing Talk, Text and Interaction* (2nd edn). London: Sage.

Thakar, R., Stanton, S. and Kane, J. (2003) Management of urinary incontinence in women. In D. Waller and A. McPherson (eds) *Women's Health* (5th edn). Oxford: Oxford University Press, pp. 322–350.

Thomas, S. (2003) *Is Policy Translated into Action?* London: Royal College of Nursing/ The Continence Foundation.

van der Vaart, C.H., de Leeux, J.R.J., Roovers, J.P.W.R. and Heintz, A.P.M. (2002) The effect of urinary incontinence and overactive bladder symptoms on quality of life in young women. *British Journal of Urology International* 90: 544–549.

Williams, S.J. and Calnan, M. (1996) The limits of medicalisation? Modern medicine and the lay populace in 'late' modernity. *Social Science and Medicine* 42: 1609–1620.

Zola, I. (1972) Medicine as an institution of social control. *Sociological Review* 20: 487–503.

16 Older women and early miscarriage: leaky bodies and boundaries

Julia Frost

Introduction

In this chapter older women's physical and psychical[1] experience of early miscarriage is explored, in the context of theoretical debates on embodiment. I will outline theories of the sociology of the body (Frank 1991; Turner 1996), and argue that the gendered and subjective nature of women's reproductive health has been overlooked. However, a re-reading of classic feminist texts finds that here the body is equally constructed as troublesome (Butler 1990) and problematic (de Beauvoir 1997). In contrast, current post-modern feminist research transcends this thinking about women's bodies – by proposing women's embodied experiences as having both *continuity* (Grosz 1994), and *leakiness* (Shildrick 1997).

This chapter presents findings from qualitative interviews with twenty-nine women who experienced a first trimester pregnancy loss, and who were over 35 years of age. The interviews were undertaken as part of a doctoral research study. I want to suggest that although notions of uncertainty, about both the process and the outcome of a miscarriage, may be distressing, notions of 'leakiness' and 'fluidity' may at the same time be useful ways of conceptualising aspects of this 'loss'. In particular, this approach allows for an exploration of miscarriage as a potentially inevitable outcome of some pregnancies. This approach does not denigrate women's individual experience of pregnancy loss, but suggests that women should be warned about the risks of early miscarriage. It also allows for the incorporation of previous and subsequent reproductive experiences into biographies of women's reproductive health, such that other reproductive events (births and deaths, menarche and menopause), and the ways in which they may frame an early pregnancy loss, are not overlooked. Finally, this approach demands that care provided to women who are at risk of, or experiencing, an early miscarriage should be women-centred.

Background

The empirical research presented in this chapter sampled twenty-nine women from a broader qualitative study that explored seventy-nine women's experience of early miscarriage (Smith *et al.* 2006). This in turn followed on from a large quantitative study concerned with women's experience of the medical management of miscarriage (Trinder *et al.* 2006). The quantitative study, the *Mi*scarriage Treatment *St*udy (MIST), took place between 1997 and 2001, was led by Dr Lindsay Smith, and involved randomising over 1,200 women across the UK to three management methods (Trinder *et al.* 2006). The women were all experiencing an incomplete abortion – whereby as well as experiencing bleeding and pain, the cervix had begun to dilate. *Surgical management* involves traditional dilatation and curettage; *medical management* consists of prostaglandins (administered both orally and vaginally); while *expectant management* involved 'watchful waiting'.

Following on from the MIST study, the qualitative investigation, led by Harriet Bradley and Ruth Levitas at Bristol University, concerned women's experience of pregnancy loss more broadly. Existing qualitative research has suggested that the effects of an early miscarriage may be long-lasting (Lovell 1983; Cecil 1994), emphasising that medical and nursing care and support can mediate what is already a potentially significant and traumatic experience (Oakley *et al.* 1990; Moulder 1998). By contrast, the typical medical view of miscarriage is as a trivial or minor event, whose outcome cannot be prevented by the application of science.

For this larger quantitative study, 146 letters were sent to a cohort of both the MIST study participants and non-participants at three hospitals within the South West of England, after ethical approval had been granted by the appropriate committees. At the time of their attendance at hospital, all of the women consented to be contacted again and letters were typically sent at six months after the pregnancy loss, with the interviews taking place between six months and one year after the miscarriage.

Between September 1999 and June 2000, sixty-three of the MIST participants, along with sixteen non-participants, were interviewed. The in-depth interviews concerned the miscarriage experience, medical management, hospital care and support, and the meaning that the women attributed to their experience.

In summary, while the randomised controlled trial was concerned with comparing the various medical treatments of incomplete miscarriage for 1,200 women, the larger quantitative study interviewed seventy-nine of those women about the medical management, their participation or not in the trial, and wider aspects of their experience. This chapter concerns only data from the women who were interviewed and who were over 35 years of age.

Analysis of the larger dataset suggested that there was something distinct about the ways in which 'older women' (that is, women who were coming to the end of their fertile years) narrated their experience of early miscarriage. This seemed interesting in the light of recent figures from the Department of Health (2003), which indicate that the trend towards deliveries at older ages, already apparent since 1975, continued throughout the 1990s. While the number of deliveries to those under 25 has declined by one-third since 1985, those for women aged over 35 have doubled in the same period (DoH 2003). However, research undertaken by Reed (1990), with over 300 nurses, suggests that nurses who care for women who experience a miscarriage see *parity* as indicative of the emotional support that should be provided, whereas increasing age is not seen as relevant.

Rather than asking the older women about their perceptions of the significance of their ageing, this was explored when raised by the women themselves, on a case by case basis, so as not to bias their response. With the women's consent, the interviews were tape-recorded, transcribed verbatim, and analysed using NUDIST software (Fielding 1993) and a voice-relational method of thematic analysis (Mauthner and Doucet 1998).

Demographically, the 'older women' interviewed were broadly representative of those who had taken part in the MIST trial and quantitative study, with reference to their occupation, marital status and parity. Eighteen of the twenty-nine women were married, ten were cohabiting and one was single. Twenty-five of the women were employed, either full or part time, in a range of occupations, while four were not in paid employment. Twenty of the women in the study had children who were now alive (ranging from one to four children), whereas nine women did not have live children. While none of these children were born after the miscarriage that was the focus of the interview, seven women reported having one or more *previous* miscarriages and six women had one or more *subsequent* miscarriages. Three women had also experienced gestationally later losses, and three volunteered that they had undergone a previous termination. Seven women had confirmed pregnancies at the time of the interviews.

However, although the quantitative and qualitative studies included women of all childbearing ages, this smaller study purposively sampled women in relation to their age. Twenty-two of these women were between 35 and 40 years of age, six were between 40 and 45 and one woman was 46.

From analysing the data, pregnancy and miscarriage appear as truly embodied – both in terms of the physical and psychical aspects of the experience. However, an initial review of the literature to inform this research identified the extent to which both the experiences of early miscarriage and women's ageing are marginal topics. As such, no unified body of research, which adequately addressed the embodied nature of older women's experience of early miscarriage, was located. Although in the course of this research several bodies of literature were studied – such as that concerning ageing and women's health – the focus of this chapter is upon situating older women's physical and psychical experience within debates regarding embodiment.

The sociology of the body

The sociology of the body literature explores the extent to which bodies are material and discursive constructs – reflecting the very tensions that exist in embodied experiences, such as pregnancy and miscarriage. Being pregnant is a *lived* experience, which, as the pregnancy continues, changes what the body is able to *do* – in terms of working, eating and sleeping. However, pregnancy is also an *identity*, and the woman increasingly becomes a 'mum-to-be', sanctioned by the health professionals whom she comes into contact with. Often the tension between *having* a pregnant body and *being* a pregnant body is compounded by the very technologies which are meant to reassure women and ensure their safety in the transition to motherhood (Katz-Rothman 1986; Bricker *et al.* 2000), and for most of the women interviewed the miscarriage was diagnosed at what was considered to be a '*routine*' ultrasound scan.

For Turner, neither religion nor science has been able to successfully account for or regulate women's sexuality and reproductive functioning, and Turner (1996) argues that in contemporary society we try to overcome the unruly nature of the body via consumer choice – from what we wear, to when we will have children. However, the uncertainties of death and degeneration remain unsettling and uncontrollable.

Thus, Turner (1996: 108–9) proposes that every society has to regulate female sexuality and reproduction. At an individual level, this might include sanctions about the right age to reproduce, and at the level of society this might involve institutions of surveillance, such as schools and health centres – responsible for health education and the provision of contraception.

But certain problems can be identified with this analysis. First, it is questionable as to how useful it is to construct women as *either* individuals *or* constituents of populations, when private and public spheres are not necessarily discrete. Second, it is unclear *which* women are included in the model, or the degree of agency that these women have. Turner's approach does not address the situations in which bodies might take issue with their *own* reproduction, restraint, regulation and representation (Frank 1991). Furthermore, Turner only makes a limited acknowledgement of recent changes in the position of some women in society. Women are constructed as a homogenous category, with limited agency, in relation to work, marriage and reproduction:

> Women now represent a significant section of the industrial work-force, albeit in the unskilled and casual sector of the market. They have inadequate but important control over reproduction through the availability of contraceptive devices. Women, as a result of legislation relating to marriage, property and divorce, enjoy juridical equality with men in principle. Finally, with the decline of the nuclear family and the growth of single parent households, women are increasingly likely to assume control of domestic space.
>
> (Turner 1996: 212)

Furthermore, in a later essay concerning 'women's complaints', Turner (1997) neither suggests the specific extent of women's medicalisation, nor provides an examination of sites of resistance, such as the self-help movement of the 1960s. Turner's analysis can therefore be seen as an oversimplification of *which* women and illnesses are constructed, and to *what* ends.

Arthur Frank is not only concerned with the *physicality* of having a body, but also the tensions between having a body and being a body – that is, *consciousness*. In relation to agency, Frank (1991: 47) proposes that any analysis must begin with an exploration of how the body is problematic *for itself* – that is, what the body *does* as well as what is done *to it*, at the level of discourse, institutions and wider society. But, like Turner, Frank sees *all* women's potential for constructing themselves as limited by their capacity to reproduce, regardless of whether or not they have children. Frank's contention is problematic, in its assumption that women's reproductive functioning is at the centre of their embodied experience. He writes that 'reproduction takes as its locus of control the potential for women's own embodied experience of birth, whether the specific woman chooses to have that experience or not' (1991: 42). Collapsing the categories of 'woman' and 'mother' has the potential to stigmatise women who, through choice or otherwise, do *not* become mothers.

While the sociology of the body literature has been at the forefront of theorising notions of *embodiment*, much of the literature fails to address the issue of women's agency – suggesting that women's bodies have things done to them, but they do not act as bodies in and for themselves. Many of the key works are either gender blinkered, or generalise the experience of women as a unified category – particularly regarding reproduction.

Feminism and the body

Writing over fifty years ago, de Beauvoir was concerned with how women had come to be constructed as the *Other* – that is, different and inferior to men. She suggested that Women-as-Mothers were seen as both close to nature, as well as dangerous, on the basis of their biology; and as such, men sought to *regulate* women (from taboos concerning pregnant women to the medicalisation of the birth process) (1997: 178). This enabled men to protect themselves from the horrors of an unpredictable nature, and constructed the foetus as something *else* that needed to be protected (from women and abortionists) and controlled (by the male medical profession). However, de Beauvoir's radical contestation that 'one is not born, but rather becomes a woman' (1997: 295), with its emphasis on social conditioning, itself constructs women's bodies as problematic. De Beauvoir suggests that in contrast to men who control their bodily emissions, when women's bodies leak (mucous, blood and other body fluids) *women do not recognise themselves*, that is to say that they feel *betrayed* by their bodies. De Beauvoir's account of motherhood suggests that biology does not *totally* explain women's subordinate position; with motherhood constructed as a 'calling', those who do not reproduce – through miscarriage, infertility or choice – are all assumed to suffer their loss; whereas those who *do* give birth, are *also* assumed to experience an 'emptiness' once a baby has been born. Thus, even when a pregnancy is successful, a woman's agency is *leaky*:

> But pregnancy is above all a drama that is acted out within the woman herself. She feels it at once an enrichment and an injury . . . but this very opulence annihilates her, she feels that she herself is no longer anything.
> (de Beauvoir 1997: 512)

But, for de Beauvoir, *all* women's bodies are problematic and 'a burden' (1997: 630). This is reflected in the claim that 'almost all spontaneous miscarriages are of psychic origin . . .' (1997: 516). What for de Beauvoir is seen as the subconscious rejection of motherhood is also, symbolically, an act of rebellion against the *burden* of the female body.

More recently, Butler has proposed that, rather than the socially constructed *nature* of female bodies, the issue is one of the *matter* of bodies – and in *Gender Trouble*, she frames gender as *only* a *performance* of corporeal acts (1990: 136). However, in the later *Bodies That Matter*, Butler rethinks this analysis, such that the 'acts' of being a body now take second place to the *physicality* of being a body (1993: 2). What Butler proposes is a rethinking of the assumption of bodily norms:

> What I would propose . . . is a return to the notion of matter, not as a site or surface, but as *a process of materialization that stabilizes over time to produce the effect of a boundary, fixity, surface we call matter.*
> (Butler 1993: 9)

But, in contrast to de Beauvoir, Butler *downplays* the reproductive functioning of women's bodies, rather than addressing it, and her concentration on materialisation allows whole areas of female bodily being to slide out of view (Hughes and Witz 1997: 56). Therefore, whereas with de Beauvoir we are left with an attempt to reinstate female subjectivity within a body that is deemed to be 'in trouble' and problematic, with Butler we are presented with the physical nature of bodies, at the expense of their gender.

Hughes and Witz (1997) have emphasised the utility of the theoretical space between the work of de Beauvoir and Butler, and have proposed the construction of a theory of women's embodiment that acknowledges *both* gender and the body, *and* the subjectivity of embodiment. It is argued that such an approach can be found in post-modern feminist analyses – regarding continuity and leakiness.

Post-modern feminism

In *Volatile Bodies*, Elizabeth Grosz (1994: 15) is critical of the extent to which de Beauvoir assumes that women's bodies are in some way more 'natural' than men's – which leads de Beauvoir to conclude that women are prisoners of their body. Furthermore, Grosz (1994: 18) is also wary of Butler's concerns with sexual difference, at the expense of the meaning of the lived body. Grosz (1994: 19) proposes that feminists need to think beyond traditional narratives, in order to articulate the specificity of the female body, and female subjectivity. In contrast to the models and agendas proposed by Turner *et al.*, Grosz (1994: 22–24) believes that in order to rethink the body we must problematise existing *presumptions* of the body that rest upon essentialist dualisms. Thus, Grosz emphasises that the *meaning* that women attribute to their embodied experiences can include both physical and psychical constructs:

> The body image is as much a function of the subject's psychology and socio-historical context as anatomy. The limits or borders of the body image are not fixed by nature or confined to the anatomical 'container', the skin. The body image is extremely fluid and dynamic; its borders, edges, and contours are 'osmotic'- they have remarkable power of incorporating and expelling outside and inside in an ongoing interchange.
>
> (Grosz 1994: 79)

Grosz's own metaphor of the body, as a Mobius strip,[2] is particularly illuminating. With this metaphor, Grosz (1994: 36, 116) is able to note the importance of the skin, as both a boundary (receiving information from both the inside and the outside) and a surface (on which a text can be inscribed). Furthermore, the Mobius strip is a continuous entity, unbroken and flowing, linking the body and the psyche as one, continuous with its historical and social context, and, as such, critical of binary modes of thinking (Grosz 1994: 116–117).

Similarly, in Shildrick's (1997) analysis, the notion of fluidity is central. By deconstructing the false binaries of inside/outside and self/other, this permits a new way of thinking about boundaries – both physical and ontological. Currently, pregnancy loss is seen as pathological and therefore marginalised; but viewing this experience as in many cases *inevitable* and to be expected may permit new ways of thinking and talking about this experience, enabling us to identify the needs of women, and provide adequate care and support.

Shildrick also proposes a new ethic of health care that incorporates women's agency as well as their bodies. She proposes that a way forward is found by exploring the meanings that individuals give to their material (embodied) practices, reconstructing women as their individual narratives (1997: 104–117). This in turn may remove women from their (medically) marginalised position. Shildrick (1997: 169–170) seeks to move beyond the ontological devaluation of embodiment, which sees women's normal bodily processes (menstruation, pregnancy, menopause, and – to an extent – miscarriage) as engendered *and* pathological:

What matters, in bioethics, and more generally for the ethical affirma-
tion of the feminine, is that acceptance of the leakiness of bodies and
boundaries speaks to the necessity of an open response. The other
within the same is far more than a metaphor for the reproductive potential of women's bodies; it is an expression of the discursive interplay
between bodies and all subjects.

(Shildrick 1997: 217)

However, while Grosz and Shildrick pay attention to notions of subjectivity and agency, leakiness and continuity, as well as the tensions between
material and discursive constructs, it appears ironic that although these
notions of rupture and leakiness have been applied to various aspects of
women's reproduction, they have not been applied to women's experience
of miscarriage – which is indeed a truly leaky experience. It is with this oversight in mind that older women's experience of early miscarriage can be
viewed.

Discussion

Within the twenty-nine interviews, over half of the women suggested that
the miscarriage had resulted from a planned pregnancy; and their decision
was typically framed in relation to their increasing age:

> R: We wanted a family, and we got married about a year ago, about
> eighteen months ago now, about a year ago when we got pregnant, and
> we just wanted to start a family . . . and a lot of it had to do with my
> age, obviously . . .
>
> (Interview 50, age 36)

However, planning was not perceived as an either/or decision, and most
women emphasised some ambivalence regarding their perception of ageing:
psychically – the ability to cope with a new baby – but also *physically* –
concerning the risk of complications, although this was typically the risk of
Down syndrome, rather than early pregnancy loss. This finding is in keeping
with that of Barrett and Wellings (2002) who, from interviews with pregnant
women, suggest that notions of planning are indeed fluid rather than fixed.

Ideas about the meaning of the miscarriage and reproductive planning
were also contextualised in relation to *other* pregnancies – both previous
successful and unsuccessful pregnancies, as well as an orientation towards
possible future pregnancies. Motherhood, even when previously achieved, is
receptive to ebbs and flows, and many of the women further defined their
status in the light of other reproductive experiences – including infertility,
new reproductive technologies, other pregnancy losses, and birth. Also, for
some women, this failed pregnancy is indicative of the end of menstruation
and the onset of menopause, a finding overlooked in the existing literature:

> R: It's actually worse now . . . 'cos . . . it's not grieving for a lost child, or nothing like that, it's just a sadness that I've never got pregnant again . . . I haven't been able to get pregnant since . . .
>
> (Interview 53, age 37)

What this suggests is that, for some women, early miscarriage is not only indicative of *a* failed attempt at motherhood, but also represents how the ability to mother is *itself* flowing away. Furthermore, as existing research has found that having children does not compensate for the loss of a pregnancy (Slade 1994), it can also be argued that having children does not diminish the loss associated with not becoming a mother *with this pregnancy*. Miscarriage is not viewed as an isolated event, but rather as symptomatic of the leakiness of the category 'mother', and women's reproductive experiences more generally (Shildrick 1997: 179).

Writing twenty years ago, Lovell (1983) suggested that staff typically worked with a 'hierarchy of sadness' – which wrongly assumes that a gestationally later pregnancy loss is automatically more significant than an earlier miscarriage. But, many of the women interviewed proposed that although their pregnancy had been cut short, they still considered what they had been carrying as *a baby*:

> R: In the past, I'd heard about women having miscarriages, and to be honest, I was totally ignorant of . . . I used to think: well, you know, just get on with your life, but it's not that simple, that feeling of loss, erm, at losing a baby that was growing inside you, I don't think . . . is something I ever . . . ever think I could image how it would feel . . .
>
> (Interview 51, age 35)

This demonstrates the fluidity between the physical and psychical construction of the pregnancy, such that despite the obvious rupture – here both the physical rupture of a miscarriage and the theoretical rupture in assuming that a miscarriage is a minor event – women fill this (literally) empty signifier with their own interpretation of events.

As Letherby (1993) has noted, sometimes women struggle to give meaning, both to their pregnancy, and to their own identity, which is betwixt and between that of Mother and Other. For some, this sense of uncertainty occurs while waiting for the pregnancy to be expelled:

> R: I just felt in limbo, just waiting for whatever was going to happen . . .
>
> (Interview 53, age 37)

Whereas for others, this category rupture can be far longer lasting, and invade the woman's long-held sense of self:

R: I think you feel like you're in limbo . . .

(Interview 30, age 37)

These women were universally critical of the platitude, 'never mind, you can try again'; and for some of these *older* women, this insensitivity magnified the sense that they probably would *not* be able to try again. Seeing themselves in limbo is indicative of the difficulty that some women experience in attempting to *stabilise* their subject position following a miscarriage (Shildrick 1997: 112–113).

Metaphors of continuity and leakiness can also be extended to the care and support that these older women receive, and several described unsympathetic health professionals, such as the GP in this account, who told the woman (then 37) that she was *too old* to become a mother:

R: I had an appalling doctor in [place], who said: I don't know why you want to have babies anyway, erm, you know, you're far too old! And was just absolutely disgusting . . .

(Pilot 8, age 45)

This is despite extensive research (Oakley *et al.* 1990) which suggests that the meaning attributed to a pregnancy loss can be mediated by the attitudes and beliefs of the GP, as well as the provision of services locally.

Where women are located within the hospital can also be a source of distress and, in part, this reflects the ambivalent status of a woman whose pregnancy is unsuccessful (are they obstetric or gynaecology cases? mothers or non-mothers?). Lovell (1983: 757) noted that having no designated place to treat these women often leads to them being inappropriately placed on gynaecology wards (with women who are undergoing terminations), or maternity units (along with mothers and young babies):

R: [I was admitted to] a sort of a gynae, antenatal ward, yeah . . . over the hospital entrance. It's quite horrible actually, because it's actually in the maternity hospital . . . and, again, I sat there . . . you know, and you're looking out over the entrance, at all the Dads coming in . . . and you know, you're right opposite the postnatal ward, with all the Mums . . . with all the Mothers and babies having sleepless nights, that hurt . . .

(Pilot 1, age 40)

New hospital protocols often treat all women under twenty weeks of gestation on gynaecology wards, whereas those over twenty weeks (when a pregnancy is potentially more viable) are treated on obstetric wards (Littlewood 1999: 220). This dualist thinking, though, ignores the subjective sensibility of the pregnant woman, and negates the meaning that she gives to *her* pregnancy. While Yudkin (1989: 59) considers that the lack of a designated space is indicative of the way in which medicine views early miscarriage as 'trivial', Littlewood (1999: 220) proposes that recent protocols ignore the wishes of the would-be-mother.

However, although there were many examples where care was perceived as fractured and discontinuous, the women typically spoke favourably of the new Early Pregnancy Assessment Clinics, which were seen as providing continuous and fluid care (Moulder 1998):

> R: It was helpful to see the *same* doctor throughout the process [at the hospital]. That was a concern, that I would see different doctors, and that I wouldn't get continuity . . . and she was just very thorough in explaining what was happening . . .
>
> (Interview 39, age 36)

This reflects Casey's (2003) view that the impact of care upon the body is dependent upon the space, time and place of care. However, a woman's sense of identity and worth is also influenced by what Edvardsson *et al* (2003) describe as the '*atmosphere*' – the people and language that are used in particular places (mothers or others, cared for by nurses or midwifes, in obstetrics or gynaecology). Edvardsson *et al.* propose that an atmosphere that is perceived as *negative* 'obstruct[s] the ability to stay whole' (2003: 379).

Conclusions

This chapter has explored theoretical debates and empirical examples in order to examine the utility of notions of leakiness. Many of the women interviewed suggested that they were ill prepared for the *possibility* of a miscarriage. With modern pregnancy care prohibiting contact with a midwife until 12 weeks, few knew of the risks of early miscarriage, and the extent to which those risks increase with age. Indeed, many women could not understand the lack of information, since as many as 20 per cent of pregnancies end in miscarriage. Making miscarriage less taboo, perhaps through a public awareness campaign, might normalise women's experience, rather than ignoring or belittling what happens, and might encourage people to better support those who have experienced early miscarriage.

Most of the women interviewed did not see miscarriage as a one-off event, but rather contextualised this experience in relation to other reproductive experiences. For example, the pain of miscarrying was described as 'like period pains' (Interview 12, age 35), while the accompanying emotions were viewed as 'like postnatal depression' (Interview 19, age 37). Those who already had children talked of not having achieved motherhood with *this* pregnancy, whereas others suggested that the miscarriage had *also*, in some way, *constituted* mothering for them.

In the 1990s Christine Moulder (1998) proposed that women who experience an early miscarriage benefited when health care was individualised;

when care was negotiated rather than imposed; when professionals engaged with them; and when the emotional aspects of miscarriage were acknowledged rather than avoided. The research findings concerning the specific experience of 'older women' suggest that while some staff work very hard to provide individualised and flowing care, existing structures within the health care system, which promote discontinuous care and the lack of a special place for women who miscarry, may further compound the experience of an early pregnancy loss. Where a specific space is provided, such as an Early Pregnancy Assessment Unit, and staff actively include the woman in the planning and implementation of her care and treatment, this is typically perceived by the women as an acknowledgement of the potential continuities and ruptures to notions of selfhood (as both *Woman* and *Mother*).

Recent post-modern feminist theory has sought to rethink ontological and epistemological issues regarding women's embodied experience. However, it is argued that the experience of miscarriage is missing from the theoretical literature. By contrast, this chapter has proposed that if we view early miscarriage as leaky, we can expand our understanding of the experience of miscarriage, pregnancy and motherhood.

Acknowledgements

The larger qualitative study was funded by the NHSE S&W Executive (Project Grant R/17/12.98/Bradley). JFs Postdoctoral Fellowship was funded by the ESRC (Award no.: PTA-026–27–0062). Thanks are due to the research team (Harriet Bradley, Ruth Levitas, Lindsay Smith, Jo Garcia and Gayle Grant), Vieda Skultans, Catherine Pope, and all of the women who participated in this study at a difficult time in their lives.

Notes

1 Following Adrienne Rich's definition of *psychical* as the 'transition of the woman's character' (1979: 12).
2 Mobius strip: surface with only one side and edge formed by joining ends of rectangle after twisting one end through 180 degrees (*Oxford English Dictionary*, 2001).

References

Barrett, G. and Wellings, K. (2002). What is a 'planned' pregnancy? Empirical data from a British study. *Social Science and Medicine* 5: 545–557.
Bricker, L., Garcia, J., Henderson, J., Mugford, M., Neilson, J., Roberts, T. and Martin, M.A. (2000). Ultrasound screening in pregnancy: a systematic review of the clinical effectiveness, cost-effectiveness and women's views. *Health Technology Assessment* 4: 16.
Butler, J. (1990). *Gender Trouble*. London: Routledge.
Butler, J. (1993). *Bodies That Matter*. London: Routledge.

Casey, S. (2003). From place to space in contemporary health care. *Social Science and Medicine* 56: 2245–2247.

Cecil, R. (1994). Miscarriage: women's views of care. *Journal of Reproductive and Infant Psychology* 12: 21–29.

de Beauvoir, S. (1997). *The Second Sex*. London: Vintage (first published 1949).

Department of Health (2003). NHS maternity statistics, England: 1998–9 to 2000–1. http://www.dh.gov.uk/assetRoot/04/08/21/66/04082166.pdf 19.08.05

Edvardsson, D., Rasmussen, B.H. and Reissman, C.K. (2003). Ward atmospheres of horror and healing: a comparative analysis of healing. *Health* 7(4): 377–396.

Featherstone, M. and Turner, B.S. (1995). Body and society: an introduction. *Body and Society* 1(1): 1–12.

Fielding, N. (1993). Analysing qualitative data by computer. *Social Research Update*. Issue 1. http://www.soc.surrey.ac.uk/sru/SRU1.html. Accessed 19.08.05

Frank, A.W. (1991). For a sociology of the body: an analytical review. In M. Featherstone, B. Hepworth and B.S. Turner (eds) *The Body: Social Process and Cultural Theory*. London: Sage.

Friedman, T. and Gath, D. (1989). The psychiatric consequences of abortion. *British Journal of Psychiatry* 155: 810–813.

Frost, J. (2004). Uncertain age: late motherhood and early miscarriage. PhD thesis, University of Bristol.

Grosz, E. (1994). *Volatile Bodies*. Bloomington: Indiana University Press.

Hughes, A. and Witz, A. (1997) Feminism and the matter of bodies. *Body and Society* 3(1): 47–60.

Katz-Rothman, B. (1986). *The Tentative Pregnancy: Amniocentesis and the Sexual Politics of Motherhood*. London: Pandora.

Lee, R. (1993). *Doing Research on Sensitive Topics*. London: Sage.

Letherby, G. (1993). The meanings of miscarriage. *Women's International Forum* 16(2): 165–180.

Littlewood, J. (1999). From the invisibility of miscarriage to the attribution of life. *Anthropology and Medicine* 6(2): 217–230.

Lovell, A. (1983). Some questions of identity: late miscarriage, stillbirth and perinatal loss. *Social Science and Medicine* 17(11): 755–761.

Matheson, J. and Babb, P. (2002). *Social Trends*. No. 32. London: HMSO.

Mauthner, N. and Doucet, A. (1998). Reflections on a voice centred relational method. In J. Ribbens and R. Edwards (eds) *Feminist Dilemmas in Qualitative Research: Public Knowledge and Private Lives*. London: Sage.

Moulder, C. (1998). *Understanding Pregnancy Loss: Perspective and Issues in Care*. London: Macmillan.

Oakley, A., McPherson, A. and Roberts, H. (1990). *Miscarriage*, 2nd edn. London: Penguin.

Reed, K. (1990). Influence of age and parity on the emotional care given to women experiencing miscarriages. *Image: Journal of Nursing Scholarship* 22(2): 89–92.

Rich, A. (1979). *Of Woman Born: Motherhood as Experience and Institution*. London: Virago.

Shildrick, M. (1997). *Leaky Bodies and Boundaries*. London: Routledge.

Slade, P. (1994). Predicting the psychological impact of miscarriage. *Journal of Reproductive and Infant Psychology* 12: 5–16.

Smith, L.F., Frost, J., Levitas, R., Bradley, H. and Garcia, J. (2006). Women's experience of three early miscarriage management options. *British Journal of General Practice* 56(524): 198–205.

Trinder, J., Brocklehurst, P., Porter, R., Read, M., Vygas, S. and Smith, L. (2006). Management of miscarriage: expectant, medical or surgical? Results of a randomised controlled trial (miscarriage management (MIST) trial). *British Medical Journal* 332: 1235–1240.

Turner, B. (1996). *The Body and Society: Explorations in Social Theory*, 2nd edn. London: Sage.

Turner, B. (1997). *Medical Power and Social Knowledge*. London: Sage.

Yudkin, G. (1989). From home to hospital and back. In V. Hey, C. Itzin, L. Saunders and M.A. Speakman (eds) *Hidden Loss: Miscarriage and Ectopic Pregnancy*, 2nd edn. London: Women's Press, pp. 53–65.

17 Sexually transmitted infections and dirt

Hilary Piercy

Introduction

The aim of this chapter is to consider the association between sexually transmitted infections (STIs) and the concept of dirt. This discussion is founded upon a qualitative research study undertaken in central England which explored the experiences of individuals who had contracted genital chlamydial infection. In this study, data collection was by means of single, stand-alone, in-depth, unstructured interviews. Whilst both males and females were included in the study, in this chapter I will confine the discussion to the female experience and draw upon the data derived from interviews with the forty females aged 16–29 years who participated. The majority of the interviews were conducted in a genitourinary medicine (GUM) clinic based within a medium-sized district general hospital and took place approximately four weeks after diagnosis. A small proportion of interviews were conducted in a town centre family planning clinic serving the same population. For these individuals the infection was a less recent experience, and therefore their inclusion provided a longer-term perspective.

The findings from the study indicated that dirt is a central concept which impacts upon all aspects of this infection. It affected the way that the women felt about themselves and the degree to which they were prepared for a positive diagnosis. It also impacted upon their interpersonal relationships with others: with the health professionals involved in diagnosing and treating the infection, with friends and family. In particular it influenced the extent to which they felt able or willing to disclose their diagnosis to others, including partners. The consequences are therefore far-reaching and multifaceted. This chapter will examine the impact of the infection at the point of diagnosis in terms of the women's responses.

These responses have particular significance in relation to the current situation with regard to chlamydia. As the most commonly diagnosed STI in England at present, chlamydia is attracting considerable attention. I will therefore first outline the key aspects of this infection and the policy and practice responses that have been developed as a means by which to tackle rising incidence rates. The impact of this infection derives from its categorisation as an STI, the implications of which are historically grounded. Consequently a historical overview of STIs will provide a context within which to discuss individual reactions to the infection experience and the implications of emergent health policies. All the names used for the respondents are pseudonyms.

Chlamydia

Chlamydia trachomatis has a relatively short history as a recognised STI. Although human diseases caused by this organism have been recognised since antiquity, the body of knowledge relating to this infection has increased rapidly from the 1970s onwards. In 1989 it was added to the list of infections routinely recorded in the genitourinary medicine clinic.

A number of factors have contributed to the current situation where considerable health efforts are being directed towards the detection and treatment of chlamydial infection. First, the number of people identified as being infected with this organism has increased steadily over the past decade. This has resulted in a situation where chlamydia is currently the most commonly diagnosed STI in England, with the highest rates of infection in those aged 16–25 years (HPA 2004). In the majority of cases this infection is asymptomatic and therefore it is considered that diagnoses represent a small proportion of the actual cases of infection. Despite the frequent absence of symptoms, this is not an inconsequential infection as the potential sequelae may be considerable. The organism can ascend to the upper genital tract and infect the epithelial cells of the salpinx causing pelvic inflammatory disease (Qvigstad *et al.* 1983; Westergard *et al.* 1982) which in turn may result in tubal infertility and ectopic pregnancy.

Concerns about the current infection rates and the consequent health implications, together with the development of sensitive tests which use samples collected through non-invasive methods, have collectively contributed to health policies designed to tackle infection rates. These have been realised primarily through the testing of identified populations and the establishment of a national chlamydia screening programme. This opportunistic screening programme, which is expected to achieve national coverage by 2007, operates predominantly through primary care facilities such as general practice and sexual health clinics. Although it targets both males and females aged under 25 years, experience from the first year of the programme indicates that the vast majority of screening is being conducted on women, and consequently over 90 per cent of diagnoses are occurring in women (LaMontagne *et al.* 2004).

A historical overview of sexually transmitted infections

The association between dirt and sexually transmitted diseases has a long history that originates in the original venereal diseases of syphilis and gonorrhoea. The historical position that these infections occupy was shaped and formed through the legal structures and social controls that emerged in the eighteenth century. These contributed to a situation whereby STIs came to be increasingly and inseparably associated with social attitudes and values, both in considerations of hygiene and as representations of morality, of sin and punishment, blame and retribution. With the passage of time, these infections became increasingly associated with specific people and activities, becoming synonymous in the eighteenth and nineteenth centuries with women, and more specifically with prostitutes, who came to be constructed as pathologised female and contaminated other (Spongberg 1997).

Syphilis

The origins of syphilis are contested. Whilst there are references in early writings to symptoms that could be attributable to syphilis, this infection made a significant appearance in the literature in the early to mid-1500s, suggesting that it spread throughout Europe in epidemic proportions (Davenport Hines 1990). From the outset, its connection with sexual activity was recognised and provided the facility to see syphilis as the evidence of divine retribution. In his edict of 1495, Emperor Maximilian declared syphilis to be God's punishment for the sins of man (Andreski 1989). Allen (2000) suggests that this fearful disfiguring condition spread through Europe on an epidemic scale producing widespread panic; the spread of infection caused increasing levels of fear and, with it, blame on a national and a personal level. On a national level it produced theories that explained the origins of this disease as located anywhere as long as it was 'other', for example the idea that it originated in America and was brought from the New World to Europe by Columbus. This explanation is attributed to the testimony of Ruy Dias de Isla who in his account 'Tractado contra el mal Serpentino' documented how he had treated a number of Columbus's sailors for this disease after they had returned to Barcelona in 1493 from Hayti (Abraham 1935). Another example is found in the writings of the sixteenth-century Venetian physician and poet Fracastoro. His lengthy poem in three parts, 'Syphilis sive morbus Gallicus' (Syphilis or the French disease), recounts how the disease was inflicted on the shepherd Syphilus as punishment by the Gods (Fracastoro 1935). This title is attributable to the first definite evidence of syphilis in Europe which dates from the capture of Naples by Charles VIII of France in 1495 (Abraham 1935). The poem, which was extremely well received in its time, not only gave rise to the name of the disease but also gave support to the common practice of attributing it to another, the beginnings of a history that variously described it as a French, Italian or Neapolitan disease, as European pustules or the ulcer of Canton (Crosby 1977). The labelling of syphilis as a foreigner's disease is considered to be a product of its abrupt appearance (Crosby 1977); however it also represented the way in which the disease was located in wrongness, conceptualised as archaically identical with the non-us, the alien. As a person judged to be wrong, a foreigner is regarded as, at least potentially, a source of pollution (Sontag 1991).

On a personal level, blame was reflected in increasingly punitive measures that castigated and persecuted those afflicted with the disease, denouncing them from the pulpit, banishing them from settlements and refusing them hospital care and treatment (Allen 2000). This approach was already well established in the treatment meted out to those with leprosy in which the outward decay of the flesh was considered a sign of inner promiscuity. Lepers were considered a moral and physical threat to the community and required to be separated from the rest of the population by ritualistic means (Turner 1996). With the appearance of syphilis, the focus of attention simply shifted to the syphilitic, who adopted the social script that had been written for leprosy, as the visible and outward manifestation of inner corruption (Spongberg 1997).

Gonorrhoea

Gonorrhoea has a much longer history than syphilis. Descriptions of symptoms attributable to the disease are recognisable in Assyrian tablets that referred to cloudy and thick urine, whilst Hippocrates described urethral strictures or strangury (Rosebury 1972). The word itself is derived from the Greek term meaning 'flow of seed' (Spongberg 1997) and this is further reflected in the Roman name of *seminis efusio* (Foucault 1986). These names reflect the ancient understanding of gonorrhoea as a relatively minor condition of little consequence, exclusively associated with males.

By the thirteenth century, the occurrence of gonorrhoea in men was attributed to impurities retained under the prepuce after exposure to an unclean woman (Rosebury 1972; Worboys 2004), a viewpoint which persisted for centuries. In the 1860s, medical textbooks described it as a specific contagious disease whereby gonorrhoeal poisons were spread to men by healthy women as a result of sexual contact with their genital fluids (Worboys 2004). This understanding reflected in part the mainly asymptomatic nature of infection in women, but was largely derived from and served to reinforce representations of the pathologised female body. The usual source of gonorrhoeal poison was considered to be that which had been deposited in the vagina of an 'unsound woman' by the man that she had previously had intercourse with. These theories positioned prostitutes as reservoirs of infection. Having become habituated themselves to its effect, they were not themselves harmed by it, but they served as a source of infection to those men with whom they had sex (Spongberg 1997). Although there was a growing real-isation in the 1870s that gonorrhoea caused infection in women, this aspect of the disease received little serious attention until the late 1890s (Worboys 2004).

The feminisation of venereal disease

In the sixteenth century, gonorrhoea was subsumed in the interest that syphilis attracted; it became gradually entangled with and incorporated into the treatises on syphilis which dominated considerations and represen-tations of venereal disease. There was considerable confusion between the symptoms of one and the other and they were increasingly understood and presented as different manifestations of the same disease. Although this view-point was challenged by some, it was apparently confirmed in the eighteenth century by the ill-fated experiment of John Hunter; he inoculated him-self with a discharge considered to be due to gonorrhoea and subsequently developed symptoms of syphilis. Hunter was chiefly responsible for the single disease theory which persisted until the mid-nineteenth century, and for the gendered interpretations of the infection that stemmed from under-standing the disease chiefly in terms of the discharge produced. Gonorrhoea was considered primarily in relation to men; however those infected were not considered a threat to others, on condition that they took trouble to remove all discharge prior to intercourse (Spongberg 1997). A focus of attention on discharges translated into a focus upon female discharges; danger was located in vaginal secretions and menstrual fluid and contact with any of these fluids was considered to produce urethral inflammation in men (Walkowitz 1982). Women's bodies therefore came increasingly to be pathologised, viewed as innately diseased. Simultaneously, however, it was considered that women could carry the disease without damage to themselves. They were, however, contagious and consequently served as a source of contamination to men (Brandt 1987).

   In the eighteenth and nineteenth centuries, attitudes towards venereal disease largely reflected the decorums of class and gender, and were them-selves reflected in the provision and availability of medical treatment. A disease that was considered an unfortunate but almost inevitable aspect of manhood was viewed as a source of disgust in women (Rizzo 1996). To seek treatment was therefore considerably more acceptable for men and collusion by doctors to keep the infection secret from prospective and current wives was common (Stewart 1996; Walkowitz 1982). There was a dichotomous split in the portrayal of women: either as dangerous sources of infection, or innocent victims of the infection, that is, the wives of those men who had been infected by the dangerous prostitutes. Whilst those women who had been infected by their husbands were expected to be submissive to male prerogatives, they were considered innocent victims and merited preferential admission for treatment in the venereal hospital, known as the London Lock (Williams 1995).

By contrast, the focus of attention came to rest increasingly on specific people and activities. STIs became synonymous with women of lower classes and more specifically with prostitutes, such that this group of women came to be constructed as contaminated, separate and distinct from other women (Spongberg 1997). This was exemplified in the three successive Contagious Diseases Acts of 1864–1899. At the time, the level of venereal disease was such that it threatened the economic stability and the fighting capacity of the nation (Walkowitz 1982). The Contagious Diseases Acts were a systematic attempt to contain venereal disease by the regulation and control of the body of prostitutes, who were viewed simply as containers of infection. The original act provided for the compulsory examination of any woman suspected of being a prostitute with a venereal disease, and for enforced hospitalisation and treatment of those considered to be infected. Two subsequent acts further extended the level of surveillance with the introduction of compulsory registration and fortnightly examinations of those presumed to be prostitutes. By the later act, the accusation of prostitution was sufficient to carry the presumption of disease (Keogh *et al.* 1913). Prostitution was taken as evidence of the existence of disease, and disease was taken as evidence of immoral behaviour. Venereal disease and prostitution had by this time become entirely synonymous, the two terms being used interchangeably.

Prostitutes had not only come to be viewed as existing outside the ordered structure of society, they had also ceased to exist as women. William Acton, one of the foremost authorities of the time, described them thus:

> She is a woman with half a woman gone and that half containing all that elevates her nature, leaving her a mere instrument of impurity: degraded and fallen she extracts from the sin of others the means of living, corrupt and dependent upon corruption and therefore interested directly in the increase of immorality – a social pest carrying contamination and foulness to every quarter to which she has access.
>
>   (Acton 1968: 119; text written in 1857)

Responses to a diagnosis of chlamydia

This is the history of STIs that locates them in otherness, the social origins which have caused them to be associated in the public consciousness with those people and behaviours that are outside the moral code and therefore represent a threat to the social order. This viewpoint may seem to be confined to the history books, a relic of past times with little currency in the present time; however the data from this study indicated that it is far from redundant and has extended beyond the traditional venereal diseases to

262   *Sexually transmitted infections and dirt*

encompass other STIs. Despite the passage of time and the relatively recent categorisation of chlamydia as an STI, these representations were clearly evident when the women in this study discovered that they had chlamydial infection.

Their overwhelming reaction to the diagnosis of chlamydial infection was horror and disgust and the predominant feelings that it generated were those of dirtiness and bodily pollution. This was most commonly described as a feeling of bodily discomfort. Although this was often a relatively transient feeling, the strength of response and the sense of discomfort were commonly profound. A number of the respondents described such feelings in conjunction with expressions of upset and distress and several of them were reduced to tears on discovering the diagnosis. This was commonly experienced and expressed as a strong sense of contamination. Jenny described herself as feeling 'unclean and not nice', whilst Michelle explained it as feeling 'eurghhhh'. The discovery that they had contracted an infection presented a direct challenge to their theoretical perception of STIs as something that other people get; this was problematic because it conflicted with their perception of self and those things that should and do happen to oneself. This feeling of contamination and the challenge that it represented to her sense of self was clearly expressed by Paula:

> 'I felt dirty, I just felt really dirty and that it shouldn't have happened to me.'

Some did link this feeling to the concept of pathogenicity, within which the source of the discomfort was the fact that 'you've caught something', something that Kelly described as being both 'disgusting and repulsive'. The concepts of dirt and disease are tightly linked, associated with the existence of micro-organisms and pathogenicity, with ideas of aesthetics and hygiene. The majority of diseases, however, are not presented as being dirty, even though they may be considered to result from unhygienic and therefore 'dirty conditions'. The women may have attempted to explain the source of their feelings in terms of pathogenicity, but they simultaneously acknowledged that such explanations were unsustainable in the face of logic and reason. Zoe recognised the non-specific and non-discriminatory nature of such an infection; however this did little to diminish her sense of contamination:

> 'I know that the bacteria's not picky who it goes to, but it just makes you feel so dirty.'

Even though the feelings of dirtiness may have been described in terms of pathogenicity, it was specific to this type of infection and the means of transmission, a distinction that Michelle made in identifying the difference between infection types:

'Because it's sexually transmitted, I think, if it had been a water infection or like, I don't know, it's just the stigma, that's what it is, people
think you're dirty or something.'

The primary response to diagnosis was an internalised distinct and identifiable feeling of bodily discomfort that simply escaped further elucidation.
Central to this feeling is the internalisation of the anthropological concept of
dirt, described by Douglas (1966) as 'matter out of place'. Dirt in this sense
is matter that exists outside of, or which confuses and challenges, the existing
structures and classifications within society. The feeling of dirtiness in relation to chlamydia reflects the internalisation of those structures and the
sense that one has done wrong, either by moving outside the boundaries, or
by transgressing an internal line. The sense of disgust, which comes from
feeling that one's body boundaries have been breached by the pathogenic
organism, reflects the internalisation of social values designed to uphold the
moral code. The breaching of the physical boundary which has been realised
through the diagnosis of infection indicates a breaching of social boundaries.
The feeling of dirtiness that results represents an internalisation of the prevalent socio-cultural view of STIs as a demonstration of breaking the pollution
rules. It is by implication an indication of transgressing the moral order,
and much of the discomfort that results is associated with attaching meaning
and significance to the resultant social situation, in relation to one's own
behaviour and that of others who are implicated. This was apparent in the
way that the women spoke of those who they considered to be associated
with STIs. In many of the accounts these were described as synonymous
with 'slappers', 'promiscuous behaviours', 'tarting around' and 'those who
were scruffy'. Similarly, expressions of feeling dirty were extended to considering and rejecting the possibility that one was 'a dirty cow'. These were
the categories that provided a source of comparison with self-perceptions of
type and behaviour. The bodily discomfort that was generated as a response
to infection reflected a sense of discordance between one's virtual and actual
identity: the discrepancy between seeing STIs as something that happen to
other people and the reality that they can and do happen to oneself.

Lees (1993) identifies how widely used and pervasively abusive terms,
such as 'slag' and 'slut', have a shared understanding of meaning; although
they are primarily related to accusations of 'sleeping around', these terms
are commonly used to describe appearance and behaviours which in reality
bear little relation to that central meaning. These terms are gendered in so
far as they have no male equivalent; derogatory terms for boys are milder
because they do not refer to social identity. Such terms function as a continual threat to a girl's moral reputation, about which she has to be ever mind-
ful, and therefore position girls in a state of continual vulnerability, in terms
of what they do and also who they associate with.

These terms are unique as deviant categories in so far as they are never
accepted by the recipient themselves or applied to their social circle (Lees

1993). Similarly promiscuity is a term in common usage, but it is itself a subjective and pejorative label. It is applied to the behaviour of others and has
little personal meaning. Whilst being promiscuous is perceived as risk behaviour in relation to STIs and specifically HIV, few young people associated
such behaviour with themselves or anticipated participating in such activity
(Breakwell 1996). Such categories are always applied to others, the shifts
invariably being socially downwards; therefore mixing with those whose
reputation is suspect represents a potential source of contamination (Lees
1993). They are therefore 'dirty categories' located in otherness and it is on
this basis that they form a suitable reservoir within which to locate STIs and
from which to distance oneself.

The implications of chlamydia as a polluting infection

One of the consequences of locating STIs in otherness is the impact that
diagnosis of the infection in oneself produces. For the majority of the respondents in this study, the diagnosis of chlamydial infection was unexpected
and unanticipated, even though the majority of them had presented with
symptoms suggestive of infection, and this was the primary reason for which
they had consulted a health care practitioner. It was clear that most, although
not all, of the women had known that one of the primary purposes of the testing to which they had submitted themselves was the detection of an STI.
This situation would suggest that they might have had a heightened awareness of the possibility of infection, which would modify the impact of diagnosis. However, this situation did little to counter the feelings of shock which
stemmed from facing up to the knowledge that they had an infection. Thus,
whilst it may have been considered a possibility in an abstract sense, to be
faced with a positive diagnosis remained unexpected. In part, this was based
upon the use of the test for ontological security and the consequent anticipation of a negative result, as Jodie explained:

> 'I'd been tested last week, didn't expect to find anything . . . as I say,
> I was hoping that they were going to be all clear.'

Even when it was the presence of symptoms that led to the request for testing, there was little indication that a clear link had been made between the
symptoms and infection; the hope was that they were due to something else.
In part this may have been due to the vague nature of symptoms, suggestive
of a deviation from normal rather than something highly untoward and
sinister. Consequently they were not evaluated as the type of symptoms associated with infection. The primary reason, however, for the degree of shock
that many respondents experienced emanated from a discrepancy between
preconceptions of the types of behaviours and people associated with STIs,
and their perception of self, their own behaviour and relationship status.
The reactions that occurred were the result of coming face to face with the

reality that they had this infection. If STIs are clearly located in other people and other behaviours, then there is a fundamental difficulty in accepting that you can become infected yourself. The categorisation system established and maintained to ensure the proper ordering of things, in which STIs are clearly other, has been challenged. The sense of personal vulnerability, promoted through increased public awareness, for which testing is supposed to produce a counter-offensive in the form of a negative result, is instead confirmed through those means that were intended to refute it. As a consequence, the women were confronted by the discrepancy between their virtual identity as someone who does not get STIs and their actual identity as someone who has an STI. The reality provided a direct challenge to their classification system, forcing a reappraisal of the situation and a re-evaluation (Strauss 1959).

A discrepancy between willingness to be tested for infection and an expectation of receiving a positive result as a consequence of that testing is a recognised phenomenon. The large Department of Health (DoH) funded study of opportunistic screening for chlamydia infection, which was undertaken between 1999 and 2000, reported similar findings. In the qualitative interviews conducted as part of that study, the majority of those interviewed expressed shock and distress at their result, despite the fact that they had been clearly aware of the purpose of testing and had consented to the test (DoH 2001).

The authors of the DoH study highlighted a paradox in the discrepancy between acceptance of a test, and the apparent lack of understanding of the consequences of a positive test result. Such a conclusion suggests that when people submit themselves to medical investigations for a specific condition, they do so in anticipation or expectation that such a condition will be identified. However, this is an oversimplification of the situation. People consent to testing and even request testing for a range of other reasons. In routine testing instigated by the health service, as in the case of cervical screening, many women conform to the programme largely as a result of normalcy and correctness, because it is the expected thing to do (Bush 2000). Their actions are founded upon a sense of responsibility and obligation to self and others (Howson 1999). Even in relation to patient-requested testing, for example in the case of HIV antibody tests, the justification for such a request relates to a variety of reasons, the majority of which are largely symbolic, associated with the commencement or closure of relationships, in conjunction with discontinuation of condom use in a developing relationship, or as a demonstration of personal responsibility (Lupton *et al.* 1995a).

In a climate of increased public and personal awareness of infection, fuelled by media campaigns, there is an increased sense of personal vulnerability which may be further heightened if acquaintances are known to be infected. Within this context, testing provides a means by which to re-establish control in the face of danger. However, whilst testing is viewed as the 'rational' thing to do, it is done in the expectation of a negative result with little anticipation of the unthinkable, namely a positive result (Lupton *et al.* 1995a, 1995b). On this basis, it suggests that for many, the purpose of a chlamydia test is to provide the security of demonstrating that the infection is not there, not to prove that it is.

The creation of a climate where testing for infection is represented as the socially responsible thing to do, the means by which to safeguard the sexual health of self and others, is contributing to an increased willingness to discuss testing with others. A number of the women in this study described how they had discussed the possibility of testing with friends, the pressure that had been exerted upon them to be tested and the pressure that they had subsequently exerted upon others to undergo testing. However, whilst it may be considered acceptable to tell others that you have been tested for infection because it is a responsible thing to do, this information sharing does not necessarily extend to sharing a positive result with friends or family, largely because it carries the fear of social sanctioning, as 17-year-old Beccy explained:

> 'We do talk about the possibility of getting checked out but I never told anyone that I did have chlamydia, we don't talk about it but we did talk about testing . . . I suppose it's not OK [to tell them that you have an infection] because I think people will think that it's dirty, that they'll look at you differently, and they'll think she's a slag or whatever because she's dirty, I don't want people to know that.'

This situation parallels that associated with cervical screening, a procedure that is now so widespread that it is the majority experience. Testing in this respect is largely considered a moral obligation and non-compliance is viewed as deviant (Howson 1999). However, the high level of acceptability of the test does not extend to the disclosure of abnormal results, which are commonly associated with a range of negative feelings including self-blame and social recrimination (McKie 1995; Quilliam 1992).

Conclusion

As identified at the outset, current practice focuses screening activities almost exclusively on women, even though the target population includes both males and females and the testing processes can be used as easily with men and women. The primary reasons reside in the organisational structure of the programme and particularly the use of existing contraceptive and sexual health consultations. Whilst this may be unavoidable given that the majority of these consultations involve women, nevertheless such an approach has the potential to perpetuate the representation of women as transmitters and contractors of infection and continues to pathologise the female body.

The purpose of the National Chlamydia Screening Programme is to identify infection in those who do not have symptoms. It will therefore lead to an increasing number of diagnoses in those who lack any physical sense of having an infection. The conceptual difficulties of considering the possibility of having this infection that were evident in those with symptoms are likely to be even more apparent in those who are asymptomatic. Additionally, the non-invasive sampling methods that have resulted from the development of testing techniques have been associated with an increased acceptability of being screened for this infection (Pimenta *et al.* 2003). However, agreeing to be tested for an infection does not necessarily prepare someone for the theoretical possibility of a positive result. Even if they have considered the possibility in theoretical terms, this does not necessarily reduce the personal impact when such a possibility becomes a reality, because of the role that social structuring and categorisation systems play in defining that individual experience.

The increased amount of testing activity that is occurring as a result of the screening programme will increase the normalcy of testing for patients and health professionals alike. It is likely therefore to further increase the social acceptability of testing. However, this will not inevitably result in an increased social acceptability of receiving a chlamydial diagnosis. Whilst it will become an increasingly common experience for health professionals to inform individuals that they have been diagnosed with this infection, it is imperative that they do not underestimate the impact of such an approach upon the individual women themselves, who struggle to deal with the spoiled identity that commonly results from the diagnosis of an infection whose roots are so deeply embedded in social and cultural attitudes and values. This places a consequent burden of responsibility upon the health professionals to ensure that whilst they may increasingly view this infection within the concept of normalcy, they do not expect the women who are facing such a diagnosis to be equally likely to do so.

References

Abraham, J. (1935) *Introduction to Syphilis or the French Disease*. London: William Heinemann.

Acton, W. (1968) *Prostitution*. London: Macgibbon & Kee.

Allen, P.L. (2000) *The Wages of Sin: Sex and Disease, Past and Present*. Chicago: University of Chicago Press.

Andreski, S. (1989) *Syphilis, Protestantism and Witch Hunts*. Basingstoke: Macmillan.

Brandt, A. (1987) *No Magic Bullet*. Oxford: Oxford University Press.

Breakwell, G. (1996) 'Risk estimation and sexual behaviour: a longitudinal study of 16–21 year olds'. *Journal of Health Psychology* 1(1): 79–91.

Bush, J. (2000), '"It's just part of being a woman": cervical screening, the body and femininity'. *Social Science and Medicine* 50: 429–444.

Crosby, A. (1977) 'The early history of syphilis: a reappraisal'. In D. Landy (ed.) *Culture, Disease and Healing: Studies in Medical Anthropology*. New York: Macmillan.

Davenport Hines, D. (1990) *Sex, Sin and Punishment: Attitudes to Sex and Sexuality in Britain Since the Renaissance*. London: Collins.

Department of Health (2001) *A Pilot Study of Opportunistic Screening for Genital Chlamydia Trachomatis Infection in England (1999–2000). Evaluation of Public and Professional Views*. London: Department of Health.

Douglas, M. (1966) *Purity and Danger*. London: Routledge.

Foucault, M. (1986) *The Care of the Self: The History of Sexuality*. London: Penguin Books.

Fracastoro, G. (1935) *Syphilis or the French Disease: A Poem in Latin Hexameters*. London: William Heinemann.

Health Protection Agency (HPA) (2004) 'Diagnoses of selected STIs, by region, age and sex seen at GUM clinics'. London: HIV and Sexually Transmitted Infections Department, Health Protection Agency.

Howson, A. (1999) 'Cervical screening: compliance and moral obligation'. *Sociology of Health and Illness* 21(4): 401–425.

Keogh, A., Melville, C., Leishmann, W. and Pollock, C. (1913) *A Manual of Veneral Diseases*. Oxford: Oxford Medical Publications.

LaMontagne, D., Fenton, K., Randall, S., Anderson, S. and Carter, P. (2004) 'Establishing the National Chlamydia Screening Programme in England: results from the first full year of screening'. *Sexually Transmitted Diseases* 80: 335–341.

Lees, S. (1993) *Sugar and Spice: Sexuality and Adolescent Girls*. London: Penguin Books.

Lupton, D., McCarthy, S. and Chapman, S. (1995a) '"Doing the right thing": the symbolic meanings and experiences of having an HIV antibody test'. *Social Science and Medicine* 41(2): 173–180.

Lupton, D., McCarthy, S. and Chapman, S. (1995b) '"Panic bodies": discourses on risk and HIV antibody testing'. *Sociology of Health and Illness* 17(1): 89–108.

McKie, L. (1995) 'The art of surveillance or reasonable prevention? The case of cervical screening'. *Sociology of Health and Illness* 17(4): 441–457.

Pimenta, J., Catchpole, M., Rogers, P., Perkins, E., Jackson, N., Carlisle, C., Randall, S., Hopwood, J., Hewitt, G., Underhill, G., Mallinson, H., McClean, L., Gleave, T., Tobin, J., Harindra, V. and Ghosh, A. (2003) 'Opportunistic screening for genital chlamydial infection. 1. Acceptability of urine testing in primary and secondary healthcare settings'. *Sexually Transmitted Infections* 79(1): 16–21.

Quilliam, S. (1992) *Positive Smear* (2nd edn). London: Charles Letts.

Qvigstad, E., Skaug, K., Fridtof, J., Fylling, P. and Ulsrap, J. (1983), 'Pelvic inflammatory disease associated with *Chlamydia trachomatis* infection after therapeutic abortion'. *British Journal of Venereal Disease* 59: 189–192.

Rizzo, B. (1996) 'Decorums'. In L. Merians (ed.) *The Secret Malady: Venereal Disease in Eighteenth Century Britain and France*. Lexington: University Press of Kentucky.

Rosebury, T. (1972) *Microbes and Man: The Strange Story of Venereal Disease*. London: Secker and Warburg.

Sontag, S. (1991) *Illness as Metaphor and AIDS and its Metaphors*. London: Penguin Books.

Spongberg, M. (1997) *Feminizing Venereal Disease: The Body of the Prostitute in Nineteenth-century Medical Discourse*. New York: New York University Press.

Stewart, M.M. (1996) '"And blights with plagues the marriage hearse"'. In L. Merians (ed.) *The Secret Malady: Venereal Disease in Eighteenth Century Britain and France*. Lexington: University Press of Kentucky.

Strauss, A. (1959) *Mirrors and Masks: The Search for Identity*. Glencoe, Ill.: Free Press of Glencoe.

Turner, B. (1996) *The Body and Society: Explorations in Social Theory* (2nd edn). London: Sage.

Walkowitz, J. (1982) *Prostitution and Victorian Society: Women, Class and the State*. Cambridge: Cambridge University Press.

Westergard, L., Philipsen, T. and Schiebel, J. (1982) 'Significance of cervical *Chlamydia trachomatis* infection in post abortal pelvic inflammatory disease'. *Obstetrics and Gynaecology* 60(3): 322–325.

Williams, D. (1995) *The London Lock: A Charitable Hospital for Venereal Disease, 1746– 1952*. London: Royal Society of Medicine Press.

Worboys, M. (2004) 'Unsexing gonorrhoea: bacteriologists, gynaecologists, and suffragists in Britain, 1860–1920'. *Social History of Medicine* 17(1): 41–59.

18 Genetic traits as pollution: 'White English' carriers of sickle cell or thalassaemia

Simon Dyson

Introduction

In this chapter, we will consider a particular instance of 'matter out of place' (Douglas 1966), namely the occurrence of genes associated with particular diseases in populations where, according to popular and professional discourses, they 'ought not to be' (Tapper 1999). The chapter commences with a brief description of sickle cell and thalassaemia and reports on interviews undertaken with twenty-seven specialist haemoglobinopathy counsellors about their experiences of asking ethnicity screening questions in connection with sickle cell/thalassaemia risk. 'White English' carriers of sickle cell or beta-thalassaemia are reported to react badly to news of their genetic status, considering themselves 'unclean', 'tainted', or 'contaminated' by a condition that, for them, has strong connotations of being 'black'. The counsellors, themselves largely of African/Caribbean descent, are obliged to absorb the racism implicit in these reactions, but develop some interesting strategies for 'cooling out' such White English carriers.

Sickle cell and thalassaemia

Sickle cell, the thalassaemias and other haemoglobinopathies are inherited blood conditions that mainly affect people of African, Caribbean, Middle Eastern, South Asian, South East Asian and Mediterranean descent (Serjeant and Serjeant 2001; Weatherall and Clegg 2001). They are also found, though more rarely, in populations of Northern European descent (Lehmann and Huntsman 1974). The NHS Plan for the UK stated a commitment to provide 'a new national linked antenatal and neonatal screening programme for haemoglobinopathy and sickle cell disease by 2004' (Department of Health 2000).

At the time of the interviews, ante-natal screening for haemoglobin disorders was selective (targeted at groups deemed most at risk by means of asking an ethnicity screening question) in nearly all health districts of England outside London (Sedgwick and Streetly 2001). However, since then, universal neonatal screening has been implemented for England, and, in 2005, around half of the population in England was covered by a universal ante-natal screening policy for sickle cell and thalassaemias, with the remaining areas covered by a selective ante-natal screening policy. The extension of sickle cell and thalassaemia screening to groups not previously covered will undoubtedly increase the number of 'white' carriers requiring support, and this is but one of several dilemmas inherent in screening for haemoglobinopathies (Dyson 2005).

Methods

Ten interviews were conducted with individual counsellors and six with two or more counsellors present. The interviews explored with the counsellors issues concerning the collection of good quality information on ethnicity and the haemoglobinopathies. The interviews were tape-recorded and transcribed in full. The interviews lasted between 25 and 75 minutes, with a mean of 45 minutes. All the counsellors interviewed were female, and two had sickle cell anaemia. Their average work experience as a counsellor was eight years. Their stated ethnicity was Black British (African or Caribbean) (24), British Asian (2) and White British (1).

'Isn't that supposed to be among black people only?' – the reported reaction of white carriers of haemoglobinopathies

Eighteen of the twenty-seven counsellors interviewed referred to the particular reactions they reported 'white' carriers to exhibit. By 'white' we are referring to those who self-describe as White English/Scottish/Welsh/Irish and *not* to those who self-describe as 'white' but who are in generally recognised risk groups for sickle cell/thalassaemia (e.g. those of Mediterranean, North African, Arab and Iranian descent or those of mixed heritage).

All eighteen counsellors referred to the surprise exhibited by white carriers when informed they carry genes associated with sickle cell or thalassaemia. The origins of this surprise are reported by the counsellors to lie in the strong association of sickle cell as a condition only affecting black people. However, the reaction of white carriers is more than surprise. Twelve of the counsellors reported that this reaction was both strong and negative, and examples of the types of reaction are summarised below.

The reported range of reactions of white carriers of haemoglobin disorders to information about their carrier status

'Tainted'; questioning of their parentage; putting questions to their parents!; annoyed; 'freaking out'; 'not white after all'; 'I'm not black'; 'I'm not Asian'; disbelief; client demands further tests; client does not accept results; client asserts there must have been an error; amazed;

resentful; 'created in the waiting room'; felt contaminated; 'gave her husband a hard time'; the test reveals non-paternity; 'flew off the chair'; go red; very puzzled; shock; 'put [the secret of the family ancestry] in a box for a hundred years'; 'how dare you ask me where my parents are from!'; the client didn't want to say she was half African; felt she was pure Aryan race; screwed (the test results) up and threw them in the bin; anger, denial; 'are you taking the mickey?'; fear; unclean.

To deal with the negative reaction of one of the carriers in greater detail, counsellor M2 suggests that the white person felt tainted by their association with 'black' people by virtue of their sickle cell carrier status.

M2: [We point] out that it's not an illness that it's never going to cause an illness. That it's not just the black population that it's found, it can be found in the white population albeit in a much smaller number. And it doesn't mean that somewhere in your background, because I think that's where sometimes they are a little bit worried, somewhere, somebody in my background that was black that I didn't know about, you know, and it's about the tainting of them. [. . .] Because if you always knew that you were white British or Caucasian and, you imagine you have feelings of what it means to be black. And then to find out that you might have something in you that could suggest that you've got black in your ancestry, that's what they're worried about. And that can cause problems and that's why I say, it can and does occasionally occur in the white population without there having been anything in the ancestry. And that's what that is.

M1: Isn't that weird, that their parents aren't their parents almost.
        [. . .]

M3: But you know you can't actually go out and say what you feel like saying about the group. It may be you're, somehow linked to that group.

The counsellors imply that part of what it means to be white is to have pre-conceptions about what it means to be black and, given that the person feels 'tainted', presumably these preconceptions are tantamount to racist views. Indeed the final comment suggests that the realisation that the white person is, as they put it, 'tainted' means that their previous racist attitude is no longer congruent with their personal experience because they now have to acknowledge a link to the black population.

F1: [. . .] We actually had about four or five Caucasian with sickle haemo-globin [. . .] And it's very interesting; there was one that was a more positive response. In fact the woman had this as her party piece, you know. Ooh I've got sickle. You know, it was like a party piece to tell her friends. It's like being cool, you know, I've probably got a bit of black somewhere. You know, because she wanted me to make sure to send her the letter, to show her the card, and that sort of like, and lots of leaflets. So that was like a cool thing. [. . .] We had another, this was a D in a Caucasian and the woman reacted so badly that we said look, you weren't a carrier when you were pregnant, it's your husband that's a carrier, don't worry about it it's not an illness. And the way she responded, it's as though the baby was contaminated in some respect. And she insisted that she wanted to know which of the husband's parents had it. And these parents were retired, but she insisted, I mean she gave the husband such a hard time, that the parents had the blood test. And it turned out that his father wasn't his father. And so we're talking about a retired couple, that's now found out that, you know, the man just realised that this man who he raised all his life isn't his son.

Here, the counsellor recalls one client who adopted a different outlook when informed she was a carrier. Her reaction was to regard her new-found status as 'cool'. This suggests the client is conceptualising minority ethnic groups as 'Other', with the 'Other' being constructed as different and exotic (Rosenblum and McTravis 1999). As such, it is a reaction that draws upon dominant discourses of the 'normality' of whiteness and the 'Otherness' of the factor (sickle cell) associated with being black. Finally we have a further example of the more overtly negative reaction of clients to the information that they are carriers. Once more the correlation with a condition held to be linked to black populations produces the notion of being contaminated by this association. The consequence of this revelation of genetic information is that the family is pressured to be tested and an instance of non-paternity is revealed to an elderly man and his son.

In another instance, knowledge of Black African ancestry is held by the mother but not her male partner.

F2:   And do you remember me saying, she came in and the partner is Italian or mix, sort of, and then I would say to you, where are your Grandparents from and everything, and she said, South African, and she turned round and said, Oh I think my Great Grandmother is coloured. And he nearly flew off his chair. He didn't realise. It's a big issue for them.

Here the issue that is raised is not one of non-paternity, but one in which the ethnic origin of ancestors on one side of the family is not known to the other. One interpretation of this is that because the mother can 'pass' (Goffman 1968) for someone who is 'white' the father has not recognised this aspect of her ancestry. The counsellor hints at some racism in the father's reaction, though whether the mother has deliberately hidden her ancestry or simply did not realise the extent of his prejudice is not clear.

In another case it is someone other than the client who has knowledge of the family's genetic ancestry and who has already taken steps to protect the family members because of his perception that this knowledge would lead to them being stigmatised.

M2:   Sometimes I've found people have been a little bit you know, where did that come from? How could that have happened? and you just smooth it as best you can. Especially when it's a carrier, you say well it doesn't mean it's an illness it's never going to be an illness. You know, it's the genetic implications, why I think it's important. But they do sort of go very, very red and puzzled. But there's a particular client in fact they were twin sisters, and they've got thalassaemia trait. And, one of the sisters did actually say that her uncle had done some studies and he's actually put some information in a box that's not to be opened for another hundred years. So I think there's something probably [laughter from other respondents] talk about family history. [Laughter] Something's going on. Most of the time it's a great shock as to, I can't imagine where this could have come from. And some people have actually said, but I always understood that this was something from the black population. You know, how could it be part of me?

Once more, the reaction of the white carriers is one of shock and embarrassment at being identified with a condition they associate with the black population. The uncle is reported to have conducted some investigations into the family history and it seems that he has discovered something (presumably some minority ethnic ancestry he thinks the family would not welcome), such that he has adopted a strategy of controlled release of information.

White carriers not only have to confront their own feelings about carrying genes they misconceive as restricted to black people. They also hear this news from counsellors who are themselves mainly of African descent. If the uneasy reaction of some white carriers betrays their own racism, so does their reported reaction to receiving the information from a minority ethnic professional.

F2:   Well I feel sometimes they make you feel uncomfortable or they feel uncomfortable. Here I am an African or an African Caribbean asking someone who believes they're Caucasian [. . .] you know, they can't get round that. It's almost like, how dare you ask me where my parents are from, I've said I'm British. You know, you get this [. . .] They just feel uncomfortable coming you know, that sort of question coming from you. I don't have problem with an African saying where you from, the only funny problem we have is when you ask, have you got any Chinese or Asian, as sisters, and they burst out laughing. Oh my goodness, I'm from Ghana, you know, but we have to ask sometimes, you know. They find it funny, but they have no problem with that ethnicity issue. So I find the Caucasian or people of mixed race have a problem with that. Because [. . .] some don't want to have said that they [are] half African or half Caribbean and half English and you're asking them, they would rather say they are Caucasian and leave it at that.

An exchange between a black counsellor and a white carrier potentially disturbs several taken-for-granted aspects of power relationships. First, it represents a professional knowing more about one aspect of the client's family than they do. Second, it is a reversal of the more usual discomfort visited upon minoritised ethnic groups when they are the ones who have to account for their ethnicity to a professional from an ethnic majority (a majority usually both in a numerical and a power sense). It is a double discomfort for someone with racist beliefs to have to account for their ethnicity to a person from a minority group whom the client is more used to 'racialising'. Third, an exchange may also raise issues of gender, with the black female counsellor in control of information and the white male client for once more vulnerable.

The following quotation encapsulates many of the issues raised in this chapter. The white carriers are reported to exhibit anger or disbelief at their newly discovered status. They associate the concept of sickle cell with the 'black' population. It is received as information that changes their lives and may produce a crisis in their self-identity. It may have considerable repercussions in terms of intra-family accusations.

H1:   [. . .] Usually, the reaction is, well this is usually a black blood problem, so how comes you're telling me, I'm white, that I'm a carrier for this thing? And usually shock. And in some cases it's anger, disbelief, denial. In some cases people accept what you say and because they understand history and, and gene mixing etc. So you have to assess each case and work with their reaction. And try and explain to them that it's mainly black people that are affected, but there are other communities that are affected by it. And it's not something to be ashamed of. I've had some clients who've said, I wonder who's been playing away. [Laughing] I wonder what's happened here, you know. So it's difficult for the white population because it has been promoted as black disorders, and something that only black people carry. So I think from an educational aspect, this universal screening programme really has a large task on its hand in educating the white community [. . .] I had a young man, I think he was in his early twenties, was diagnosed with beta thalassaemia trait through a full blood count. The haemoglobinopathy testing wasn't selective, so there wasn't any informed consent. So that was an issue. So he came to us very surprised that he's come through with this beta thalassaemia trait which was a black or

Mediterranean disorder. So that was the first issue. Why was I screened? Why wasn't I told? So we had to explain the MCV, the MCH and all this and why he was screened. Then there was the issue of race. And, I'm white so how can I carry this thing are you sure you've got the diagnosis right? So we had to get out the ethnic picture really and explain that beta thalassaemia trait affects a wide variety of people. Although it is mainly Asian people that carry this, you are at risk as well and we explained the screening process that we are going to start finding a lot more white people because our screening criteria had changed. And that you're not a rare case, it's just that we're not really looking at the wider population in more detail, which we will be in the future. Therefore people start to calm down [. . .] you have to be very calm and try and answer their questions and try and be respectful of their fears. It's a job that we do every day but this information is new to them and it changes their lives. And once you've given them that information, you can't take it back. So you have to try to put yourself in their situation. It's not just another case and it's not just information that you're giving, that they can just take away. It's something that they may have to go home and explain to their relatives, which is what happened with this young man. So I think the other family members got screened as well. And they had mum in and sister and dad. And they had counselling sessions and by the time they came in they were a lot calmer and a lot more aware and a lot more accepting. But it did cause some issues when he was first diagnosed with his parents, and how the family accepted the diagnosis of something that mainly affects black people. So there was like an identity crisis I felt. Issues of, are you sure you've got the diagnosis right, are you taking the mickey? Are you saying that my family have done something that they shouldn't have done? Are you saying that there's a dark secret in our family and if the other members in the white community knew this, would they see us as mixed race, different?
[. . .]

H2:   Yea I've had some cases like that as well. It was a white couple and mum was screened during pregnancy because her iron levels were very low, we couldn't state anything. So she was quite alarmed by the letter we sent her. And she gave birth, baby got screened, baby had alpha thalassaemia trait, and it caused a lot of frustration in their family. Both couples were very upset. When they came to see me, the husband was very, very, he was accusing her of having an affair, all sorts [. . .] he was questioning about whether the baby was his. [. . .] They were quite angry; they were very, very angry and very, very upset. And I did explain to them all the processes and then we eventually found out, we traced it back to the mum. And it was from the mum. It was from her side of the family. It was following on from her and, but she came round eventually but it took her husband a little while to come round. And he did admit that he, you know, it was lack of education. And so, I think that seems to be the case. Even amongst Asian communities as well. And I think that, that communities it is the lack of education. This is not in our family, what are you trying to say?

H1: Especially . . .

H2: Where's this come from? [. . .] Especially being a trait, it's hidden. It's not a disability, there's no symptoms, they all think, sudden[ly] think, why are you telling me now, I'm twenty so and so years old or whatever, why wasn't it picked up x number of years ago? So that seems to be the main problem.

H1: We have a lot of problems with women who are on their third pregnancy and the other two children previously hadn't been screened and they want to know why.

There are two particular issues the quotations raise with regard to the implementation of a screening policy. One is the anger clients are reported to exhibit when they discover that they have been screened opportunistically without explicit consent for the particular test. The other problem reported is where a mother has been through one pregnancy before the implementation of a particular policy for either ante-natal screening or neonatal screening. She then wishes to know why the precautions now in place were denied during her earlier pregnancy. This may have implications for the introduction of new screening policies as part of current NHS Screening Programme initiatives.

'They don't know about their history': 'cooling out' white carriers

Thus far in this chapter, we have examined the reactions of 'White English' carriers to the news that they carry genes associated with sickle cell/ thalassaemia. In this section we look at the skills exhibited by the counsellors in dealing with these reactions. These skills are characterised as 'cooling out' the white carriers, calming them down and, by skilful face-to-face work, moving them to an acceptance of their situation. These responses by the counsellors are especially adroit, as they require the counsellor to suspend their own distress in relation to the implicit racism of the client.

In this first extract, Counsellor D1 recounts her experiences with white carriers of beta-thalassaemia. She recalls that a GP of South Asian descent had told the clients that the condition only affected black people. When the couple arrive for haemoglobinopathy counselling they are blaming each other. The counsellor's strategy for dealing with their reaction was to fill in their lack of historical knowledge and suggest that the wrecks of the Spanish Armada may have been one mechanism for the assimilation of people of Mediterranean descent into the general population.

D1:   [. . .] we've got white families now with beta thalassaemia [. . .] and some of them [are] negative. [They were told] it's a condition that affects black people, by their GP, who was Asian as well, you wouldn't believe it. And they come here sort of thinking, where did this come from? And the blaming started. [. . .] the last lot I had actually was quite horrendous because I had to sit there and sort of explain to them what was the Spanish Armada, you know, sort of history. So you're really in this, you have a sort of global view of what happened historically so that you're able to explain or educate people. Because many people don't know actually what happened. They don't know about their history, so that, that can cause quite a bit of a problem.

Interviewer: Right. Why do you think it bothers them so much, that they carry beta thalassaemia?

D1:   Oh it's race isn't it. It's the way that we're told. And remember you know, they've looked at people that are still sort of full [inaudible] you know have, and to be told you know sort of. And when they come and see you, what I find, the dynamics within that is very interesting actually as a professional black woman sitting there; they don't see me as a black woman [. . .] well that's the impression I get, because the things that were said there. But it's actually when everything is finished, sitting there professionally explaining things to them they said, when they're going said, oh I hope you didn't mind? I said mind in what sense? You know you're, you know, black and we did say some stuff [. . .] Oh no, as far as we are concerned we've got no Germans, no foreigners, in our family, not unless there is something in yours, that's the other side of the family, because they had two families here at the time. You know, sort of no, no, no foreigners at all. They tend to mix it with the Germans. It's always this bit about [chuckle] the Germans and foreigners. Possibly they didn't say black because I might have been there [. . .] I'm really fascinated actually sometime just sitting there watching that kind of embarrassment, it's quite interesting. There's quite a lot learning from it as well. And you as a professional person [. . .] if you're not very grounded actually it can really undermine you. [. . .] I could say the negativity that comes out can impact on you and you couldn't respond if you're not professionally grounded.

Furthermore she implies that it is ironic that she has to teach white people their own history. Counsellor D1 goes on to make the assertion that the reason behind the discomfort of the client is the issue of 'race'. She implies that the white carriers have previously looked at black people in a negative way, and are thus confronted with the need to re-assess their own identity as comprising a genetic component they associate with this 'blackness'.

Moreover, she suggests that their reaction to her as a professional black woman is that they 'don't see her as a black woman'. She implies that they speak in negative terms about what it means to be a carrier of genes they associate with being black. In doing so they first put to the background the fact that Counsellor D1 is black in the sense that they initially do not acknowledge that their negative reaction to association with 'blackness' is highly insulting, not only in and of itself, but because it is expressed in the presence of a black woman. Subsequently the couple realise they have been expounding racist sentiments in front of a black woman, and distance themselves by expressing the hope that the counsellor does not mind. This is a very invidious linguistic strategy, for it would be difficult for the counsellor to say she does mind. It is also very reminiscent of the manner in which racist views are projected onto a group, but where the person doing the projecting excuses an individual minority ethnic person from that association.

Counsellor D1 further implies that the couple have chosen to express their xenophobia by referring to foreigners or Germans rather than black people, since she feels the couple may feel less accountable for their comments by adjusting the target of their expression in this way.

Finally, Counsellor D1 expresses interest in the phenomenon she is experiencing. She notes the clients are embarrassed, presumably because they have to confront their own racism. She feels that she has to be very 'grounded', both in terms of her professionalism, and in terms of her self-identity as a black woman, in order not to let the negative experience shake her self-esteem and her belief in her work.

In the next example, counsellor F1 recounts an experience with a white mother of a baby who is a sickle cell carrier. She states that the mother immediately became very angry and threatened to sue the counsellor for suggesting that her baby carried this gene:

F1:   [. . .] we appointed this baby for counselling and for blood test and the first thing that I got on the form was a mother that was very upset, very angry and telling us, she's going to sue me, because the letter also went on headed paper, Sickle Cell and Thalassaemia Centre. [. . .] First thing she said, my baby hasn't got any sickle cells. And it really got very, very difficult. So I said, well look come down and we [can] talk about it and you know, it's just sort of routine and, we could have made an error and we'd like to just check again. And interesting she brought her husband, her mother, her father, his mother, his father. It's like saying, look at all of us, can you see black in any of us? [. . .] And it's interesting because as a counsellor [chuckling], you're meant to be professional but you can be quite intimidated by that. And I can remember saying to her things like, you might have had a great grandfather from India. He might have been a Raj in the British, British army, and that sort of went down well. [Still chuckling] The thought that she had a great grandfather who might have been a Raj or a Colonel in the British army in India. And she responded to that, but I felt I couldn't touch on anything to do with black or ethnicity. I had to treat it in terms of, maybe her forebears lived in an area, and this to him, of course, was a form of defence against malaria. You know, and this is how I was more counselling the woman about her not having any black in her than around the baby's haemoglobin.

The counsellor clearly has to undertake a great deal of work in calming the client, since she reports three strategies in one sentence that she replied to the mother with. First, she suggests, 'Let's talk', the implication being that what is at stake can still be the subject of negotiation. Second, the issue is referred to as just routine, again arguably an attempt to de-sensitise the mother by suggesting that the issue is not extraordinary. Third, she suggests that the whole situation may be the result of an error that may be resolved by a re-test.

The client, however, raises the stakes by bringing her extended family to the counselling centre as (in her view) a graphic demonstration of the pure white lineage of her family, but actually revealing that she, like most of the population, does not appreciate the tenuous link between skin colour and risk of carrying sickle cell/thalassaemia genes. The counsellor again refers to being potentially intimidated. This raises issues of the health and safety of the haemoglobinopathy counsellors. The invidious position they are placed in has led to the counsellors being directly exposed to the racial (some might argue racist) views of the clients, a position equal opportunities employers would not wish to permit to continue.

The multiple strategies employed by the counsellor are again interesting, and involve distancing the information as far as possible from an association with Black African heritage. The counsellor suggests the gene may derive from India. Moreover, she speculates that it might be because the client's ancestors were high status citizens within the British Empire in India. She mentions the protection against malaria thought to be associated with the selective advantage of sickle cell/thalassaemia carriers (Allison 2002). In short she claims that her counselling work is to moderate the shock of being thought 'black' more than to address the genetic consequences of being a carrier.

Counsellor K independently recounts very similar problems and strategies. She reports that a number (unspecified) of white couples start from the position of denial that they 'have any black in their family'. It becomes apparent that these couples feel 'contaminated' and feel 'unclean' at the idea that they have genes that they perceive as associated with black people.

K: [. . .] it's more confusion 'cos where people are aware of the whole background of the haemoglobin status, they're a lot more at ease, they've investigated the family tree and they'd be able to tell you. [. . .] especially if they're Caucasian couples, when they come in the first thing they'll say is, I haven't got any black in my family. And you've got to try and break down that barrier so that they realise we're talking about the blood, we're not talking about the colour or the wrapping. As I say to them, we're not on about the wrapping, we're on about blood and blood is one colour. So it's trying to get them to think it through. And once they relate it to the history of the country and the history of the family, they can go back and then ask the relevant questions of their parents and find out where it originated from.

Interviewer: [. . .] what is it that troubles them so much do you think?

K: The fact that you're telling them they've got black in their family. You know, as if it's something unclean or, or not spoken about because it's a contaminate. So if you're telling them that's there, where did it come from because they know for sure that it's not in their family. But then when you can say, but not all people who carry this trait are black. They can look very Mediterranean; they can accept it better coming from that perspective. And when you look at the Roman times they find it easier coming from that route than they do coming from the slavery route and the mixing of blood from there. So it's just finding a way that they're comfortable with approaching the subject.

Again, the counsellor tries a number of approaches to desensitise the white clients. Of particular interest is the manner in which she again distances the relationship from Black African heritage, and in particular from any association with slavery, and suggests Mediterranean ancestry and the Roman Empire occupation of Britain as possible routes by which the gene may have passed into the 'white' family.

Conclusion

In this chapter we have examined the reported reactions of 'White English' carriers of sickle cell/thalassaemia genes. In many cases this reaction was negative, the carriers exhibiting anger at being 'tainted', as they saw it, with a condition that supposedly only affects black people. This leads in some to a crisis of identity, in which they are compelled to face up to their previous assumption of a 'pure' white identity that gives them an insider status in society, and confront their new status as someone with links to an outsider group. Their previous racist characterisation of black people comes back to haunt them. Even those who take the news calmly still construct their experience as having been exposed to an exotic 'Otherness'. The assumption of some white carriers that they are insiders to society makes the task of a black professional, whom the carriers construct as an outsider, very challenging.

These accounts by the counsellors indicate that they deal with such situations very skilfully indeed, adopting a variety of strategies for addressing the negative reactions of white carriers. First, they have to suspend any professional or personal reaction to the racism implicit in the reaction of the white carriers. Second, they provide the client with other possibilities (they can see a geneticist, they can have a re-test). Third, they distance the information as far as possible from Black African ancestry and slavery, focusing on ethnic groups which, whilst still minoritised ethnic groups in UK society, are perceived to be relatively less threatening to the self-identity of the White English carrier, such as Mediterranean, high status Indian, or Roman. Moreover, the reaction of white carriers raises health and safety issues for counsellors. For it is not clear what personal cost to their well-being is incurred by absorbing the racism of clients and by 'cooling them out' through studiously avoiding an association of sickle cell with ethnic groups to which the counsellors themselves belong.

Universal neonatal screening is a major route through which white carriers are identified. The implementation of a national universal neonatal programme in England in 2005 suggests that the issues raised here will become much more prevalent in the future, and suggests an urgent need for both professional and community education. It further suggests that haemoglobinopathy counsellors need the support of managers and their own professional development initiatives to help them in this work. Meanwhile, the counsellors deserve our respect for the skilful manner in which they carry out the messy, emotionally toxic, work of responding to clients whose 'racial' views are foregrounded by the unexpected results of screening.

Acknowledgements

The author would like to thank the twenty-seven specialist haemoglobinopathy counsellors for their generosity in giving these interviews.

The research was funded by the NHS Sickle Cell and Thalassaemia Screening Programme, with additional funding from the Unit for the Social Study of Thalassaemia and Sickle Cell. The views expressed here are those of the author alone and do not necessarily represent those of the NHS Sickle Cell and Thalassaemia Screening Programme.

References

Allison, A.C. (2002). The discovery of resistance to malaria of sickle cell heterozygotes. *Biochemistry and Molecular Biology Education* 30(5): 279–287.
Department of Health (2000). *The NHS Plan: A Plan for Investment, a Plan for Reform.* London: HMSO.

Douglas, M. (1966). *Purity and Danger: An Analysis of Concepts of Pollution and Taboo.* London: Routledge & Kegan Paul.

Dyson, S.M. (2005). *Ethnicity and Screening for Sickle Cell and Thalassaemia.* Oxford: Churchill Livingstone.

Goffman, E. (1968). *Stigma: Notes on the Management of Spoiled Identity.* Harmondsworth: Penguin.

Lehmann, H. and Huntsman, R.G. (1974). *Man's Haemoglobins*, 2nd edn. Philadelphia: J.P. Lippincott.

Rosenblum, K.E. and McTravis, C.T. (1999). *The Meaning of Difference: American Constructions of Race, Sex and Gender, Social Class, and Sexual Orientation.* Boston: McGraw Hill.

Sedgwick, J. and Streetly, A. (2001). *A Survey of Haemoglobinopathy Screening Policy and Practice in England.* London: NHS Sickle Cell/Thalassaemia Screening Programme. http://www.kcl-phs.org.uk/haemscreening/publications.htm# EQUANS%20Review (accessed 5 November 2003).

Serjeant, G.R. and Serjeant, B.E. (2001). *Sickle Cell Disease*, 3rd edn. Oxford: Oxford University Press.

Tapper, M. (1999). *In the Blood: Sickle Cell Anaemia and the Politics of Race.* Philadelphia: University of Pennsylvania Press.

Weatherall, D.J. and Clegg, J.B. (2001). *The Thalassaemia Syndromes*, 4th edn. Oxford: Blackwell Science.

Zeuner, D., Ades, A.E., Karnon, J., Brown, J., Dezateux, C. and Anionwu, E.N. (1999). Antenatal and neonatal haemoglobinopathy screening in the UK: review and economic analysis. *Health Technology Assessment* 3(11).

19 Women out of place

Mavis Kirkham

This book is about leakage: of body fluids, genes, micro-organisms, knowledge and people. If dirt is 'matter out of place' (Douglas 1966), the categorisation of place and the rigidity of its boundaries are very important for the women studied here. Some categories are imposed upon women, though it is a long time since I heard women or children told to keep their place. Mostly we want to belong, to claim a place which is ours. The categories/places from which leakage occurs are seen differently and valued differently from within and without.

My changing place

Long ago, I worked briefly as a cleaner in a cancer hospital. Twice a day, when the nurses were busy elsewhere, the cleaners congregated behind the door in the ward kitchen and drank tea. We used the crockery used by the patients, those were the days when patients drank from crockery, but we always drank from milk-jugs, not cups. Recounting this to my partner, a social anthropologist, I first encountered the concept of pollution and taboo in a healthcare setting. We belonged to the place, but only hidden behind the door when the nurses weren't using the kitchen. Our use of the jugs identified us as separate from the people with cancer who drank from the matching cups. Thus, we acknowledged and observed our lowly place in the hospital hierarchy and our separation, being healthy, from users of the service. Ironically, it was much later that I understood the more physical dangers I ran in cleaning under the beds of old ladies during their radium treatment and chatting with them as they seemed so lonely.

I drank out of a milk-jug when I was a cleaner because that was what cleaners there did. By the time I trained as a midwife, previous work as a social scientist had trained me to observe as an outsider and this ensured that much of my professional socialisation did not 'take'. It has been important to me, as a midwife, to cultivate the observant outsider part of my own vision. This means I never truly belong but I enjoy being able to observe and analyse what we do as midwives and I have been a midwife long enough to be able to pass as such.

Now, as an organic gardener, who has long cultivated a plot where compost, hens and vegetables rotate and the fruit trees were planted upon the placentae of my grandchildren, it seems normal to me that fertility, growth and beauty originate from what is seen as most dirty. The compost heap transforms waste and muck into nutrients. Concepts have to be fluid because the transformation can be seen. Humble labourers – worms, micro-organisms and to some extent myself – transform the muck into compost. The toxicity of muck is also chemically relative: a mulch which would delight some plants will kill or damage others. Skill, knowledge and diligence endlessly serve the transformation of potentially corrosive muck into food and flowers.

Training as a nurse and midwife gave me clear concepts of physical cleanness and therefore of dirt. Over time, I have watched the right place for challenging matter change with social change. We no longer make a bit of money for the hospital by selling placentae to cosmetics companies. Threat of disease brings an imperative to burn, as seen in cattle diseases. Maternity hospitals have struggled and produced organisational responses as parents sought to hold and bath their dead baby or carry from the hospital their aborted foetus. Maternity care has changed, though slowly, in response to articulate and persistent service users; ironically we did not seek to learn from gynaecology nurses (see Chapter 14), since professional midwifery has sought to separate itself from nursing. Attitudes to the socially polluting change more slowly than attitudes to problematic physical matter. As a midwife, I found myself confronting actions and responses which classify birth as dirty and midwifery as socially polluted when working within a modern hospital with high standards of hygiene and surgical sterility. As a researcher and a midwife working mainly with home births, I find the concepts persist. In symbolism and in language used, concepts of dirt seem much more rigid and less capable of recycling than in the garden. Yet for women, birth, especially homebirth, can be an occasion when barriers are dissolved and new ways of seeing are developed. Sometimes this happens for midwives too.

Wanting to belong

Mostly we want to belong, especially at the beginning of a chosen career. Student midwives want to be able to do the things that midwives do, to pass as part of the community of midwives and to cope with the uncertainties around them. This can lead them to embrace the visible actions of midwives, such as 'doing the obs' (Davies and Atkinson 1991), rather than the studied, quiet inaction which creates safe space within which childbearing women can choose their own paths. Doing professional acts, such as clinical observations, reinforces our professional status. Such acts tend to keep others in their more humble place, as patients or as women who do not want to trouble the midwife because she is so busy (Kirkham and Stapleton 2001).

Professional status is important here. Mary Smale describes the 'unspoken rules' developed to keep embodied breastfeeding knowledge from contaminating professional knowledge concerning breastfeeding (Chapter 10). Professional knowledge carries status for those who use it, but personal experiences influence attitudes and can therefore be ignored but not eradicated. Women want to know the personal experiences of their midwives and denying them this knowledge ensures professional dominance. Knowledge probably flows best in a relationship of equality where personal experience is used wisely and mindfully (Smale 2004). Thus the protection of professional knowledge and status limits both the knowledge and relationships available to midwives and their clients (Kirkham 1996).

Is this rigidity of thought and categorisation more likely with groups, such as midwives, with relatively little power relative to medicine or general management in hospitals? It is logical that professionals with more autonomy themselves would feel more able to facilitate choice for their clients. The relationship between professional autonomy and facilitative practice has been observed in medicine (Kaplan *et al.* 1996). This may also account for the greater job satisfaction experienced by community or case-holding midwives compared with their hospital colleagues (Kirkham *et al.* 2006). This may be yet another example of professionals' inability to facilitate for their clients what they do not themselves experience. It is also likely that those who feel their professional position is threatened are likely to resist inputs into their professional body of knowledge from sources which are seen to be of lower status. Midwifery has experienced over two hundred years of medical encroachment, though some midwives have latterly learnt to gain a degree of status from technical work cast off by medicine. The perception of threat and the pressure to 'go with the flow' of organisational systems and powerholders (Kirkham and Stapleton 2001) may well account for the rigid and brittle nature of many midwifery concepts and categorisations, as well as tendencies to stereotype (Kirkham *et al.* 2002) and ensure conformity by bullying (Curtis *et al.* 2006; Mander 2004).

As midwives, we may see ourselves as oppressed and threatened, but the attitude of gynaecology nurses to midwives, as conveyed by Sharon Bolton (Chapter 14), is very different. The gynaecology nurse's description of midwives certainly made me think twice.

> Midwives deliver live healthy babies in a routine way and get the title of 'practitioner' and are seen as being superior to us and yet they won't do what we do.

The description of respectful care of a dead or dying and/or malformed foetus and its parents is a clear example of what society sees as dirty work made significant and honourable. There is much that midwifery could learn here, but we have tried so hard to hold ourselves separate from nursing that this area of learning has not even been considered. Fear of pollution blocks the potential gains of lateral and collegial thinking here, just as admitting our embodied knowledge and that of mothers could enlarge and extend, but deprofessionalise, our knowledge of breastfeeding.

Rites of passage

Key changes in social state, which most chapters in this book address, are seen as rites of passage. The classic anthropological study of rites of passage by Van Gennep (1960) highlighted three stages: separation, liminality and incorporation. 'Embedded in his vision is the concept of the threshold' (Kenworthy Teather 1999), *limen* in Latin. Turner (1969) described the stages as pre-liminal, liminal and post-liminal. Pre-liminal and liminal stages involve seclusion.

The attributes of liminality are ambiguous, the individual is between social states and belongs neither to their 'old world' nor to their 'new world' (Van Gennep 1960). This is a time of change and creativity where, held in the safety of seclusion and rite, firm categorisations become fluid, normal status can be reversed, profound contradictions are contemplated and considerable vulnerability is experienced.

There are other views of rites of passage. Wilson (1980) speaks of the complete rite of passage as involving movement through the 'preparatory stage', into 'the play' and ending when the individual was fully incorporated into 'the game'. Again, there is potential for flexibility and change in the central stage of play. This is followed by acceptance of the rules of the game in 'an orderly change from one reference group to another' (Wilson 1980: 140).

Female rites of passage?

Returning to liminality

People cannot always move smoothly between the stages and sometimes stay in a state of liminality (Turner 1969). It is across thresholds that leakage occurs unless containment is strictly practised. Mahon-Daley and Andrews note that,

> there are various taboos and spatial restrictions associated with breastfeeding, which serve to position breastfeeding space as liminal space . . . which women move into to breastfeed and out of to reintegrate with society and 'normal' daily activities.
>
> (2002: 70)

Whether the liminal space is sought because breastfeeding in the normal world is unacceptable (see Chapter 7), or to protect the child from the evil eye (see Chapter 9), the need remains. Nevertheless, the constant supply and demand nature of breastfeeding as food, comfort and relationship means that there is an ever-present danger of leakage of the activity of breastfeeding, as well as of milk itself.

The maintenance of 'normal' life alongside breastfeeding makes such liminal practices difficult. Maher (1992) describes how, despite legal rights to take time during the working day to breastfeed, few mothers do this, due to practical difficulties and the fear of provoking resentment from employers and colleagues.

It may be that women are more likely to experience liminality alongside normal life, stepping frequently between these states, nurturing different relationships and maintaining different social states simultaneously, rather than progressing smoothly 'from one reference group to another' (Wilson 1980: 140). Or this may be seen as an aspect of modernity: the expectation that a normal life in a bounded body is maintained alongside the leakages, which are part of being female.

Time and liminality

In the liminal state, time can be experienced in different ways from the linear concept of time that prevails in industrial societies. Women's embodied experiences of time tend to be cyclical. 'Women, grounded whether they like it or not in cyclical bodily experiences, live both the time of the industrial society and another kind of time that is often incompatible with the first' (Martin 1989: 198).

Caring also takes place in non-linear time, focused upon the needs of the person cared for which may be linked to their embodied cycles or very immediate and seemingly outside time. Studying hospice care of the dying, Julia Lawton found that focus upon the present, in the non-linear temporal framework of liminality, makes equality, rather than dependence, possible. 'Relationships of equality are reflected and reinforced through the construction of cyclical, non-progressive time' (Lawton 2000: 66). Time so experienced is defined as 'polychronic', by Hall (1983). In this state, 'personal relationships and interactions take precedence over the rigid time schedules of the calendar and the clock. Time is not experienced as a line, but as a point in which relationships or events converge' (Helman 2000: 23).

Unless conducted according to a medicalised model, this description fits labour, dying and many other transitions. It also fits supportive care focused upon the needs of the other: the work of those who are with women in life's transitions. 'Caring time is cyclical and rhythmical allowing for relationality, sociality, mutuality and reciprocracy' (Dykes 2006: 182). Frequently repeated liminal states such as breastfeeding, focused upon the baby who does not know of linear time, also fit this description.

Thus women experience polychronic time in relationships and in embodiment. But the construct of time which dominates western life and healthcare is solely linear and closely measured. Caring and relationship, which focus on the person cared for rather than efficient linear timing, tend to be discounted within such a construct. Within healthcare, the denial of relationship and its implications can be experienced as damaging by workers and their clients (Kirkham *et al.* 2006; Edwards 2005). This is one factor in the frustration of healthcare workers in many contexts (e.g. Lipsky 1980; Ball *et al.* 2002). It is also a factor for those women who seek a deviant, but personally safe setting for a major life transition (e.g. Edwards 2005).

Concealment

The pressure to lead a normal life may also lead to concealment. Adaptation to incontinence and its concealment with pads and other devices may be more acceptable than confronting the dangers of leakage and accepting the dirty identity of being incontinent in order to embark upon a treatment regime (see Chapter 15). The women interviewed by Hilary Piercy did not discuss their chlaymidial infection with their friends, though the infection is common and easily treated (Chapter17). Their silence thus left others unaware how common this infection is and did not challenge its association with those who are seen as both dirty and other. Similarly, the possibility of miscarriage was not in the minds of many of the women interviewed by Julia Frost until their own experience of it (Chapter 16), but the frequency of miscarriage makes it likely that they all knew women who had had this experience.

Women's frequent need to conceal polluting states, such as menstruation and lactation, also has commercial implications. The production of 'sanitary' products and equipment for the concealment of lactation has expanded greatly in recent years and new products constantly aim to enhance 'invisibility' (Bramwell 2001). Thus advertising constantly emphasises the importance of concealment of these body fluids and their attendant status.

Where leakage cannot be concealed, real social isolation follows, as experienced by the women with 'too much milk' studied by Cheryl Benn and Suzanne Phibbs (Chapter 8).

Some women experience contradictory needs for such concealment. Helen Stapleton describes how mothers with eating disorders experience considerable problems in public places. They need to conceal both breastfeeding and self-induced vomiting, which latter practice must also be concealed from the infant (Stapleton 2006).

Concealment of liminal states may make 'normal' life possible for many women. Yet such concealment must constitute denial of that state to a considerable extent. By its nature, concealment cannot provoke support or discussion of the experience. Concentration upon concealment may limit the experience, as for those women who give up breastfeeding on returning to work, or distract from the personal change and growth which transitional experiences could engender.

A safe place

Citing the work of Bruce Lincoln (1981), Virginia Beane Rutter (1993) observes that, in contrast to male initiation patterns, which reflect 'a process of separation, liminality and reincorporation', women's rites tend to follow a pattern of 'enclosure, metamorphosis (or magnification) and emergence' (Rutter 1993: pxvii). 'Containment, transformation and emergence form a ritual pattern of renewal for women' (1993: 225). There are differences in how these stages could be applied. Rutter, for instance, sees breastfeeding as evidence of emergence: 'During lactation her milk flows, opening her physical boundary into the world, into relationship in a new way' (1993: 226). This is true in terms of relationship with the baby. Yet her social position may be more liminal than emergent (see Mahon-Daly and Andrews 2002), unless she copes well with censure or mixes largely with other breastfeeding mothers (see Chapter 7). Nevertheless, the concept of containment is of importance.

The concept recurs, from the term 'confinement' for the childbearing period which, in many societies, includes a month of postnatal rest and nurturing, to the best-selling story of *The Red Tent* for menstruation, story telling and female withdrawal from the social world (Diamant 1997). Such confinement does more than conceal the liminal state.

Carol Lees Flinders surveys a number of cultural practices and concludes: 'In every instance with which I am familiar these ceremonies involve ritual enclosure, and in these contexts enclosure connotes, not imprisonment or limitation of any sort, but a symbolic gestation' (Flinders 1998: 152).

Rutter (1993) sees the containment of liminality as 'therapeutic enclosure' which 'can be a place of self-realization'. She describes Navarro women's rites of passage in terms very similar to those used by the dais quoted in this book (see Chapters 11, 12 and 13). The women involved feel themselves to be part of 'the power of change and fecundity in all things' (Rutter 1993: 66–67). Rutter draws parallels with western women's experiences in psychotherapy. In such processes the women's 'sense of self is not assaulted; it enlarges . . . she is becoming one who can feed and heal others . . . she is acquiring power' (Flinders 1998: 155).

The need for a safe, contained space comes up repeatedly in this book and other writings. For instance, women who had experienced miscarriage wanted 'a specific space' as well as continuing support from staff (see Chapter 16). It may be that in the concealment of contained rites of passage, the care and support between women, as well as the polluting body fluid, become invisible.

Trudy Stevens sees the process of birth as something,

> very precious that needs protection. It needs the creation of a very particular type of cocoon. Today such a cocoon is comprised of hygienic factors and risk management, of particular competencies, responsibilities

defined by Agenda for Change concerns about potential litigation and the expectation of perfection.

(Stevens 2004)

Those of us who heard Trudy Stevens' paper certainly identified with the rites of purity and danger now being associated with hygiene and risk management. Whilst a 'cocoon' is certainly needed and is always created within the values of its society, the one spun from concepts of hygiene and risk management offers little by way of self-actualisation for midwives (Ball *et al.* 2002; Kirkham *et al.* 2006) or mothers (Edwards 2005; Kirkham and Stapleton 2001). Some women in traditional societies may also experience dissonance within their rites of passage but their words go unrecorded.

Adjusting to early motherhood traditionally involves a degree of segregation from normal life and its tasks (as shown in several chapters in this book and Stevens 2004). During this time the mother is cared for and concentrates upon her baby. The breastfeeding mothers observed by Fiona Dykes drew the curtains round their beds (Chapter 6). The matron of Wellington St Helens Hospital in 1918 suggested that women were tethered to their beds for ten days postnatally to ensure the only rest they had 'from one confinement to the next' (see Chapter 2). In the UK, professional postnatal care is now very much seen as the Cinderella of understaffed maternity services. Society presses women to get back to normal and carefully conceal the bodily leakages, which would previously have merited seclusion, rest and support.

There is also a need for safe space in which to reflect upon and learn from our work. The community midwives, studied by Ruth Deery and me (see Chapter 5), lacked even the concept of such space and suffered because of this. The pressures for productivity, contained within an industrial model of healthcare, emphasise measurable input and output. Action and linear time are measurable; relationships and cyclical time are not. As caring is devalued (Davies 1995), so safe space for caring or for reflection upon caring is increasingly unlikely to be seen as part of healthcare professionals' work.

Yet, safe spaces have a place in modern management thought. The 'creative compartments' advocated by Gerard Fairtlough have the flexibility, openness, trust and communication characteristic of liminal states: 'With this combination of features, there can be an explosion of innovation . . . in which the creative capacity of human beings is unlocked' (Fairtlough 1994: 89). These words echo the rhetoric of the NHS but not its increasingly rule-governed reality.

Birth as a rite of passage

The entrance to society most clearly demonstrates the nature of a rite of passage and the strangeness and contradictions of the liminal state. In western society 'the bounded body, as a literally physical condition, is both central and fundamental to selfhood' (Lawton 2000: 133). Yet, in birth, the body opens, or is surgically opened. The boundedness of the maternal body is breached, as the newborn moves from within the mother into the social world. This is the most dramatic of all leakages across body boundaries and happens via an orifice deemed to be particularly dirty; it is at the same time the ultimate act of creativity. The baby is dirty and must be cleaned, is new and must be blessed as the society endorses. The baby is reached for only by the mother and the go-between, who deals with birth dirt (see Chapter 1), and is cleaned before being handed to the father, priest or paediatrician. Thus, the journey is negotiated from the body, through dirt and pollution, to social acceptance of the newcomer. The baby once cleaned and claimed by its society is seen as a separate creature. In western medical systems the newborn is in many ways classed as a product of the hospital (see Chapter 1), and must then be protected from contamination, even from its mother. This is especially true if the baby is premature or sick. Restrictions on visiting babies in hospital are justified as protecting the baby from infection, and mothers of premature babies often feel that they are seen as polluting what lies within the clean field of the incubator (Taylor 2006).

Surgical deliveries contain secretions by mechanical means, are technically controlled and are therefore seen as cleaner. This is held to be imperative, for instance where the mother might infect the baby with HIV. Helen Callaghan described elective caesarean section as 'the ultimate method of sanitisation' of birth (see Chapter 1).

It is rare for hospitals to treat the newly delivered mother and baby as a unit. After the baby has been cleaned, the mother remains polluted. The fine nuances and changing nature of the ongoing dirt are described by Pamela Wood and Maralyn Foureur (Chapter 2).

Place, power and the labelling of dirty workers

Women withdraw to the appointed place during labour. Each society manages birth according to its values:

> birth and the immediate post-partum period are considered a time of vulnerability for mother and child – indeed, frequently a time of ritual danger for the entire family or community. In order to deal with this danger and the existential uncertainty associated with birth, people tend to produce a set of internally consistent and mutually dependent practices and beliefs that are designed to manage the physiologically and socially problematic aspects of parturition in a way that makes sense in that particular cultural context. It is not surprising therefore that – whatever the details of a given birthing system – its practitioners will see it as the best way, the right way, indeed *the* way to bring a child into the world. For these reasons, we find that within any given system,

birth practices appear packaged into a relatively uniform, systematic, standardised, ritualised, even morally required routine.

(Jordan 1993: 4)

Brigitte Jordan's anthropological insight explains much about birth and the behaviour of its practitioners. It explains medical opposition to homebirths in the UK more clearly than any clinical argument, as response to a profoundly wrong place and therefore to extreme pollution. It also explains the difficulties of obstetricians and hospital workers in Pakistan (see Chapter 13) who are committed to a western medical model in a country where most births are not in hospital or medically attended. For them, the attendant dai epitomises all that is deviant, dangerous and dirty and she is therefore blamed. Similarly, in nineteenth- and early twentieth-century England, the working-class midwife or handywoman became a convenient scapegoat and means of sidestepping the possibility that other factors, such as poverty, influenced women's health (Mander and Reid 2002). In William Arney's (1982) view, midwives offer an alternative to medical services for birth and therefore must be controlled, symbolically and organisationally.

The attendant during a rite of passage is also themselves polluted (see Chapters 3 and 12), though for a lesser period of time. They attend the transformation and as such are essential to the rite and gather some of its pollution, as shown in several chapters in this book and in studies of those who work around death (e.g. Lawton 2000). They do what others shrink from doing.

Those who work to support others during rites of passage may valorise their dirty work, or they may resist society's categorisation of them. The specialist continence nurses interviewed by Joanne Jordan saw their work as liberating women from both their incontinence and a healthcare system which trivialises their experience and places an over-medicalised emphasis upon surgery (Chapter 15). 'For the gynaecology nurse it is the "dirty" nature of their work that makes it special' (Chapter 14). Their support can transform women's experience.

The dais interviewed by Subadhra Rai felt that, in handling the placenta and cord, they were in touch with the divine in the midst of pollution, as well as providing their service as an act of selfless duty (Chapter 12). In presenting dais' understanding of 'narak', Janet Chawla described how the land and women 'partake of the same nature of fecundity'. The dais speak reverently of the placenta as life-giving, as well as polluted (Chapter 11). Thus the dais reverently embrace the contradiction that, in order for new life to emerge, that which produced and nurtured it also emerges and is classified as filthy and polluting. Janet Chawla notes that this very pollution 'has allowed for abiding female spaces and birth cultures In the "male" or "dominant" view these female times are "filthy" or polluted, but they are also times when masculine, social and even familial demands on women are suspended' (Chapter 11). The safe space for change and creativity thus springs from its associated pollution. In western industrial society the transition, along with the pollution, is controlled as it is denied.

Margaret Chesney (2004) recounts dais' stories of how 'the dirt must come away' (that was the original title of her chapter for this book). These heroic tales of cleansing and life-saving echo the pride of gynaecology nurses and dais, working and building their skills in safe, if polluted places.

The pollution of those who work with women in transitional states appears to be linked with their relationship with the contradictions and creativity of the liminal state. It is also inversely linked with power, as Helen Callaghan observes, 'the theory of birth dirt is about power relationships in childbirth' (Chapter 1). Those who see themselves as attending the state of transition in a support role but not as the main actor tend to be viewed as dirty and identified with the liminal state, waiting upon it and cleaning up. More technical and powerful workers who conduct or control changes in social state, such as obstetricians, are not identified as dirty workers. Their work carries status, controls rather than attends uncertain events and is attended by another profession, which 'acts as a protective layer' (see Chapter 1) and deals with much of the actual dirt. Both types of workers may undertake some tasks in common – vaginal examinations for obstetricians, midwives and dais; handling the dead and body products for doctors and nurses – but it is the lower status group which carries the pollution. This may change with context: the trained midwife does the dirty work in Australia (see Chapter 1), relative to the status of the obstetrician; in Pakistan the trained woman is called a 'lady' health worker, relative to the dai (Chesney 2004). It is also important to note that where high status and technical action identify a role as that of primary actor, rather than polluted attendant, the woman herself lacks power. Rites of passage focus upon the individual in transition; the attendent dai, for instance, is relatively powerless, as shown by Margaret Chesney (see Chapter 13). In obstetric services, the obstetrician holds power, the woman can exercise 'informed compliance' (Kirkham and Stapleton 2001), the family is scarcely part of the picture.

Simon Dyson (Chapter 18) and Hilary Piercy (Chapter 17) raise another professional role, that of those who reveal to women a state, previously unknown to them, which they see as polluted. Simon Dyson examines the dilemmas and skills of black haemoglobinopathy counsellors in the face of their white clients' racist assumptions. Government proposals to deprofessionalise chlamydia testing do not address the issue that some may need similarly skilled help in adjusting to their status as 'dirty' when a test is positive. Skilled, new and demanding aspects of support are needed in such technically produced liminal states.

Enduring categorisations of dirt

One striking thing that comes out repeatedly from this book is the enduring nature of the categorisations of dirt over time, even when social change would lead us to think such categories have gone, or at least been eroded. Hilary Piercy (Chapter 17) shows how a diagnosis of chlamydia makes people feel dirty. Sexual mores have changed, yet the dirtiness of a sexually transmitted infection persists even in the absence of any symptoms or any negative feelings about the sexual relationship which led to this easily curable infection. The history of sexually transmitted disease as dirty and shameful casts a long shadow, the policy implications of which have not been acknowledged.

Simon Dyson's chapter (18) shows the lengths to which white people go to assimilate within their value system the knowledge that they are carriers of a 'black' haemoglobinopathy trait. These people would probably not see themselves as racists, yet the concept of taint persists.

This book also demonstrates skilled resistance to such categorisation. The heamoglobinopathy counsellors had strategies for 'cooling out' white people who reacted angrily to their genetic status (see Chapter 18). It is noteworthy that a black heritage was more acceptable in a distant, imperial context! The specialist continence nurses (Chapter 15) and gynaecology nurses (Chapter 14) used the specialist nature of their professional niche and demonstrated resistance to the categories that contained them, challenging the status quo, honouring and empowering the women in their care.

The need for safety and fluidity

The concept of pollution enables us to examine contradictions: the juxta-position of filth and fertility; pollution containing the potential for safe developmental space for women; the sacred and the earthy within the concept of 'narak'; the move from protecting women from infection to protecting hospitals and staff from contamination by their patients. We can peel back multiple meanings within elements usually measured in linear fashion, such as time and space, or explore the relationship between power and pollution. We can even contemplate pollution flowing against the flow of power, as explored by Kuldip Bharj (Chapter 4) and reported to me by a number of women over the years, not all of whom were Muslims. It is in the fluidity of the liminal state that such contradictions and complexities can be contemplated and new roles and relationships developed with support.

Concepts of pollution also create the concept of leakage and the need to prevent it. Many dilemmas of leakage for women are explored in this book. The prevention of leakage so often also prevents growth, in our body of knowledge or circle of support, for instance. Sometimes the effects of leakage prevention work are themselves toxic for the self, as when we are required to handle the toxic waste of others without the potential for recycling. Leakage is essential for health, development and fertility, in our embodied selves and in our thought.

Leakage is particularly needed in professional thought. The sealing out of embodied knowledge from professional practice concerning breastfeeding

(Chapter 10), or any other aspect of health, demonstrates professional insecurity, and cannot make for good practice. It must limit the knowledge and help available to women and the support available to professionals. Ruth Wilkins sees the professional outlook as conceptually blind to relationship and process, divorcing mothers and midwives from themselves (Wilkins 2000: 29), alienating them from their own experience and denying points of connection between mothers and midwives (2000: 32). In order to accept the leakage that could bring connection, professionals need to feel safe. This is likely to come in different ways: such as by celebrating their dirty work as skilled and requiring uniquely women's knowledge (see Chapter 14), by building peer support through enabling education (Smale 2004), or other strategies to enable constructive use of the professional's embodied experience (e.g. Battersby 2006).

Women need safe places for relationships, reflection and transition and for the development and celebration of caring roles. Productive containment has to be controlled by women, not a site of enforced isolation. Thus it is possible to create a situation where we feel 'safe enough to let go' (Anderson 2000) of what prevents birth, change or relationship. Sometimes this can be done with appropriate support within healthcare settings (Anderson 2000), sometimes the safe place is a geographical choice. For the women studied by Nadine Edwards who sought home births, 'home was a metaphor for control and connection and hospital a metaphor for loss of control and separation' (Edwards 2005: 17). The safe place always includes safety within relationships.

Rites of passage contain such places in their liminal states. As well as the transitions of women's lives, health workers experience transitions in understanding and knowledge, which need reflective time. Although modern healthcare does much to remove rites of passage, or time within the liminal state, concepts of pollution remain and can be used as sites of resistance. In the most dirty, physically and socially tainted situations, 'spaces are created where the status quo can be challenged and, however gradually, ultimately changed' (Chapter 14). Margrit Shildrick sees such leaks and flows as a 'resistance to closure' with massive potential for change (Shildrick 1997: 43). 'An acceptance of the leakiness of bodies and boundaries speaks to the necessity of an open response' (1997: 217), a mindfulness, not falling back on professional rules or formulas but ensuring ongoing relationship.

Fiona Dykes urges us to 'accept leaky distinctions'. Her call to 'acknowledge complexity, difference, and diversity . . . while avoiding disembodiment' (Chapter 6) could be applied to all the situations explored in this book.

Within current systems and power-structures it is inevitable that women will be seen as out of place, together with our knowledge, bodily fluids and other attributes. However, it would be possible to use the generosity of spirit shown in the MATRIKA project (see Chapter 11) to address the world of professional healthcare. Dirt is a useful concept with which to strategically address this, to embrace the contradictions involved and to plan resistance from common, if polluted, ground.

References

Anderson, T. (2000) Feeling safe enough to let go. In M. Kirkham (ed.) *The Midwife–Mother Relationship*. Basingstoke: Macmillan.

Arney, W.R. (1982) *Power and the Profession of Obstetrics*. Chicago: University of Chicago Press.

Ball, L., Curtis, P. and Kirkham, M. (2002) *Why Do Midwives Leave?* London: Royal College of Midwives.

Battersby, S. (2006) Exploring attitudes towards infant feeding. In V.H. Moran and F. Dykes (eds) *Maternal and Infant Nutrition and Nurture: Controversies and Challenges*. London: Quay Books, pp. 202–229.

Bramwell, R. (2001) Blood and milk: constructions of bodily fluids in Western society. *Women and Health* 34(4): 85–96.

Chesney, M. (2004) Birth for some women in Pakistan, defining and defiling. Unpublished PhD thesis, University of Sheffield.

Curtis, P., Ball, L. and Kirkham, M. (2006) Bullying and horizontal violence: cultural or individual phenomena? *British Journal of Midwifery* 14(4): 218–221.

Davies, C. (1995) *Gender and the Professional Predicament in Nursing*. Buckingham: Open University Press.

Davies, R.M. and Atkinson, P. (1991) Students of midwifery: 'doing the obs' and other coping strategies. *Midwifery* 7: 113–121.

Diamant, A. (1997) *The Red Tent*. London: Macmillan.

Douglas, M. (1966) *Purity and Danger*. London: Routledge.

Dykes, F. (2006) *Breastfeeding in Hospital*. London: Routledge.

Edwards, N. (2005) *Birthing Autonomy*. London: Routledge.

Fairtlough, G. (1994) *Creative Compartments: A Design for Future Organisation*. London: Adamantine Press.

Flinders, C.L. (1998) *At the Root of This Longing*. San Francisco: HarperCollins.

Hall, E.T. (1983) *The Dance of Life: The Other Dimensions of Time*. Tiptree: Anchor Press.

Helman, C. (2000) *Culture, Health and Illness*, 4th edn. London: Butterworth-Heinemann.

Jordan, B. (1993) *Birth in Four Cultures*. Prospect Heights, Ill.: Waveland Press.

Kaplan, S.H., Greenfield, S., Gandek, B., Rogers, W.H. and Ware, J.E. (1996) Characteristics of physicians with participatory decision making styles. *Annals of International Medicine* 124(5): 497–504.

Kenworthy Teather, E. (1999) *Embodied Geographies*. London: Routledge.

Kirkham, M. (1996) Professionalisation: midwives with women or with the powers that be? In D. Kroll (ed.) *Midwifery Care for the Future*. London: Bailliere Tindall.

Kirkham, M. and Stapleton, H. (eds) (2001) *Informed Choice in Maternity Care: An Evaluation of Evidence Based Leaflets*. York: NHS Centre for Reviews and Dissemination.

Kirkham, M., Stapleton, H., Curtis, P. and Thomas, G. (2002) Stereotyping as a professional defence mechanism. *British Journal of Midwifery* 10(9): 509–513.

Kirkham, M., Morgan, R. and Saul, C. (2006) Why midwives stay. Unpublished research report, University of Sheffield.

Lawton, J. (2000) *The Dying Process*. London: Routledge.

Lincoln, B. (1981) *Emerging from the Chrysalis: Studies in Women's Initiations*. Cambridge, Mass.: Harvard University Press.

Lipsky, M. (1980) *Street-Level Bureaucracy*. New York: Russell Sage Foundation.

Maher, V. (1992) *The Anthropology of Breastfeeding*. Oxford: Berg.

Mahon-Daly, P. and Andrews, G.J. (2002) Liminality and breastfeeding: women negotiating space and two bodies. *Health and Place* 6: 61–76.

Mander, R. (2004) The B-word in midwifery. *MIDIRS Midwifery Digest* 14(3): 320–322.

Mander, R. and Reid, L. (2002) Midwifery power. In R. Mander and V. Fleming (eds) *Failure to Progress*. London: Routledge.

Martin, E. (1989) *The Woman in the Body*. Milton Keynes: Open University Press.

Rutter, V.B. (1993) *Woman Changing Woman: Feminine Psychology Re-conceived through Myth and Experience*. San Francisco: Harper.

Shildrick, M. (1997) *Leaky Bodies and Boundaries*. London: Routledge.

Smale, M. (2004) *Training Breastfeeding Peer Supporters: An Enabling Approach*. Sheffield: WICH Researsh Group, University of Sheffield.

Stapleton, H. (2006) *Childbirth and Eating Disorders: A Qualitative Study of Some Women's Experiences*. Sheffield: University of Sheffield.

Stevens, T. (2004) Pollution and safety – controls of a secular world. Paper given at *'Pollution and safety: exploring the "dirty" side of women's health'*. Conference, University of Sheffield.

Taylor, L. (2006) personal communication on work in progress.

Turner, V. (1969) *The Ritual Process: Structure and Anti-structure*. London: Routledge & Kegan Paul.

Van Gennep, A. (1960) *The Rites of Passage*. London: Routledge.

Wilkins, R. (2000) Poor relations: the paucity of the professional paradigm. In M. Kirkham (ed.) *The Midwife–Mother Relationship*. Basingstoke: Macmillan.

Wilson, B. (1980) Social space and symbolic interaction. In A. Buttimer and D. Seamon (eds) *The Human Experience of Space and Place*. London: Croom Helm, pp. 135–147.

Index